AAL-8763

D1035115

AAL-8763

# SKIN
# SURGERY

*A Practical Guide*

# SKIN SURGERY

## *A Practical Guide*

WAGGONER LIBRARY
DISCARD

**Richard P. Usatine, M.D.**
Associate Clinical Professor
Department of Family Medicine;
Director, Predoctoral Education
UCLA School of Medicine
Los Angeles, California

**Ronald L. Moy, M.D.**
Associate Clinical Professor
Department of Medicine/Dermatology;
Director, Dermatologic Surgery
VA West Los Angeles Medical Center
UCLA School of Medicine
Los Angeles, California

**Edward L. Tobinick, M.D.**
Assistant Clinical Professor
Department of Medicine/Dermatology
UCLA School of Medicine
Los Angeles, California

**Daniel Mark Siegel, M.D.**
Associate Professor of Clinical Dermatology
Director, Division of Dermatologic Surgery
Vice Chairman, Department of Dermatology
Stony Brook School of Medicine
State University of New York at Stony Brook
Stony Brook, New York

**MACKEY LIBRARY**
**Trevecca Nazarene University**

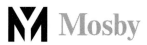 Mosby

St. Louis   Baltimore   Boston   Carlsbad   Chicago   Minneapolis   New York   Philadelphia   Portland
London   Milan   Sydney   Tokyo   Toronto

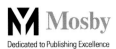
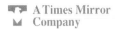

*Publisher:* Susie H. Baxter
*Developmental Editor:* Ellen Baker Geisel
*Project Manager:* Carol Sullivan Weis
*Production Editor:* Karen M. Rehwinkel
*Composition Specialist:* Terri Knapp
*Designer:* Jen Marmarinos
*Manufacturing Manager:* Karen Lewis

**Copyright ©1998 by Mosby, Inc**

All rights reserved. No part of this publication may be reproduced, stored in a
retrieval system, or transmitted in any form or by any means, electronic, mechanical,
photocopying, recording, or otherwise, without written permission of the publisher.

Permission to photocopy or reproduce solely for internal or personal use is
permitted for libraries or other users registered with the Copyright Clearance
Center, provided that the base fee of $4.00 per chapter plus $.10 per page is paid
directly to the Copyright Clearance Center, 222 Rosewood Drive, Danvers, MA
01923. This consent does not extend to other kinds of copying, such as copying for
general distribution, for advertising or promotional purposes, for creating new
collected works, or for resale.

Printed in the United States of America
Composition by Mosby Electronic Production
Lithography/color film by Graphic World, Inc.
Printing/binding by Grafos

Mosby, Inc.
11830 Westline Industrial Drive
St. Louis, Missouri 63146

ISBN 0-8151-7362-8

98 99 00 01 02 / 9 8 7 6 5 4 3 2 1

# Preface

We have written this book for primary care physicians and residents in primary care fields and dermatology to improve their knowledge and skills in skin surgery. It is a practical guide for learning the many basic procedures of skin surgery (including shave and punch biopsies, suturing techniques, elliptical excisions, cryosurgery, electrosurgery, incision and drainage, and intralesional injections). Experienced physicians, midlevel practitioners, residents, and medical students will find valuable learning opportunities throughout the text and in the illustrations.

What makes this book unique is that it was produced by the cooperative efforts of a family physician and three dermatologists. The goal of this joint effort was to create a book that brings together the experience of the writers and translates that expertise into a very practical approach to learning skin surgery for primary care physicians. The final product is a book that will help you learn time-efficient, cost-effective, curative, and cosmetically excellent skin surgery.

We demonstrate a step-by-step approach to skin biopsies, excisions, and other skin procedures using photographs, illustrations, and narrative descriptions. The book is more than a how-to guide because we have provided the rationale and supporting literature to help you choose and perform the appropriate type of skin procedure for many common malignant, premalignant, and benign skin lesions. We teach you to biopsy suspicious lesions with the goal of producing an adequate specimen for pathologic diagnosis while obtaining the best cosmetic result.

As the prevalence of skin cancer increases in the population, many physicians will be called on to diagnose skin cancers. Therefore we have provided the reader with photographs and information to facilitate the early diagnosis and curative treatment of skin cancers. We teach the reader to perform early diagnostic biopsies and to perform the definitive surgical treatment. We also provide rationale for deciding when to refer difficult cases.

Using this book will help you develop the confidence to do basic skin surgery and provide you with knowledge about when to refer cases that are beyond your expertise.

Richard P. Usatine

# Acknowledgments

We are grateful to our patients for generously allowing us to photograph their skin conditions and surgeries. We thank our staff members and colleagues for helping us collect the photographs that are essential for this book.

We would like to acknowledge Debbie Kafka and Betty Chu for their support in putting this book together, including their many trips to the film processing store. We also thank Dr. Susan Stangl, Dr. Norman Solomon, Dr. Martin Smietanka, and Dr. Lesley Wilkinson for their feedback on the manuscript.

- Dr. Usatine would like to thank his family, for graciously allowing the slides and manuscript to take over their dining room table for months at a time. Specifically he would like to thank his wife Janna Lesser for her support and love and his children Rebecca and Jeremy for the joy they bring to their parents.

- Dr. Moy would like to acknowledge Dr. Usatine's enthusiasm for keeping this project alive and his wife Lisa and daughters Lauren and Erin for their support.

- Dr. Tobinick would like to thank his parents, Sidney and Odelle; his brothers, Arthur and Matthew, for their love, support, and encouragement; and Alan Weinberger and Peter Rainer for their friendship and support.

- Dr. Siegel would like to thank his parents Al and Judy for sharing their love of the printed word with him.

Finally, we wish to express our thanks to Mosby, especially Susie Baxter, Editor; Ellen Baker Geisel, Developmental Editor; Karen Rehwinkel, Production Editor; and Jen Marmarinos, Designer.

Richard P. Usatine

Ronald L. Moy

Edward L. Tobinick

Daniel Mark Siegel

# Contents

# CHAPTER I

# Facilities, Instruments, and Equipment

*Richard P. Usatine    Ronald L. Moy*

Simple surgical procedures can be performed in almost any office if the lighting is adequate. Standard office lighting is often too dim to allow proper visualization of the operative field. When a physician is setting up a new facility, he or she should consider using parabolic reflectors rather than plastic diffusers on fluorescent lights placed in the ceiling. The number of fixtures used in a standard clerical setting should be increased (up to double the number of fixtures is advantageous and worth the extra cost). For many physicians, this will provide adequate lighting for performing simple surgical procedures.

Adequate lighting can also be achieved by using office surgical lights that are either ceiling mounted or on a rolling base. One of the least expensive sources of light is an incandescent gooseneck lamp. Halogen lamps provide the brightest light but cost the most to purchase and maintain. Fluorescent lights are thermally cool and may have a central magnifying area that facilitates visualization of the operative site. Headlamps can also be used to illuminate the operative area; when used in conjunction with loupes, headlamps are invaluable when performing finely detailed procedures.

It is helpful to have a surgical table with a height adjustment. Individual preferences will determine if a physician performs most procedures while sitting or standing; however, bending often over the surgical table will lead to acute and chronic back or neck problems for the physician. If a physician spends a significant amount of time operating, this becomes critical. Alternatively, a physician's stool height can be adjusted so that the physician does not need to bend over a patient.

It is not necessary to have elaborate operating room facilities to do any of the procedures described in this book, although one might wish to perform most of these procedures in a "clean" room that is not also being used for "dirty" procedures such as sigmoidoscopies.

To summarize, basic surgical or examination room components should include the following:

- Surgical or examination table
- Adjustable stool
- Adequate lighting
- Mayo stand to hold surgical instruments during surgery

## SMALL INSTRUMENTS

Small surgical instruments can be categorized by their purpose in surgery, such as the following:

- Cutting: scalpels, scissors, punches, curettes
- Tissue holding: forceps, skin hooks

- Undermining: scissors
- Hemostasis: hemostats
- Suturing and wound closure: needle holders, scissors, staplers

## Cutting

Instruments required to perform excisions include scalpel handles with No. 15 blades (although No. 11 and No. 10 blades are useful to have in stock for various procedures), forceps with one or two teeth, a skin hook, iris scissors to cut sutures, a Webster needle holder that does not have teeth (smooth), and small undermining scissors (usually tenotomy or Gradle scissors). Kelly or mosquito clamps—curved or straight—are also useful for clamping and tying bleeding vessels.

It is best to purchase high-quality instruments that will last and perform better during surgical procedures. It is very important to have a high-quality needle holder because a poorly manufactured one will not hold needles properly. The best surgical instruments are often made in Germany, England, and the United States. Some of the less expensive surgical instruments are manufactured in countries such as Pakistan, and the quality of these instruments can vary.

### Scalpels

A scalpel has two parts, the handle and blade. The most commonly used blade for skin surgery is a No. 15. A No. 11 blade is pointed and is useful for incision and drainage of an abscess. A No. 10 blade is larger than a No. 15 blade and has the same shape. The No. 10 blade is useful for doing a shave biopsy of a large lesion or for cutting thicker skin (Fig. 1-1).

Blades are disposable and can be purchased separately or preattached to disposable plastic handles. The advantage of a totally disposable scalpel is it elimi-

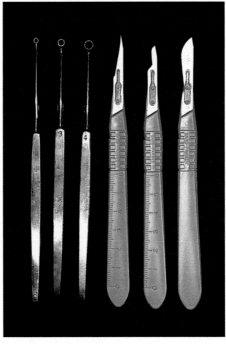

**FIG 1-1**
Curettes (2, 3, and 4 mm) and scalpels (Nos. 11, 15, and 10 blades).

nates the risk of being cut while attaching or removing a disposable blade from a nondisposable metal handle. The extra cost of the fully disposable scalpel is small when the potential risk of being cut by a contaminated instrument is considered. Although risk of being cut can be minimized by using a blade-removal instrument (Miltex makes one), disposable scalpels also save time by avoiding the need to clean and autoclave a reusable handle. The disadvantage of disposable scalpels is that they are not as stable or as sharp as a metal scalpel handle with a disposable blade. Personna makes particularly sharp Teflon-coated blades. However, sharp disposable blades are also available from Bard-Parker and Cincinnati Surgical. Delasco sells all three of these blade types as well as fully disposable scalpels. It may be worthwhile to try out more than one type to determine which one meets your personal needs. Although some physicians believe that a metal scalpel handle allows them to make more precise incisions on delicate as well as thick skin areas, others use completely disposable scalpels and believe that these serve their needs.

### Scissors

The most useful scissor for snip excisions and cutting the base of a punch biopsy is the iris scissor, a small, sharp-tipped scissor that may be straight or curved. Use of the straight or curved iris is a matter of personal preference. Scissor length varies from $3\frac{1}{2}$ to $4\frac{1}{2}$ inches. The iris scissor can be used for suture removal and cutting sutures. It can also be used for blunt dissection and undermining, although a blunt tenotomy scissor is recommended for these procedures.

Scissors need periodic sharpening, but properly cleaned and treated instruments will generally last a long time and are worth the investment.

### Punches

Punches come in sizes ranging from 2 mm to 8 mm. Physicians may choose between disposable, one-use punches and reusable steel punches (See Fig. 9-5). Disposable punches are presterilized and need no maintenance. Reusable punches, although initially far more expensive, will last longer but must be maintained by proper, skilled sharpening and require sterilization between procedures. We use disposable punches for the majority of procedures because of convenience.

### Curettes

Dermal curettes are useful for excising seborrheic keratoses, molluscum contagiosum, and many basal cell and squamous cell carcinomas. The head of the curette may be round (Fox curette) or oval (Piffard curette). One side of the curette head is dull. The other side has a semisharp blade that is designed to cut through friable or soft tissue (such as in the lesions mentioned above) but is not sharp enough to cut normal skin.[1] This allows the curette to distinguish between abnormal and normal tissue and to selectively remove the abnormal tissue.

Curettes range in size from 1 to 7 mm. Nondisposable and disposable curettes are available. We use nondisposable curettes. The size and shape of the curette used are in part determined by personal preference. Larger curettes allow for removal of larger lesions with fewer strokes. Smaller curettes are more precise and can be used on smaller lesions and for curettage of small pockets of tumor that are more difficult to reach with larger curettes.[2] It is helpful for a physician to have a range of curettes available in the office. The 3-mm curette is probably the most commonly used size, and a range of 2 to 4 mm is adequate for most procedures (Fig. 1-1).

## Tissue Holding

A large variety of forceps and skin hooks are available that enable a physician to handle skin in a means that facilitates cutting, undermining, and suturing. The goal of tissue holding is to provide the most stability during these procedures while minimizing skin trauma and scarring.

### Forceps

Basic types of forceps include tissue forceps, dressing forceps, and splinter forceps. To aid in removing splinters, splinter forceps have sharp tips and no teeth. Dressing and tissue forceps are available with and without teeth. Forceps with serrated tips are better used for handling sterile dressings because the serrations can crush tissue. There are varying opinions on the value of teeth on forceps. Some physicians believe that they can handle skin more atraumatically when forceps have teeth, whereas others believe there is less tissue trauma without teeth. This is probably an issue that may be determined by personal preference.

The most commonly used forceps in skin surgery is the Adson forceps, which has a broad handle and a long, narrow tip. One common configuration of teeth is one tooth on one tip fitting into two teeth on the other tip. Many variations of this configuration exist. We suggest you start with the basic 4¾-inch Adson forceps, with or without teeth, and experiment with others as needed.

### Skin hooks

Skin hooks are capable of holding tissue in the least traumatic manner. They are better than any forceps and do not crush skin edges, which increases the risk of infection and scarring. Skin hooks are especially useful for holding skin while placing deep sutures (see Fig. 8-5).

Therefore the hooks are worth purchasing and learning to use. Skin hooks are available with single- or double-pronged hooks and with sharp or blunt prongs. We recommend the single, sharp-pronged hook.

Skin hooks may be used for many of the same purposes as forceps and for additional procedures such as the following:

- To lift out a punch biopsy specimen
- To hold a wound edge while undermining the skin
- To retract a skin edge to expose bleeding sites and to obtain hemostasis
- To evert the skin edge while placing deep and superficial sutures
- To determine the degree of skin redundancy while treating dog-ears (See Chapter 10)
- To put traction on the corners of an ellipse while placing staples

## Undermining

The skin is best undermined with blunt-tipped scissors. Blunt tips cause less trauma to the tissue and are more likely to displace vessels and nerves than to cut through them.[1] Undermining with a scalpel is most likely to cut vessels and nerves, but sharp-tipped scissors can also cut vital structures.

Blunt-tipped scissors come in many shapes and sizes. Blunt tenotomy scissors are most useful for undermining skin. They are available with curved or straight blades. Personal preference determines the size and shape used. However, smaller scissors are better for more delicate work.

## Hemostasis

Hemostats are primarily used to clamp bleeding vessels selected for electrocoagulation or ligation. Hemostats may also be used to break up loculations after opening an abscess or for blunt dissection around cysts and lipomas. The best hemostats for skin surgery are small instruments known as *mosquito forceps*. Personal preference determines the size and shape used.

## Wound Closure

### Needle holders

Needle holders for skin surgery should be short and small enough to hold small needles with 4-0 to 6-0 sutures. Because the suturing is not being done in a deep cavity, the needle holder does not have to be long. A shorter handle allows for more precise handling. We prefer smooth rather than serrated jaws on needle holders to avoid fraying sutures while doing instrument ties. The Webster needle holder with smooth jaws is most commonly used in skin surgery and is available in 4¾-inch and 5-inch sizes. Larger and heavier needle holders may be helpful when suturing tougher, thicker skin (e.g., on the back). Small, fine needle holders are useful for finer work on the face and other more delicate areas. It is important to have good quality needle holders. Needle holders with gold-plated finger rings and tungsten carbide inserts are also available. Although these items are not necessary, physicians should not purchase poorly made, cheap instruments with the objective of saving money in the short term.

### Suture-cutting scissors

Virtually any type of scissor may be used to cut sutures during surgery or to remove sutures after some wound healing has occurred. There may be an advantage to using a designated pair of scissors for suture cutting because tissue-cutting scissors will become dull if used often to cut sutures. Iris scissors work well to cut sutures during surgery or to remove sutures postoperatively. These fine, sharp-tipped scissors can easily go under the suture to cut it for removal. There are special suture-removal scissors that have a hook on the end of one blade that is designed to slip under the suture and cut it without traumatizing the underlying skin. Examples of scissors include the Spencer, Shortbent, and Littauer stitch scissors.

### Staplers

Wounds can be closed more rapidly with staples than sutures. Staples are more expensive and are generally not used in cosmetically sensitive areas. Staples are best applied to long incisions on the scalp, trunk, or extremities. Staplers may be reusable or disposable. Reusable staplers are autoclavable and are used with sterile staple cartridges. An example of using staples on the scalp is found in Chapter 15.

## Small Instrument Sets

To save time and packing materials, it helps to establish standard small instrument sets for use in the office. Suggested sets for different surgical needs include the following:

### Basic instrument set

- Adson forceps (with teeth)
- Iris scissors (straight or curved): useful for snip excision (e.g., skin tag), with 2-mm punch if not suturing the defect, and for suture removal

### Small excision set

- Adson forceps
- Iris scissors

- Webster needle holder (smooth)
- Designated suture scissors (optional): useful for punch biopsy to be sutured and small elliptical excision

### Large excision set

- Adson forceps
- Iris scissors
- Webster needle holder
- Blunt tenotomy scissors
- Mosquito hemostat
- 2 skin hooks (single, sharp prong)
- Designated suture scissors (optional)
- Add cotton-tipped swabs, metal basin, and blade handle as needed

Sets of cotton gauze and cotton-tipped swabs may save time and money over individually packaged gauze and swabs. Cotton gauze and swabs purchased in bulk may be autoclaved in packs to be used for moderate to large skin procedures.

## Surgical Skin Markers

It is extremely helpful to mark the lines or area that you intend to cut. This is true for simple elliptical excisions and shave biopsies, and not just for flaps and grafts. It is best to mark the skin before administering anesthesia because the anesthesia may distort the lesion or make it less visible.

There are a number of types of surgical markers available. The standard markers use gentian violet and are nontoxic. Preoperative prepping with alcohol will rub off the gentian violet, but Betadine and Hibiclens may not. These markers can be purchased in sterile packages for single use in a sterile procedure. However, for procedures such as shave biopsies and snip excisions that will not be sutured, the marker need not be sterile. A fine-point marker is most useful. For slightly more money (about 10% more), twin-tipped markers are available that have a broad tip on one end and a fine tip on the other. A sterile marker costs approximately $1 to $2. A nonsterile marker is often less expensive. There have been no reported cases of tattooing.

## MAGNIFICATION DEVICES

It is helpful to have at least one device available to magnify lesions. There is a wide range of magnifying lenses available, from inexpensive hand-held magnifying lenses to expensive binocular loupes. Good quality magnification with good resolution will allow the physician to see small features, such as telangiectasias, that may not be visible to the naked eye.

The advantage of loupes that are mounted to eyeglasses or a headband is that the physician is able to use both hands in a procedure while getting the benefit of magnification. Magnification levels range from two to six times normal. Two times magnification should be sufficient for most skin lesion diagnoses and procedures and provide a comfortable working distance from the lesion in focus (about 10 inches). The Opti-Visor is a good starting device; the Heine binocular loupe is an expensive, high-quality optical instrument.

## PROTECTIVE GEAR

To be protected from blood and fluids during surgery, it is essential to wear surgical gloves. Surgical masks and eye protectors should be available for surgeries on known high-risk individuals or for surgeries in which the risk of exposure to blood or fluid is greatest. See Chapter 2 for further information on universal precautions.

## TOPICAL ANESTHETICS

- EMLA (Eutectic Mixture of Local Anesthetics) cream
- Topical lidocaine jelly or ointment
- Cetacaine spray

## CRYOANESTHESIA (REFRIGERANTS)

- Ethyl chloride
- Medi-Frig or Fluoro Ethyl

## CHEMICAL HEMOSTATIC AGENTS

- Aluminum chloride
- Monsel's solution (ferric subsulfate)
- Trichloroacetic acid
- Silver nitrate sticks

## EQUIPMENT

### Shave Equipment

- No. 15 (or No. 10) blades with scalpel handles
- 3-ml syringe and needle for local anesthesia
- Cotton-tipped swabs for hemostasis

### Punch Equipment

- Punches: 2 mm to 8 mm
- Fine, sharp scissors
- Forceps
- Needle holder and sutures or hemostatic solution

### Cryotherapy Equipment

#### Liquid nitrogen

- Storage dewar (tank) (See Fig. 11-1)
- Cryogun (See Fig. 11-2)
- Cotton-tipped swabs

- Cotton balls
- Styrofoam cups

## Electrosurgery Equipment

### Solid state electrosurgical units

- Hyfrecator Plus* (by ConMed, previously by Birtcher) (See Fig. 12-2)
- Delasco 734*: a newer version of the discontinued Hyfrecator 733
- Surgitron Radiofrequency Unit (by Ellman) (See Fig. 12-5)
- Surgistat (by Valley Lab)

### Hyfrecator Plus Accessories

- Disposable electrodes (See Fig. 12-4)
- Electrolase blunt tips
- Electrolase sharp tips: beware of the fact that these tips can cut tissue when you are not intending to do so (inadvertently)
- Metal hubbed needles with adapter
- Epilation needles
- Sterile sleeves for switching handles: sterile gloves or 12-inch sterile Penrose drains can be used to cover handle in a sterile field

### Smoke Evacuators

- Con-Med Hyfre-Vac
- Delasco SaftEvac†
- Ellman Vapor-Vac
- Accuderm-Vac
- Buffalo filters

### Thermal Pencil Cautery

- Available with sterile or nonsterile tips

## Equipment for Incision and Drainage

- Lidocaine with epinephrine, needle and syringe
- Scalpel with No. 11 blade (essential for the incision)
- Cotton-tipped swabs
- Hemostat, preferably curved
- Forceps (for packing the dead space)
- Scissors (to cut the gauze [Nu-Gauze])
- 4 × 4 gauze pads to remove pus from field
- Nu-Gauze (width based on size of abscess; comes in ¼-inch and ½-inch, iodinated or noniodinated)

## Equipment for Intralesional Injections

- Injectable steroids (triamcinolone acetonide 3 mg/ml, 10 mg/ml, 40 mg/ml)
- Needles (25 gauge to 30 gauge)
- Syringes (1 ml or 3 ml, Luer Lok preferable)
- Vials of sterile saline for injection (for dilutions)

---

*Least expensive models.
†Least expensive unit.

## CONCLUSION

To do skin surgery well, it is important to have the appropriate instruments for the procedure. Good instruments that are well maintained will facilitate the diagnosis and treatment of skin disorders. The following resource list provides sources for the best instruments, supplies, and equipment at the best price.

## RESOURCES

- Acuderm: 800-327-0015 (a good selection of disposable punches, curettes, and other instruments; they also sell skin-marking pens)
- Bernsco: 800-231-8409
- Delasco Dermatologic Buying Guide: 800-831-6273 (the most comprehensive catalogue of dermatologic supplies, equipment, and dermatology books)
- Henry Schein: 800-772-4346
- Miltex: 800-645-8000
- Moore Medical: 800-234-1464
- Padgett Instruments: 800-842-1029
- SSR Surgical Instruments: 800-932-7364

Local medical supply companies can usually offer less expensive prices than any of the mail order companies

### Internet Addresses

Internet addresses for the companies listed above include the following:

- **www.delasco.com:** This site offers a comprehensive home page with online catalog and order entry form. The Delasco home page also has a hotlinks page that has links to other Web sites for these topics: dermatology organizations and sites, medical sites, general information, academic dermatology departments, dermatology news, and humor.
- **www.henryschein.com:** You can order products online, but there is no online catalog at this time. More than 12,000 products are contained in the printed Henry Schein Medical Catalog. These products include pharmaceuticals, vaccines, diagnostic tests, gloves, paper products, and examination room supplies.
- **www.mooremedical.com:** You can order products online, but there is no online catalog at this time. Headquartered in New Britain, Connecticut, Moore Medical is a national distributor of brand name and generic pharmaceuticals and medical and surgical supplies.

## REFERENCES

1. Diwan R: Instruments for dermatologic surgery. In Lask G, Moy R, editors: *Principles and techniques of cutaneous surgery*, New York, 1996, McGraw-Hill.
2. Krull EA: Surgical gems: the "little" curette, *J Dermatol Surg Oncol* 4:656-657, 1978.

# CHAPTER 2

# Preoperative Preparation: Universal Precautions, Sterilization, and Medical Evaluation

*Edward L. Tobinick   Ronald L. Moy   Richard P. Usatine*

The practice of skin surgery in the physician's office requires familiarity with surgical technique, careful planning, instruction of ancillary personnel, patient education, and proper preparation of the surgical site, the surgical instruments, and the patient. Universal precautions to prevent the transmission of infectious diseases are paramount to protecting the physician, the medical staff, and the patient.

## UNIVERSAL PRECAUTIONS

With the identification of AIDS in the 1980s, measures to prevent the transmission of contagious diseases to medical personnel gained wide support from those who work in the surgical suite.[1-4] Blood-borne diseases continue to be a hazard to surgical personnel, despite the availability of serologic tests to detect the presence of many infectious diseases.[5-8] Diseases of chief concern are hepatitis B, hepatitis C, and HIV/AIDS. However, other contagious diseases, such as tuberculosis and syphilis, also present some potential risk to medical personnel.

The first prerequisite for the proper maintenance of universal precautions is education of all office staff who may potentially be exposed to infectious material, particularly blood. We make a concerted effort in our offices to educate all employees. All personnel who may come in contact with blood should be vaccinated against hepatitis B.[3] All personnel must also be advised of the necessity of informing their supervisor if a needle-stick injury or other exposure to blood occurs. Office protocols vary, but we usually recommend testing the patient for serologic evidence of potential infectious disease, testing the employee, and administering the appropriate preventive measures if definite exposure has occurred. We recommend checking with the Occupational Safety and Health Administration (OSHA) and the Centers for Disease Control and Prevention (CDC) to confirm the current recommendations for blood or other body-fluid exposure.

The basics of universal precautions include the use of surgical gloves and the use of barrier clothing, such as gowns, face masks, and eye protection when appropriate; proper disposal of sharp, disposable surgical instruments, such as needles and scalpel blades, in special puncture-proof containers; disposal of all contaminated drapes and other soft items in specially marked containers; and collection and disposal of this material by professional hazardous-waste removal companies. Recommendations for the use of gloves are presented in detail the *Morbidity and Mortality Weekly Report* dated June 24, 1988. This publication is available by calling the National AIDS Information Hotline at 1-800-342-2437 or the National AIDS Information Clearinghouse at 1-800-458-5231. In addition, OSHA has published a brochure on "blood-borne pathogens." To obtain this document, call 202-219-7157. The CDC recommendations are listed in Box 2-1.

In our office we add to these basic universal precautions. We have found it especially helpful to practice choreographed surgery, with particular attention paid to any sharp instruments. We handle only one sharp instrument at a time

---

**BOX 2-1    Universal Precautions**

1. All health-care workers should routinely use appropriate barrier precautions to prevent skin and mucous-membrane exposure when contact with blood or other body fluids of any patient is anticipated. Gloves should be worn for touching blood and body fluids, mucous membranes, or nonintact skin of all patients; for handling items or surfaces soiled with blood or body fluids; and for performing venipuncture and other vascular access procedures. Gloves should be changed after contact with each patient. Masks and protective eyewear or face shields should be worn during procedures that are likely to generate droplets of blood or other body fluids to prevent exposure of mucous membranes of the mouth, nose, and eyes. Gowns or aprons should be worn during procedures that are likely to generate splashes of blood or other body fluids.
2. Hands and other skin surfaces should be washed immediately and thoroughly if contaminated with blood or other body fluids. Hands should be washed immediately after gloves are removed.
3. All health-care workers should take precautions to prevent injuries caused by needles, scalpels, and other sharp instruments or devices during procedures; when cleaning used instruments; during disposal of used needles; and when handling sharp instruments after procedures. To prevent needle-stick injuries, needles should not be recapped, purposely bent or broken by hand, removed from disposable syringes, or otherwise manipulated by hand. After they are used, disposable syringes and needles, scalpel blades, and other sharp items should be placed in puncture-resistant containers for disposal; the puncture-resistant containers should be located as close as practical to the use area.
4. Although saliva has not been implicated in HIV transmission, to minimize the need for emergency mouth-to-mouth resuscitation, mouthpieces, resuscitation bags, or other ventilation devices should be available for use in areas in which the need for resuscitation is predictable.
5. Health-care workers who have exudative lesions or weeping dermatitis should refrain from all direct patient care and from handling patient-care equipment until the condition resolves.
6. Pregnant health-care workers are not known to be at greater risk of contracting HIV infection than health-care workers who are not pregnant; however, if a health-care worker develops HIV infection during pregnancy, the infant is at risk of infection resulting from perinatal transmission. Because of this risk, pregnant health-care workers should be especially familiar with and strictly adhere to precautions to minimize the risk of HIV transmission.

From CDC: *MMWR* 36(suppl 2S):1S-18S, 1987.

and are aware of its position at all times. We take particular care to avoid rushing when performing surgery, and attempt to have extra help available—within earshot—at all times.

## SCHEDULING OF COMPLEX SURGERIES

Simple surgical procedures, such as shave or punch biopsies, need no special scheduling. These procedures can be done rapidly as the need arises. However, physicians contemplating performing more complex surgical procedures in the office will benefit from careful, deliberate consideration of how best to integrate the surgeries into the office schedule. Proper scheduling is critical to producing the efficient, unhurried surgical atmosphere that is reassuring to both the patient and the staff.

Some offices schedule more complex surgeries at the end of the morning or the end of the afternoon to avoid being rushed by other patient responsibilities. This allows the physician to approach surgery in an unhurried manner. It may also be helpful to do more complex surgeries at the beginning of the week and avoid surgery on Friday so patients can be seen the day after surgery for a postoperative check.

## SURGICAL PLANNING

Universal precautions are one aspect of the planning required before surgery. Other aspects include the following:

- Preoperative medical evaluation
- Informed consent
- Standby medications and equipment
- Sterile technique
- Sterilization of instruments
- Preoperative patient preparation (skin, hair, drapes)
- Preoperative medications (e.g., antibiotic prophylaxis to prevent skin infections, endocarditis prophylaxis)

## PREOPERATIVE MEDICAL EVALUATION

### Medical History

A complete medical history and review of systems before minor skin surgery may not be necessary. Items that should be included in the history include the following:

- Current medications, especially anticoagulants, aspirin, and other nonsteroidal antiinflammatory drugs (NSAIDs), cardiac drugs
- Allergies, especially to antibiotics, tapes/adhesives, iodine
- Cardiac disease (e.g., any condition requiring endocarditis prophylaxis (e.g., valve disease), uncontrolled hypertension, epinephrine sensitivity, angina, pacemaker (electrosurgery precautions)
- Other illnesses and medical conditions (e.g., seizure disorder, hematologic disorder or bleeding diathesis, joint replacement (endocarditis prophylaxis), high-risk groups [injection drug users], diabetes)
- Pregnancy
- Keloids or hypertrophic scars
- Infectious diseases (e.g., hepatitis, AIDS, tuberculosis)

For minor skin surgery under local anesthesia, blood pressure does not need to be monitored unless the patient has a history of hypertension that is not controlled. Uncontrolled hypertension may lead to increased bleeding during surgery. It is prudent to be more careful with fragile patients, such as the elderly, and to be particularly careful with the use of epinephrine-containing anesthetics in patients with a history of angina, cardiac disease, or a sensitivity to epinephrine. It may help to warn patients that they may develop an increased heart rate or a feeling of anxiety after injection of lidocaine with epinephrine.

### Informed Consent

Thorough discussion with the patient regarding the benefits and risks of the planned surgical procedure and the alternatives to surgery that are available is essential before surgery. It is always best to leave adequate time for this discussion so that all of the patient's questions can be answered in an unhurried manner. For many routine minor procedures, such as skin biopsy, a written consent may not be needed. However, written consent is always obtained for procedures that may have more significant adverse consequences, such as scarring or functional effects. Appendix A is a sample skin surgery consent form. Feel free to use or modify this form for your own office.

### Standby Medications and Equipment

It is helpful to have injectable Benadryl and epinephrine available for subcutaneous injection in case of an anaphylactic reaction to anesthesia, latex, or other medication. It may also be helpful to have an Ambu bag, an insertable airway, oxygen, a cardiac monitor, and a defibrillator in your office, but these items are not absolutely necessary.

## STERILE TECHNIQUE

Absolute sterile technique is not necessary for many of the minor skin surgical procedures performed. This is true for cryosurgery and electrosurgery, but also for shave biopsy of the skin, curettage, incision and drainage, and other small surgical procedures in which the wounds are left open to heal without suturing. Although all instruments must be sterile before use for these procedures, the physician may use nonsterile gloves. Sterile drapes are not needed. In our office, we use single-use scalpels and needles that are disposed of at the end of the procedure.

Sterile technique is necessary when performing surgery in which the wound will be closed, such as with suturing or staples. Careful instruction of ancillary surgical personnel in sterile technique is necessary.

### Sterilization of Instruments

Before sterilization, instruments must be cleaned of blood and debris. This can be done manually with a soft toothbrush or by using an ultrasonic cleaner; a combination of the procedures is often necessary.

A steam sterilizer (autoclave) is necessary to sterilize the instruments and ensure that viral diseases such as hepatitis or HIV are not transmitted from patient to patient. Holding solutions should not be used to sterilize instruments. They can only be used to temporarily hold or clean instruments and are inadequate for proper sterilization. The instruments should be placed in sterilization bags with indicator strips to ensure the sterilization process is effective. These bags come in a variety of sizes to accommodate different instrument sets. Self-sealing bags cost a bit more than those that must be taped, but the convenience outweighs the cost.

The instruments can be packaged in sets for specific procedures. Instruments can also be sterilized in other containers, but they need to be moved in a sterile manner onto the surgical table. Gauze, cotton-tipped applicators, electrosurgery tips, and glass containers can all be steam sterilized by putting them in steam sterilization bags. It can be helpful to create surgical packs that contain a number of cotton-tipped applicators and gauze. This can save you the time of opening individually sterilized packets and can save money by allowing you to buy applicators and gauze in bulk.

# PREOPERATIVE PATIENT PREPARATION

## Preparation of the Skin

The most common preoperative preparations to be used on the skin include alcohol, Betadine (povidone-iodine), and Hibiclens (chlorhexidine). The main advantages of using Hibiclens are that it has longer-lasting antibacterial effect than Betadine and the risk of contact sensitivity may be less. The disadvantage of using Hibiclens is that it is more toxic to the eye if it accidentally drops into it. However, if the eye is flushed immediately, no damage may be done. Caution must be taken when using alcohol or Hibiclens tincture to be sure that all of the alcohol has evaporated before any cautery is performed in the area. This eliminates the possibility of ignition of the solution, the surrounding drapes and gauze, and the physician.

The most important part of the preoperative preparation of the skin is the mechanical rubbing of the antiseptic onto the skin with a sterile gauze. It is actually impossible to sterilize the skin because bacteria can extend into hair follicles. The goal of the preoperative preparation of the skin is to reduce the bacteria on the skin surface by scrubbing the skin with a good antiseptic such as Betadine or Hibiclens. Betadine must be allowed to dry on the skin for its effect to be optimal. Skin preparation may be performed using sterile gauze from the operative field or Betadine swab sticks. An 8-oz bottle of Hibiclens can be kept in each examination/procedure room and can be used repeatedly by pouring the solution onto clean gauze.

## Preparation of Hair

The best method of hair removal over a surgical site is to use scissors to cut the hairs. Using scissors is preferable to using a razor because a close shave causes minute abrasions and cuts into the skin that can increase the chance of infection. For elective procedures, the site can be shaved by the patient 2 days before surgery. The scalp is the area of the body in which the hairs can most interfere with surgery. Plastering down the hair with water, petrolatum, or ointment can decrease the number of hairs that interfere with surgery without causing a noticeable loss of hair during the postoperative period.

## Drapes

The use of sterile fenestrated aperture drapes (drapes with a hole) is necessary when suturing is performed so that the sutures do not drag over nonsterile skin. Sterile drapes are not necessary for small procedures, such as a shave biopsy, where suturing is not performed. Disposable or linen-quality sterile drapes are adequate for the procedures described in this book. You can create your own aperture drapes by cutting a hole in a sterile disposable drape. This can save money and allow you to custom make the hole size you need. The paper used to wrap surgical trays before sterilization is excellent for this purpose. Drapes can be cut in a variety of sizes with a variety of holes and then sterilized alone or as part of a packet. Prepackaged disposable sterile drapes have a slight advantage in that they have adhesive around the aperture to stabilize the drape and isolate the field. This can save time and allow you to custom make the hole size you need.

## PREOPERATIVE MEDICATIONS

The most important part of medication history is to find out if the patient is taking aspirin because this drug can cause excessive bleeding in the intraoperative or postoperative period. The ideal situation is to have the patient stop taking aspirin at least 2 weeks before any surgical procedure. It is important to warn the patient about over-the-counter products that contain aspirin and NSAIDs that can also have an effect on platelet function. NSAIDs need to be stopped 2 days before a procedure because the effect of NSAIDs on platelets is reversible. However, aspirin has an irreversible effect on platelets, and its use requires that the patient wait 2 weeks after discontinuing use for new platelets to replace the old ones.

Minor procedures, such as skin biopsies, may not require stopping aspirin use. Coumadin can also be a potential cause of excess bleeding, but it does not cause the same degree of excess bleeding as aspirin. For most minor skin procedures described in this book, Coumadin does not need to be stopped before surgery. If you are not the physician prescribing and monitoring the use of Coumadin by your patient, that physician should be consulted before the Coumadin is stopped. Rather than stopping anticoagulation, alternative procedures must be considered and discussed with the patient and the prescribing physician before Coumadin therapy is altered. If the procedure is complex, stopping the Coumadin about 2 to 4 days before surgery can lessen the chance of any excess bleeding. However, the risks of stopping the Coumadin (thrombosis, embolism, and stroke) must be weighed against the benefit of surgery. Coumadin can be restarted about 2 days after surgery when the chance of hematoma formation decreases. Pressure dressings can help minimize the risk of hematoma. In general, rather than stopping Coumadin we prefer to take exceptional care in using electrosurgery for hemostasis, which does not require interruption of anticoagulation.

Other medications do not usually interfere with skin surgery. A history of an antibiotic allergy may be relevant if prophylactic antibiotics are given. Antianxiety medications such as triazolam, diazepam, or lorazepam can be useful in the very anxious patient. If these medications are administered sublingually (under the tongue), the onset of action can be quicker than when they are administered orally. These medications should not be given to a patient who will be driving home. All patients given intraoperative or preoperative sedatives must be accompanied by an adult, must be counseled not to drive on the day of the surgery, must be observed postoperatively until the sedative effect has sufficiently diminished, and must be counseled that their mental capacities may be diminished for a prolonged period after surgery.

It is not advisable to do skin surgery on patients who have unstable angina because the epinephrine in the local anesthetic can precipitate angina. Although this is unlikely, it is worth having nitroglycerin in the office to deal with this potential situation.

Patients who have uncontrolled diabetes mellitus may have impaired wound healing. Closer follow-up after surgery may help avoid potential problems with these patients.

## Antibiotic Prophylaxis

Preoperative antibiotics such as oral cephalexin, dicloxacillin, or clindamycin may be recommended for use with the patient who has a higher risk of infection.[9,10] These situations might include a patient who has a contaminated or infected lesion; a lesion in an area of increased bacteria, such as the axilla, ear, or mouth; a lesion on a hand or foot, especially in patients with peripheral vascular disease; a situation in which the operation might take more than 1 hour or if the wound was open for more than 1 hour; a patient where complete sterile technique was not optimal; or any situation in which an infection would have serious consequences, such as in a diabetic patient or a patient with neutropenia. See Table 2-1 for classification of wound infections and the need for antibiotic prophylaxis.

## Endocarditis Prophylaxis

Endocarditis prophylaxis is not recommended for incision or biopsy of surgically scrubbed skin.[10,11] However, it may be prudent to use prophylaxis before surgery involving the mucus membranes of the mouth, nose, and perirectal areas or of eroded or infected skin.[11] Patients that require preoperative antibiotics are those with prosthetic heart valves, prosthetic joints, or significant valvular heart disease. These patients often know that they have to take antibiotics before any dental procedure. Cardiac conditions for which endocarditis prophylaxis is recommended are listed in Box 2-2.

### TABLE 2-1    Classification of Wound Infections

| Class | Antibiotic prophylaxis |
|---|---|
| **Clean**<br>Noncontaminated skin, sterile technique = 5% infection | No |
| **Clean contaminated**<br>Wounds in oral cavity, respiratory tract, axilla/perineum;<br>breaks in aseptic technique = 10% infection rate | ?Yes |
| **Contaminated**<br>Trauma, acute nonpurulent inflammation, major breaks<br>in aseptic technique (intact, inflamed cysts; tumors with<br>clinical inflammation) = 20% to 30% infection rate | Yes |
| **Infected**<br>Gross contamination with foreign bodies, devitalized tissue<br>(ruptured cysts; tumors with purulent, necrotic<br>material) = 30% to 40% infection rate | Yes |

From Haas AF, Grekin RC: *J Am Acad Dermatol* 32:155, 1995.

Haas and Grekin[10] developed Table 2-2 to determine if patients with eroded or infected skin should get endocarditis prophylaxis. These are not American Heart Association (AHA) recommendations. For contaminated skin in patients at high risk for developing bacterial endocarditis, the recommended antibiotic regimens are the same as those listed in Table 2-3.

In June of 1997 the new AHA recommendations for the prevention of bacterial endocarditis were published in *JAMA*.[11] The major changes in the updated recommendations include the following:

(1) emphasis that most cases of endocarditis are not attributable to an invasive procedure; (2) cardiac conditions are stratified into high-, moderate-, and negligible-risk categories based on potential outcome if endocarditis develops; (3) procedures that may cause bacteremia and for which prophylaxis is recommended are more clearly

---

**BOX 2-2    Cardiac Conditions for Which Endocarditis Prophylaxis is Recommended***

**High Risk**
Prosthetic cardiac valves
Previous bacterial endocarditis
Surgically constructed systemic-pulmonary shunts

**Moderate Risk**
Most congenital cardiac malformations
Rheumatic and other acquired valvular dysfunction
Hypertrophic cardiomyopathy
Mitral valve prolapse with valvular regurgitation

From Dajani AS et al: *JAMA* 277(22):1794-1801, 1997.
*American Heart Association (AHA) recommendations.

---

**TABLE 2-2    Recommendations for Endocarditis Prophylaxis in Dermatologic Surgery**

| Procedure | Persons at risk | Prophylaxis |
|---|---|---|
| Surgical manipulation of intact skin | None* | No |
| Surgical manipulation of eroded, noninfected skin | AHA "high or moderate risk" | Yes |
| Surgical manipulation of infected/abscessed skin, presence of distant skin infection | AHA "high or moderate risk," patients with orthopedic prosthesis, those with ventriculoatrial/peritoneal shunts | Yes |

From Haas AF, Grekin RC: *J Am Acad Dermatol* 32:155, 1995.
*AHA*, American Heart Association.
*A subgroup of patients with prosthetic valves and who are undergoing prolonged procedures or those procedures performed in contaminated areas warrant prophylaxis.

**TABLE 2-3    Recommended Prophylaxis Regimens for Cutaneous Procedures for Prevention of Wound Infections and/or Endocarditis**

| Antibiotic | I hr preoperative dose | 6 hr postoperative dose |
|---|---|---|
| First-generation cephalosporin | 1 g orally | 500 mg orally |
| Dicloxacillin | 1 g orally | 500 mg orally |
| Clindamycin* | 300 mg orally | 150 mg orally |
| Vancomycin† | 500 mg intravenously | 250 mg intravenously |

Modified from Haas AF, Grekin RC: *J Am Acad Dermatol* 32:155, 1995.
*Suitable for patients allergic to penicillin or cephalosporin.
†For recent prosthetic valves or orthopedic prostheses (*S. epidermidis*).

specified; (4) an algorithm was developed to more clearly define when prophylaxis is recommended for patients with mitral valve prolapse; (5) for oral or dental procedures the initial amoxicillin dose is reduced to 2 g, a follow-up antibiotic dose is no longer recommended, erythromycin is no longer recommended for penicillin-allergic individuals, but clindamycin and other alternatives are offered.[11]

## CONCLUSION

Outpatient skin surgery requires careful preparation to ensure optimal results and safety of patient and medical personnel. Strict adherence to universal precautions to prevent the transmission of contagious disease is necessary. Brief medical evaluation by the physician before performing minor procedures is recommended. Sterilization of equipment, sterile technique, informed patient consent, preoperative preparation of the operative site, preoperative medications, and endocarditis prophylaxis are all areas that require preoperative consideration. Proper preoperative planning is essential, even for minor office procedures.

## REFERENCES

1. CDC: Recommendations for prevention of HIV transmission in health-care settings, *MMWR* 36(suppl 2S):1S-18S, 1987.
2. CDC: Update: universal precautions for prevention of transmission of human immunodeficiency virus, hepatitis B virus, and other bloodborne pathogens in health-care settings, *MMWR* 37:377-388, 1988.
3. CDC: Guidelines for prevention of transmission of human immunodeficiency virus and hepatitis B virus to health-care and public-safety workers, *MMWR* 38(suppl 6):1-37, 1989.
4. OSHA: Bloodborne pathogens final standard, Fact Sheet 92-46, 1992, the Administration.
5. McCray E: The Cooperative Needlestick Surveillance Group: occupational risk of the acquired immunodeficiency syndrome among health care workers, *N Engl J Med* 314:1127-1132, 1986.
6. Gerberding JL et al: Risk of transmitting the human immunodeficiency virus, cytomegalovirus, and hepatitis B virus to health care workers exposed to patients with AIDS and AIDS-related conditions, *J Infect Dis* 156:1-8, 1987.

7. McEvoy M et al: Prospective study of clinical, laboratory, and ancillary staff with accidental exposures to blood or other body fluids from patients infected with HIV, *Br Med J* 294:1595-1597, 1987.
8. CDC: Update: human immunodeficiency virus infections in health-care workers exposed to blood of infected patients, *MMWR* 36:285-289, 1987.
9. Sanford JP, Gilbert DN, Moellering RC, Sande MA: The Sanford guide to antimicrobial therapy, Vienna, Va, 1997, Antimicrobial Therapy, Inc.
10. Haas AF, Grekin RC: Antibiotic prophylaxis in dermatologic surgery, *J Am Acad Dermatol* 32:155-176, 1995.
11. Dajani AS et al: Prevention of bacterial endocarditis: recommendations by the American Heart Association, *JAMA* 277(22):1794-1801, 1997.

# CHAPTER 3

# Anesthesia

*Richard P. Usatine*    *Ronald L. Moy*

Local anesthesia is the reversible loss of sensation to a localized area achieved by the topical application or injection of anesthetic agents. Regional anesthesia involves larger areas and is achieved by nerve block and/or field blocks through the use of injectable anesthetic agents. The goal of all anesthesia is the elimination of pain caused by surgery.[1]

Local anesthetics block the pain fibers of a nerve better than those fibers that carry sensations of pressure, touch, and temperature. Therefore if the patient feels pressure or pulling but no pain, the patient should be reassured that this is not unusual.

There are many anesthetic agents that can be injected or applied topically. Table 3-1 summarizes the characteristics of many of the agents that are used today.

## SURFACE ANESTHESIA: TOPICAL AND AEROSOL

### Topical Anesthetics

- EMLA cream
- Topical lidocaine jelly
- Cetacaine spray
- TAC (tetracaine, adrenaline, cocaine)

The most effective topical anesthetic for the skin is EMLA cream (Fig. 3-1). It consists of 2.5% lidocaine and 2.5% prilocaine in an oil-in-water emulsion. This anesthetic cream requires a 1-hour application under occlusion before good anesthesia is obtained. It is useful in treating the patient who is afraid of needles, even those as small as a 30-gauge needle. Because it produces only superficial anesthesia, the EMLA cream is only useful for some laser procedures and simple curettage of molluscum contagiosum. EMLA is available in 5-g tubes with occlusive dressings or in 30-g tubes without dressings. EMLA should not be used in infants younger than 3 months because the metabolites of prilocaine form methemoglobin.

Cocaine is one of the earliest-known topical anesthetics, with the distinction of being the only topical anesthetic that also causes vasoconstriction. For this reason, its main value is for anesthesia of vascular mucus membranes, such as the nose. Although cocaine is one of the ingredients in TAC, there is no reason to use it alone for planned cutaneous surgery. TAC is used to provide topical anesthesia before suturing lacerations in small children.

Topical lidocaine is available as a 2% jelly or viscous solution, a 5% ointment, or a 10% spray. Regardless of the vehicle, topical lidocaine takes 15 to 30 minutes to produce anesthesia on mucosal surfaces. The degree of anesthesia is not comparable to injectable lidocaine, and unless it is combined with another agent

**TABLE 3-I    Common Local Anesthetics**

| Generic/trade names | Concentration available (%) | Potency | Approximate time of onset | Onset (min) | Approximate duration (min) | | Maximum dose (mg) |
|---|---|---|---|---|---|---|---|
| | | | | | Without epinephrine | With epinephrine | |
| **Amides (hepatic metabolism)** | | | | | | | |
| Lidocaine Xylocaine | 0.5, 1.0, 2.0 | Intermediate | Rapid | 5 | 30-120 | 60-400 | 300-500 |
| Prilocaine Citanest (in EMLA) | 1.0, 2.0, 3.0 | Intermediate | Rapid | 5-6 | 30-120 | 60-400 | 600 |
| Bupivacaine Marcaine/ Sensorcaine | 0.25, 0.05, 0.75 | High | Moderate | 8 | 120-140 | 240-480 | 150-250 |
| **Esters (plasma metabolism)** | | | | | | | |
| Cocaine (in TAC) | 2-10 (topical) | High | Rapid | | 45 | — | 200 |
| Procaine Novocain | 0.5, 1.0, 2.0 | Low | Rapid | 5 | 15-45 | 30-90 | 600-1000 |
| Tetracaine Pontocaine (in Cetacaine and TAC) | 0.1, 0.25 | High | Moderate | 7 | 120-140 | 240-480 | 100 |

Modified from Matarasso SL, Glogau R: Local anesthesia. In Lask G, Moy R, editors: *Principles and techniques of cutaneous surgery*, New York, 1996, McGraw-Hill.

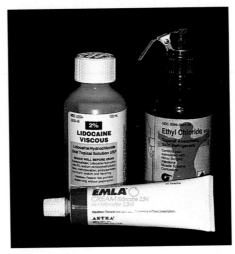

**FIG 3-1**
Topical anesthetics: lidocaine jelly, EMLA, and
ethyl chloride.

such as phenylephrine, it has no vasoconstrictive action. Therefore for mucosal surgery in the mouth, it is best to inject 1% lidocaine with epinephrine after the topical lidocaine has numbed the surface. For this purpose, it is easy to put lidocaine in the 2% jelly form on a cotton swab and have the patient hold it against the mucus membrane before the subsequent injection. This technique might be used to anesthetize a mucocele or fibroma on the lip.

Topical lidocaine jelly or Cetacaine spray can be effective for surgical procedures inside the mouth. It is usually better to use topical lidocaine in the mouth before injection of lidocaine with a needle so that painless anesthesia can be obtained.

TAC is useful in achieving anesthesia in an open laceration on a child. It is not useful for intact skin and therefore has no role in planning and executing a skin biopsy or excision.

### EMLA technique for intact skin

1. Use alcohol wipes to remove oil from the area of skin to be anesthetized.
2. Apply EMLA in a thick layer to skin, then apply occlusive dressing (Tegaderm, Op-Site, or plastic wrap) for 60 minutes; 30 minutes may be sufficient if skin is inflamed (because of increased absorption). One hour of application time should be sufficient for thin skin, such as on the face; however, thicker skin on the extremities and trunk may take 1½ hours to achieve anesthesia.
3. Remove EMLA with alcohol or with a tissue.
4. Perform additional anesthesia without delay. Topical anesthesia will last only minutes after the EMLA is removed.

## Cryoanesthesia

### Refrigerants

- Ethyl chloride
- Medi-Frig (tetrafluoroethane)
- Fluoro Ethyl (25% ethyl chloride and 75% dichlorotetrafluoroethane)
- Liquid nitrogen

Cryoanesthesia is useful before the removal of small skin lesions such as skin tags and molluscum contagiosum. For example, it can be used before a snip excision of a skin tag or curettage of molluscum contagiosum. Cryoanesthesia does not provide adequate anesthesia for the removal of larger lesions. It is slightly less effective and less expensive than EMLA, but it works much faster. The agents listed above are all inexpensive and easy to use.

Topical refrigerants can also be used to provide surface anesthesia before opening a small, superficial abscess such as a paronychia. They can also be used to numb the skin (in a needle-phobic patient) before injecting local anesthesia with a needle. These agents are sprayed on the skin until a white frost develops. The physician then has a number of seconds to perform the injection before the numbing effect wears off.

Ethyl chloride is the only one of the refrigerants listed that is flammable. Medi-Frig can be safely used before electrosurgery for small skin tags and molluscum contagiosum, whereas ethyl chloride cannot. The manufacturers of Medi-Frig claim that it is nontoxic and ozone safe, whereas the label on ethyl chloride warns against inhaling too much of the product.

Liquid nitrogen can freeze the skin to cause a numbing effect; however, its use causes immediate pain that lasts until the area thaws. For this reason, we do not recommend it for use as cryoanesthesia.

# LOCAL ANESTHESIA BY INJECTION

The two most widely used local anesthetics for injection in skin surgery are lidocaine and bupivacaine (Marcaine/Sensorcaine) (Table 3-1). Lidocaine has the advantage of having a more rapid onset (almost instantaneous) and shorter duration of anesthesia. This shorter duration is sufficient for skin surgery, especially when its use is combined with epinephrine.

## Epinephrine

With the exception of cocaine, all of the other injectable anesthetics are vasodilators. Using epinephrine with local anesthesia (1) decreases bleeding during surgery and (2) keeps the anesthetic in the area where it was injected, thereby decreasing immediate systemic absorption and toxicity and increasing duration of anesthesia. This allows greater total amounts of anesthetic to be used because the body can metabolize the anesthetic locally and reduce systemic absorption.

The vasoconstrictive effect of the epinephrine can often be seen as the skin blanches with injection; however, it may take 15 minutes to achieve maximal vasoconstriction.

## 1% Lidocaine With Epinephrine

For most skin surgery procedures, the recommended anesthetic is 1% lidocaine with epinephrine. Its advantages include only a negligible incidence of true allergies, almost immediate anesthesia, duration of about 1 hour, and decreased bleeding because of the epinephrine. The most common commercial preparation contains 1% lidocaine (10 mg/ml) with 1:100,000 of epinephrine.

## Maximal Doses

Maximal doses of 1% lidocaine as cited in the literature are found in Table 3-2. The lidocaine can be diluted with sterile water or normal saline (1:1) to a 0.5% lidocaine if volumes greater than 50 ml are needed. This does not decrease the anesthetic effect. Lidocaine dosages of up to 55 mg/kg injected

**TABLE 3-2  Table of Maximal Doses of 1% Lidocaine**

| Type of lidocaine solution | Formula by body weight | Maximal ml for weight of 50 kg | Maximal ml for weight over 70 kg |
|---|---|---|---|
| 1% lidocaine without epinephrine | 4.5 mg/kg | 22.5 | 31.5 |
| 1% lidocaine with epinephrine | 7 mg/kg | 35 | 49 |

subcutaneously are used safely with the tumescent liposuction technique so that 7 mg/kg is a safe and conservative maximal dosage. Use of 1% lidocaine is preferable to 2% in most cases because the larger volume produces greater hemostasis and makes most cutaneous surgery easier to perform. Use of 2% lidocaine without epinephrine may be useful in digital blocks when it is desirable to use less volume.

## Decreasing Pain Caused by Injection

Techniques to decrease the pain caused by injection of local anesthesia include the following:

- Inject very slowly
- Use a small-gauge needle (27 to 30 gauge)
- Pinch the skin as the needle enters it
- Distract the patient in conversation
- Inject down a hair follicle
- Use only one to two injection sites
- Add sodium bicarbonate to the lidocaine

The main technique for decreasing the pain of injection is to inject the local anesthetic very slowly using a small-gauge needle (27 to 30 gauge). The 30-gauge needles with plastic hubs are usually slightly sharper and less painful than those with metal hubs. The larger the gauge number, the smaller the needle diameter and the less painful the injection. However, needles smaller than 30 gauge are not strong enough for use in local anesthesia.

The smaller the syringe, the less force that must be used to inject the area. A 3-ml syringe is a good compromise between cost and comfort. It holds enough anesthesia for most small procedures and will not cause wrist pain to the injector. Preloading a number of syringes at the start of each day can save time if several procedures are to be done that day.

It may be helpful to pinch the skin as the needle enters it and to distract the patient in conversation. Although the needle should be inserted quickly, the injection will be less painful if the volume of anesthesia is injected slowly. The more superficial the injection, the more painful it is. For example, an injection bleb similar to that of a tuberculin skin test is more painful than a deeper subcutaneous or fat injection. It is usually less painful if the injection is done slowly and deeply at first, followed by redirecting the needle for a more superficial, dermal, blanching type of injection. In this manner, a volume of 5 ml or more can be given slowly through one injection site. Skin blanching helps determine the area that has been anesthetized. If need be, this area can be extended by reinjecting through another site that has already been anesthetized.

Some physicians will inject down a hair follicle to lessen the pain of the needle stick itself. Injection of the anesthetic into a hair follicle is less painful than a percutaneous injection; however, this is not required in most cases. Using topical anesthesia first can make the needle stick less painful. Although EMLA must be applied at least 1 hour before injection of local anesthesia to prevent the pain of a needle stick, aerosol anesthesia can work in a few seconds.

Injecting enough anesthetic so that the skin is firm (called *tumescent anesthesia*) can limit the amount of bleeding because small blood vessels become compressed by the anesthetic fluid. Waiting at least 10 to 15 minutes after injection can also limit bleeding because it takes at least 10 minutes for epinephrine to take effect. In most cases, it is not necessary to wait this long because the lidocaine and epinephrine are usually effective within 1 minute of injection.

Adding sodium bicarbonate in a 1:10 dilution to the lidocaine and epinephrine anesthetic solution markedly decreases the pain caused by injection (e.g., 1 ml of sodium bicarbonate can be added to 10 ml of lidocaine). The addition of sodium bicarbonate neutralizes the commercially available lidocaine-epinephrine solutions that have a pH of 4 to 6. One problem with adding this 1:10 dilution of sodium bicarbonate is the time required to make these syringes. The lidocaine-bicarbonate syringes need to be made at least weekly because they last 1 week at room temperature and up to 2 weeks with refrigeration.[2]

## Long-lasting Anesthetics

Long-lasting anesthetics such as mepivacaine or bupivacaine are used when it is necessary to decrease the possibility of postoperative pain for about 6 hours. The problem with using these anesthetics is that they can be more painful to inject and have a slow onset. Also, much less is known about the maximum dosage that can be used before toxicity occurs.

## Injection Technique

Draw up 1 to 2 ml of 1% lidocaine with epinephrine for shave or punch biopsies and 3 ml for larger biopsies. Insert the needle into one site of the circumference of the circle of anesthesia needed around the lesion. Because the anesthesia will diffuse throughout the tissue and the needle can be advanced while injecting slowly, most anesthesia can be done with one injection.

For shave and punch biopsies, the tip of the needle should reach the deep dermis so that a gentle elevation and blanching of the tissue occurs (Fig. 3-2). If the anesthetic is injected into the subcutaneous tissue, no elevation will occur, there is a risk of injecting directly into a vessel, and the anesthetic effect does not last as long. Injecting the anesthesic at this level is appropriate, however, if you need to remove a deep cyst or lipoma.

When an injection is superficial in the dermis, you may see an accentuation of the follicles called *peau d'orange* (Fig. 3-3). This skin distention is more painful than the pain that occurs with a deeper dermis injection. However, if you intend to do a shave biopsy, you can start with a deeper dermis injection and finish with a more superficial injection to raise the lesion for biopsy. Starting deeper and adjusting the needle to a more superficial level is an effective technique (this can be done without removing the needle from the original injection site). If the lesion to be removed is large, a second insertion site may be needed. When injecting subcutaneously with a needle larger than 30 gauge, it is important to pull back on

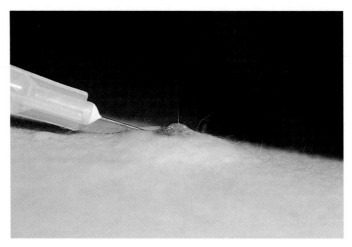

**FIG 3-2**
Elevation of tissue after injection with 1% lidocaine and epinephrine.

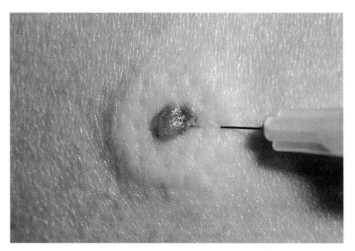

**FIG 3-3**
Superficial injection of local anesthetic in the dermis may cause accentuation of the follicles, a condition called *peau d'orange*.

the plunger before injecting at any one site to avoid injecting into a vessel. Advancing the needle and injecting simultaneously can be done in the dermis but should be avoided in the subcutaneous tissue.

## Adverse Reactions

Adverse reactions to lidocaine and epinephrine include the following:

**Lidocaine**
- Allergy to lidocaine
- Central nervous system (CNS) or cardiovascular effects from too much lidocaine (tremors, drowsiness)

**Epinephrine**
- Tachycardia
- Tremulousness
- Decreased peripheral circulation

**Needle**
- Laceration of nerve (rare but more likely during a nerve block)
- Infection or abscess from lack of sterile technique

For patients with normal circulation, it is safe to use epinephrine for local anesthesia in areas such as the tip of the nose, the ears, or the penis, despite old dogma that epinephrine should not be used in these areas. However, epinephrine should *not* be used for digital ring blocks, full ring blocks around the ear, penile nerve blocks, and other regional or field blocks in these areas. Furthermore, epinephrine should not be used in the very distal extremities of a patient with very poor circulation.

There are a few patients who ask that no epinephrine be used because it makes them anxious. It is true that some patients may get tachycardia for a few minutes along with a feeling of anxiousness shortly after the injection. This can usually be handled by warning the patient about this and reassuring him or her that the feeling will pass in a few minutes. For most patients, this may have occurred in the past during a dental procedure.

A few physicians do not like to use epinephrine because they are afraid of postoperative bleeding. By eliminating epinephrine, they believe that any bleeding vessels will be visualized and the bleeding will then be stopped with electrocoagulation. We disagree with these opinions. In reality, the only bleeding that is stopped by epinephrine is from very small vessels that cause limited oozing. These small bleeders are stopped initially by the pressure bandage and eventually stop by themselves. When epinephrine is not used, much more electrocoagulation is required, causing more thermal damage and char. This slows wound healing and creates more foreign bodies within the wound. The main disadvantages to not using epinephrine are longer surgical time and a bloodier field.

If the patient develops cyanosis, decreased pulse rate, or decreased capillary refill after receiving epinephrine, it may be helpful to apply warm compresses to the injection site to increase peripheral circulation.

Rare adverse effects associated with too large a systemic dose of injectable anesthetics (injection into a vein or too large a dose of the anesthetic) include myocardial depression and CNS effects such as light-headedness, tinnitus, perioral tingling, metallic taste, tremors, slurred speech, and seizures.[1]

## *Lidocaine allergies*

Lidocaine allergies are extremely rare. Almost all patients who report an allergy actually have had a vasovagal reaction with lidocaine injections or a sensitivity to the epinephrine effects. Other patients are actually allergic to the paraben preservative in the multidose vials of lidocaine or they are allergic to a local anesthetic ester such as Novocain. Because the paraben is not added to the single-use vials, it may be helpful to try these vials when the patient reports an allergy.

The ester forms of local anesthetics, such as Novocain, produce more allergic reactions. Fortunately, there is no cross-reactivity between Novocain and lidocaine. Therefore lidocaine use is safe in a patient with a true Novocain allergy. Even dentists are using lidocaine these days. Patients may think they are receiving Novocain in the dentist's office, but they are most likely receiving lidocaine.

The approach to a patient who reports a specific allergy to lidocaine is to take a careful history because a vasovagal or epinephrine reaction may be the actual cause of the patient's allergy. Referral to an allergist is rarely indicated, except for someone with a history consistent with a life-threatening type of allergic reaction. It is reasonable to try a test injection of a small amount of lidocaine (from a single-use vial), because true systemic lidocaine reactions are so rare.

An alternative to lidocaine is injectable diphenhydramine (Benadryl) or normal saline. Diphenhydramine provides adequate short-term anesthesia, but it may cause the patient to become drowsy. When normal saline is injected to induce a firm wheal, it provides a few minutes of anesthesia as well.

## REGIONAL BLOCK ANESTHESIA (DIGITAL AND FIELD BLOCKS)

The digital block, or ring block, is an example of a nerve block. The advantages of a nerve block are that it provides a longer duration of anesthesia and does not distort the anatomic landmarks. The digital block is also one instance when epinephrine should not be used.

The digital block injection can be less painful and more effective than a local injection on the end of a digit. Two injections along either side of the digital bones will almost always provide good anesthesia on a distal digit. Injection on each side of the digit with 1% lidocaine will anesthetize both anterior and posterior nerves on either side of the digit. A 3-ml syringe should be used with 1% lidocaine, delivering 1.5 ml on each side of the digit (Fig. 3-4).

Other regional blocks (i.e., infraorbital, supraorbital, or mental nerve blocks) are not as helpful because local anesthesia is not as painful in these areas. Penile blocks are very useful to anesthetize all but the ventral glans.

### Field Block

A field block creates a "wall" of anesthesia around a relatively small area to be anesthetized. Rather than injecting the anesthetic directly into the area to be numbed, the anesthetic is injected around it to affect the nerves that normally transmit sensations of pain and touch (Fig. 3-5). A field block is useful when it is

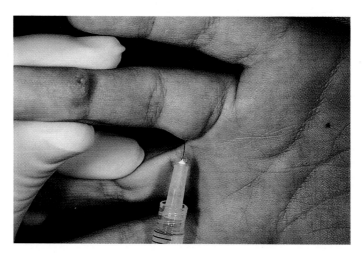

**FIG 3-4**
Digital block before electrosurgery of a wart on a finger.

necessary to avoid distorting the tissue to be cut, in cases of infection, and in locations where local anesthesia may not work adequately. Epinephrine can be used to decrease bleeding.

The field block is especially useful before draining an abscess. Because the acid environment of the abscess can hydrolyze the anesthetic, the field block allows the anesthetic to work on normal surrounding tissue and avoids the problem of distending the abscess further by keeping the anesthetic out of the abscess cavity. A 1-inch to 1½-inch needle is useful for administering a field block.

To avoid losing visualization of a small lesion after direct injection of lidocaine into the region of the lesion, an alternative to the larger field block is to mark the lesion with a surgical marker before doing the injection (Fig. 3-6).

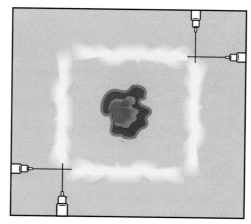

**FIG 3-5**
Field block.

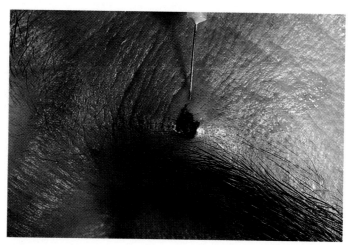

**FIG 3-6**
Skin marked with a surgical marker before injection of anesthesia.

## SUMMARY OF EQUIPMENT

### Anesthetics
- Topical anesthetics: ethyl chloride, EMLA, topical lidocaine preparations
- Injectable anesthetics, especially 1% lidocaine with epinephrine or 1% lidocaine without digital blocks

### Needles
- 18 to 22 gauge for drawing up anesthetic from vial
- 27 to 30 gauge × ½ inch is optimal for most local injections and digital blocks
- 27 to 30 gauge × 1½ inch may be useful for field blocks

### Syringes
- 3-ml syringe is optimal
- 5-ml syringe is adequate for larger areas

### Other
- Alcohol wipes
- Gloves

The skin surface can be cleared adequately with an alcohol wipe or Hibiclens rubbed on the surface for a few seconds. Gloves should be clean, but need not be sterile for the injections. Needles smaller than 30 gauge are too flexible and do not penetrate the skin well. See Chapter 1 for a list of distributors of surgical and anesthetic supplies.

## CONCLUSION

A thorough understanding of the techniques for administering local anesthesia is essential for the performance of painless skin surgery. A safely and properly anesthetized patient will allow the most controlled and highest quality surgery. Keeping the patient comfortable will create a happy customer and maximize compliance during and after surgery.

## REFERENCES

1. Fewkes JL: Anesthesia. In Robinson JK et al: *Atlas of cutaneous surgery*, Philadelphia, 1996, WB Saunders.
2. Bartfield JM et al: Buffered lidocaine as a local anesthetic: an investigation of shelf life, *Ann Emerg Med* 21(1):16-19, 1992.

## SUGGESTED READINGS

Matarasso SL, Glogau RG: Local anesthesia. In Lask G, Moy R, editors: *Principles and techniques of cutaneous surgery*, New York, 1996, McGraw-Hill.

Moy JG, Pfenninger JL: Peripheral nerve blocks and field blocks. In Pfenninger JL, Fowler GC, editors: *Procedures for primary care physicians*, St. Louis, 1994, Mosby.

# CHAPTER 4

# Hemostasis

*Richard P. Usatine*

Achieving hemostasis is an essential component of all surgery. The goal of hemostasis in surgery is to control bleeding while avoiding unnecessary tissue destruction. It is important to understand the advantages and disadvantages of all methods of hemostasis to be able to choose the appropriate method for each surgical situation.

Hemostasis can be achieved by chemical agents that produce superficial hemostasis or by electrocoagulation for deeper hemostasis. Hemostasis may also be achieved by physical methods that involve pressure, sutures, or gelatin sponges.

## TYPES OF HEMOSTASIS

- Chemical/topical
- Electrocoagulation
- Direct pressure or pressure dressing
- Sutures and ties
- Physical agents (gelatin sponge)

## CHEMICAL/TOPICAL HEMOSTASIS

Fig. 4-1 shows an assortment of chemical hemostatic agents used for superficial hemostasis. All of the chemical hemostatic agents have the advantage of being low in cost and easy to use and store.

## CHEMICAL HEMOSTATIC AGENTS

- Aluminum chloride
- Monsel's solution (ferric subsulfate)
- Trichloroacetic acid
- Silver nitrate sticks
- Phenol

### General Principles of Chemical Hemostasis

Chemical hemostatic agents work by causing protein precipitation, which stops the bleeding. These agents work best in a dry field, allowing the chemical to go directly to the bleeding tissue without being diluted by pooled blood. Chemical agents are meant to be used in open, superficial wounds that will not be sutured.

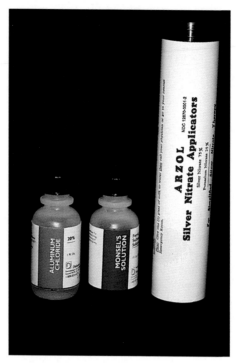

**FIG 4-1**
Chemical hemostatic agents (aluminum chloride,
Monsel's solution [ferric subsulfate], silver nitrate
sticks).

They are especially useful after a shave biopsy or a small punch biopsy. Chemical agents should not be used in deep wounds that will be closed with sutures.

When using chemical hemostatic agents after a shave biopsy, we recommend rolling a dry cotton-tipped swab with light pressure across the field before applying the chemical. The hemostatic agent should then be applied to the dry field by rolling or twisting the swab against the open wound. Although light pressure often works, sometimes it may help to use heavier pressure while twisting the swab clockwise and counter-clockwise against the area. After a 1- to 3-mm punch biopsy, a dry cotton-tipped swab can be held with downward pressure against the open hole to dry the field. If sutures are not to be used, then a chemical agent should be applied with downward pressure and held against the wound until hemostasis is achieved.

All of the hemostatic chemicals can cause damage if they get into the eye. Physicians should exercise great caution when using chemical agents or electrocoagulation after a shave or snip (scissors) biopsy on the eyelids or near the eye. The chemical from a dripping cotton-tipped swab can run into the eye when the biopsy is close to the globe. After wringing out the cotton-tipped swab against the side of the bottle or a gauze pad, the physician should carefully touch the cotton-tipped swab to the eyelid or periocular skin to avoid getting the chemical into the eye. If any chemical does get into the eye, the eye should be flushed immediately.

## Aluminum Chloride

Aluminum chloride comes in strengths from 20% to 70%. Most solutions are water or alcohol based. Alcohol alone (anhydrous alcohol) will only support a

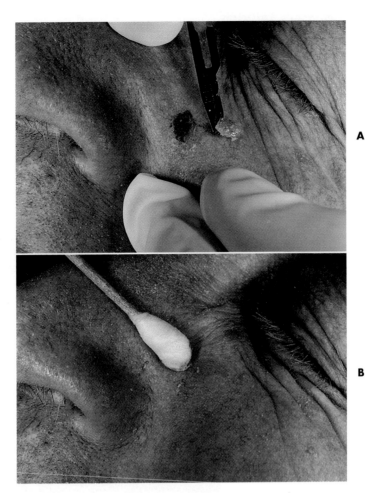

**FIG 4-2**
After a shave biopsy (**A**), aluminum chloride on a cotton-tipped swab is used to achieve hemostasis (**B**).

solution of up to 20%, so the stronger concentrations are either in water or a mixture of water and alcohol. We prefer to use aluminum chloride in an aqueous solution because it can be used safely with electrosurgery and in higher concentrations. With an alcohol-based solution, it is possible to ignite the alcohol when electrosurgery is performed in the same field. However, drying the field after applying the alcohol-based solution makes it safe to use electrosurgery.

Aqueous aluminum chloride can be purchased under the trade name *Lumicaine* or ordered as a 35% or 70% solution from Delasco. The 35% solution is excellent for hemostasis and is the most commonly used formula. *Drysol*, a brand name of 20% aluminum chloride in anhydrous ethyl alcohol that is sold by prescription to treat hyperhidrosis, also produces hemostasis.

The major advantage of aluminum chloride is that it is a clear solution that does not stain or tattoo the tissue. It does not cause tissue necrosis and does not damage the normal skin surrounding the wound. Aluminum chloride should not be used in deep wounds that will be sutured because it can delay healing and increase scarring.[1]

In Fig. 4-2, aluminum chloride is being used after the shave excision of a seborrheic keratosis. The biopsy site healed with no visible scarring or tattooing.

## Monsel's Solution

Monsel's solution is 20% ferric subsulfate. It is used to produce hemostasis after biopsies of the skin and cervix. It is applied to the skin in the same manner as aluminum chloride. Monsel's solution is just as easy to use as aluminum chloride, and there are claims that it is slightly more effective in achieving hemostasis.[2]

The major disadvantage of Monsel's solution is that there is a small risk of tattooing the skin because the iron in the solution causes it to be brown (Fig. 4-3). Tattooing may occur through iron deposition or stimulation of melanocytes.[1] This is rare, but it is of sufficient concern that we prefer to use aluminum chloride on the face. Monsel's solution can also cause minimal tissue destruction at the application site, but it has no affect on surrounding normal skin. One nuisance in using Monsel's solution is that the iron can precipitate around the bottle cap and make it difficult to open.

Monsel's solution can leave a histologic artifact in the skin. Therefore when a repeat biopsy must be done in an area where Monsel's solution was previously used, it helps to warn the pathologist.[3,4] This is rarely an issue, but for a lesion that presents a diagnostic dilemma or one that may need a repeat biopsy, it is best to avoid using Monsel's solution. Table 4-1 provides a comparison of aluminum chloride and Monsel's solution.

## Silver Nitrate

Silver nitrate comes in easy-to-use sticks and solution. It is not a particularly useful agent after a skin biopsy because its hemostatic action is slower and the response to it is more variable.[1] It also has the risk of causing scarring or tattoo-

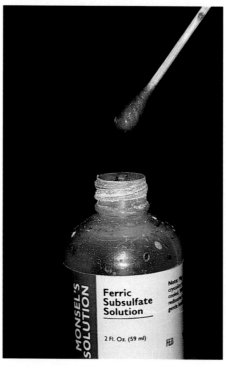

**FIG 4-3**
Because of iron in the solution, Monsel's solution is brown and may tattoo the skin.

**TABLE 4-1    Comparison of Aluminum Chloride and Monsel's Solution**

|                    | Advantages                                        | Disadvantages                                                                                   |
| ------------------ | ------------------------------------------------- | ---------------------------------------------------------------------------------------------- |
| Aluminum chloride  | Ease of use, no tattooing, no tissue necrosis     | Not for deep wounds to be sutured, flammable if using alcohol solution                         |
| Monsel's solution  | Ease of use, safe with electrosurgery             | Risk of tattooing, not for wounds to be sutured, can cause tissue destruction, bottle cap gets stuck |

ing by leaving silver in the dermis. Silver nitrate is helpful in the treatment of persistent granulation tissue that occurs sometimes in infants after the umbilical tissue falls off. As with Monsel's solution, silver nitrate can also be used on the cervix after a biopsy.

### Trichloroacetic Acid

Trichloroacetic acid (TCA) preparations come in a range of 30% to 50% strengths in an alcohol solution. TCA is useful in the treatment of condyloma acuminata on intact skin. TCA also produces hemostasis after a shave biopsy. It is a clear solution and does not cause tattooing. The major disadvantage is that TCA causes some tissue destruction of the surrounding skin. This may be desirable in some cases (e.g., after a shave excision of condyloma to ensure destruction of any remaining, nonvisible forms of the human papilloma virus). In most cases, use of TCA has no advantage over use of aluminum chloride.

### Phenol

Phenol is a caustic solution that can produce hemostasis. It causes damage to the surrounding skin, and is rarely used as a hemostatic agent.

## ELECTROCOAGULATION

When electrosurgery is used for hemostasis it is called *electrocoagulation*. Electrocoagulation is an ideal method to control bleeding during surgery. This is especially true with an excision that will be closed with sutures. Electrocoagulation is commonly used with elliptical excisions and, if needed, in a punch biopsy that will be sutured. In Fig. 4-4, the Hyfrecator is being used to control bleeding in an open surgical wound before closure. (As discussed earlier, chemical agents should not be used with wounds that will be sutured.) During surgery, electrocoagulation helps to produce a bloodless field. This allows the physician to see the landmarks better for placing both deep and superficial sutures. Often, electrocoagulation is used after undermining and before placing deep sutures (See Chapter 10).

The judicious use of electrocoagulation can prevent postoperative bleeding and hematoma formation. Because there are no guarantees, patients should be given information on what to do if postoperative bleeding occurs and a number to call if help is needed. When the surgery to be done is larger than a small shave,

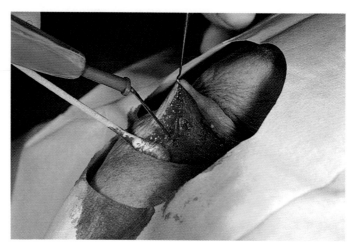

**FIG 4-4**
Electrocoagulation with a Hyfrecator in an open wound to be sutured.

punch, or excision, it is prudent to review the risks of bleeding with the patient before surgery. See Chapter 2 for discussion of preoperative screening for risk of bleeding (e.g., aspirin or Coumadin use).

Electrosurgery is useful after a shave biopsy in the rare instance in which chemical agents fail. However, the physician must remember to dry the surgical field with a cotton-tipped swab or gauze before using electrosurgery after a chemical agent in an alcohol solution has been used.

Electrosurgery is an ideal method for hemostasis when tissue destruction is desired. The best example of this is during curettage and desiccation of a basal cell carcinoma (BCC). The electrodesiccation simultaneously destroys malignant tissue and produces hemostasis. Excessive electrocoagulation may cause scarring. (See Chapter 12 for further information on this procedure.)

In surgical wounds that need closure, it is important not to use so much electrocoagulation that it produces large areas of char and tissue necrosis. This can increase the risk of wound infection.[2] When a vessel is not responding to electrocoagulation, it may require a surgical tie.

The disadvantages of electrosurgery include the following:

- It can cause unnecessary tissue destruction and scarring after a shave biopsy
- It can splatter blood and produce a smoke plume that can theoretically transmit infection to the medical personnel present
- It carries all the risks of using electrical equipment: burns, shocks, equipment malfunction (See Chapter 12)

In general, the risks of electrosurgery are minor if the safety precautions explained in Chapter 12 are followed. Burns, significant shocks, and transmission of infection during electrosurgery are very rare events that can be prevented.

## Electrosurgical Equipment and Its Use

Modern electrosurgical equipment uses an alternating current transferred to the patient through cold electrodes. The tissue is heated through tissue resistance to the current. The current used can range from 0.5 MHz to 4 MHz (radiofrequency). Two major types of electrosurgical units (Hyfrecators and radiosurgery units) are covered in detail in Chapter 12.

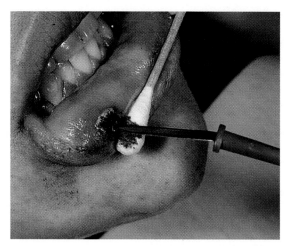

**FIG 4-5**
Electrocoagulation with a Hyfrecator for a pyogenic granuloma. Note how the swab is rolled just ahead of the electrode to provide a dry field.

Regardless of the type of unit used, there are four major ways to produce electrocoagulation:

- Electrode directly contacts the bleeding site or vessel (monoterminal)
- Electrode is touched to a hemostat or forceps that is grasping the bleeding tissue or vessel and then activated (monoterminal)
- Special bipolar forceps are used in the bipolar terminals of the Hyfrecator; the forceps grasps the tissue and is activated with the foot peddle
- Cut with coagulation; a number of electrosurgical units have a blended cur-rent setting that is used to cut tissue and to produce hemostasis simultane-ously (see Chapter 12 for further information on this process)

In Fig. 4-5, a pyogenic granuloma was just shaved off the lip of a postpartum woman. A dry cotton-tipped swab was rolled ahead of the electrode with pres-sure to dry the field for electrocoagulation with a Hyfrecator electrode. Because this was a very vascular lesion, the electrocoagulation was applied as the cotton-tipped swab was lifted from the bleeding site.

Because a shave excision is not a strictly sterile procedure, the handpiece that holds the electrode does not have to be sterile. It can be held in nonsterile, clean surgical gloves, and the power of the unit can be adjusted by the operator with-out concerns about breaking a sterile field. However, when doing an excision in which sutures will be placed, the handpiece needs to be sterile or covered in a sterile sheath or the physician can change gloves after touching the handpiece or unit.

The Surgitron Radiofrequency device has a handpiece that can be sterilized in an autoclave (although this accelerates the rate at which it needs to be replaced). Con-Med, which manufactures the Hyfrecator Plus, also produces nonsterile and sterile handpiece sheaths. Unfortunately, the sterile handpiece sheath covers the wire, is very long, and can be cumbersome to use. The most economic and con-venient sterile sheath for the Hyfrecator may be a 12-inch, sterile Penrose drain. These sell for less than $1 per drain and are the right size to cover the handpiece. A sterile surgical glove may also be used.

To summarize, electrocoagulation should be used in the following situations:

- In a wound that will be closed with sutures
- To obtain a bloodless field during surgery
- To prevent postoperative bleeding and hematomas
- When chemical hemostatic agents fail
- When tissue destruction is desired (e.g., with removal of a BCC)

If in the midst of a surgery there is a need to use the Hyfrecator, it can be poked through one of the middle fingers of a sterile glove. This is a quick and easy, immediate solution to the issue of keeping the procedure sterile while allowing the physician to hold the handpiece.

When using electrocoagulation near the eye, the physician should be aware that the spark will arc to the area closest to the electrode. Make sure that the treatment area is closer to the electrode than the globe. A spark to the globe is potentially damaging to the eye.

## MECHANICAL HEMOSTASIS: PRESSURE AND SUTURES

The direct application of pressure works to slow bleeding. A large blood vessel that does not stop bleeding with electrocoagulation can be ligated. Suturing a wound is a form of pressure application that brings the two open sides in direct opposition to each other. Packing an open wound (such as a drained abscess) also is a form of direct application of internal pressure.

After suturing an elliptical excision, it is wise to apply a pressure dressing to decrease the risk of hematoma formation. This can be left in place for 24 hours and is described further in Chapter 18. We recommend that patients apply direct pressure for 15 minutes by the clock if postoperative bleeding occurs at home.

In skin surgery, it is very rare that any blood vessels are large enough to require tying off. It is usually quicker to use the electrosurgery unit for these larger blood vessels, with the exception of superficial large arteries such as labial or temporal arteries. These vessels can be clamped with a small hemostat and tied off with absorbable sutures.

## PHYSICAL AGENTS

### Gelatin Sponge

A number of gelatin sponges are sold to produce hemostasis. These include Gelfoam, Helistat, Oxycel, and Avitene. A piece of Gelfoam can be placed into the hole of a punch biopsy that is not sutured. There are also absorbable hemostats sold (e.g., Surgicel, Collastat, and Instat). These products are expensive and have no distinct advantage over the less expensive chemical agents.

## RECOMMENDED HEMOSTASIS METHODS

Recommended hemostasis methods for various procedures are listed in Table 4-2.

## CONCLUSION

There are many techniques available to control bleeding during and after surgery. Judicious application of these hemostatic methods can save time, minimize com-

**TABLE 4-2    Recommended Hemostasis Methods for Various Procedures**

| Procedure | Hemostasis method |
|---|---|
| Shave biopsy | Chemical agent and/or light electrocoagulation |
| Punch biopsy | Sutured: may include pressure or electrocoagulation before closing with suture |
| | If not sutured: chemical agent, electrosurgery if needed |
| Elliptical excision | External pressure and electrocoagulation to produce dry field, closing with sutures and external pressure dressing |
| | Chemical agents should not be used |
| Electrosurgery | Use setting and power sufficient for electrocoagulation |
| Curettage | Chemical agents or electrocoagulation |
| Scissor surgery | Chemical agents or electrocoagulation (snip surgery) |
| Cryosurgery | Bloodless procedure |
| Incision and drainage | Electrocoagulation if needed, packing the wound produces hemostasis by pressure |

plications, and maximize the cosmetic outcome of surgery by reducing unnecessary tissue destruction. Good surgical outcomes occur when physicians pay close attention to important preoperative factors, use good surgical techniques, and provide informed and consistent postsurgical care (See Chapter 18).

## RESOURCES

Chemical agents and electrosurgery equipment can be ordered from the Delasco Dermatology Buying Guide (1-800-831-6273) and from some of the other resources listed in Chapter 1.

## REFERENCES

1. Billingsley EM, Maloney ME: Considerations in achieving hemostasis. In Robinson JK et al: *Atlas of cutaneous surgery*, Philadelphia, 1996, WB Saunders.
2. Fewkes JL, Cheney ML, Pollack SV: *Illustrated atlas of cutaneous surgery*, Philadelphia, 1992, Lippincott-Gower.
3. Habif T: Clinical dermatology: a color guide to diagnosis and therapy, ed 3, St. Louis, 1996, Mosby.
4. Olmstead PM, Lund HZ, Leonard DD: Monsel's solution: a histologic nuisance, *J Am Acad Dermatol*, 3:492-498, 1980.

## SUGGESTED READING

Larson PO: Topical hemostatic agents for dermatologic surgery, *J Dermatol Surg Oncol* 14:623-632, 1988.

# CHAPTER 5

# Choosing the Type of Biopsy

*Edward L. Tobinick    Richard P. Usatine*

Biopsy of the skin is performed to ascertain or confirm the diagnosis of skin lesions, both benign and malignant, and in many cases, to simultaneously remove them. Skin biopsies can be broadly categorized into three types: shave, punch, and excisional. Choosing which type of biopsy to perform influences the diagnostic yield, the cosmetic result, and the time required for the physician to perform the procedure.

## GENERAL PRINCIPLES

### Shave Biopsy

Choice of biopsy type has much to do with the physician's initial assessment of the lesion. It is particularly important to consider the depth of involvement within the skin. The shave technique is particularly suited to lesions confined to the epidermis, such as seborrheic keratoses or molluscum contagiosum; to small basal cell carcinomas (BCCs) (Fig. 5-1), so as not to interfere with subsequent curettage; and to many benign nevi. Important advantages of shave biopsy include the following:

- Minimal risk of bleeding (suitable for patients on anticoagulants)
- Speed (because no sutures are required)
- Rapid healing (because a full-thickness wound is not created)
- The ability to easily remove relatively large, raised lesions

Cosmetic results of a shave biopsy can be excellent; in many cases, but not all, results will be superior to those achieved with excision biopsy. Shave biopsy is also useful in certain anatomic areas, such as the back and the shin, that are difficult to suture. Disadvantages include a possible indentation, if a deep shave is performed, and recurrence of the lesion.

### Punch Biopsy

Punch biopsy is the method of choice for most inflammatory or infiltrative diseases and for other lesions in which the predominant pathology lies in the dermis, such as a dermatofibroma. Small punches are also good for use on the face because they can leave an excellent cosmetic result, especially if care is taken to produce a defect that falls within skin tension lines. Punch biopsy produces a full-thickness specimen of the skin that, when done properly, extends to the subcutaneous fat.

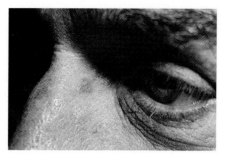

**FIG 5-1**
Nodular basal cell carcinoma on the nose.

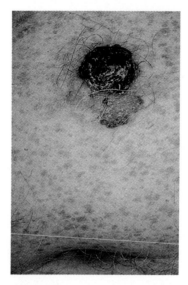

**FIG 5-2**
Malignant melanoma superior to the umbilicus.

### Excisional Biopsy

Excision is the biopsy method of choice for lesions highly suggestive of malignant melanoma (Fig. 5-2). It is also used to diagnose and remove dermal and subcutaneous cysts and tumors (epidermal cysts and lipomas) and lesions that are too large to be removed by punch (generally greater than 8 mm in diameter).

## IS IT SKIN CANCER?

### Pigmented Lesions: Melanoma and Its Differential Diagnoses

Early detection and prompt removal of melanoma can be lifesaving. It is incumbent on the physician to biopsy any suspicious pigmented lesion. Pigmented lesions highly suggestive of melanoma should be excised in their entirety, if possible, at the earliest possible time. If the lesions are large or the area has cosmetic importance, prompt referral to a dermatologist or a plastic surgeon for excisional biopsy is recommended.

Pigmented lesions that are unusual and are considered to have a low, but definite, possibility of malignancy also require prompt biopsy. If these lesions are small, total excision with small margins is the method of choice. Very small lesions, those less than 3 mm in diameter, can often be adequately excised by using a deep shave technique or a 3-mm punch to remove the entire lesion, with a 1-mm margin of normal skin both around and under the lesion. Large lesions (those greater than 1 cm in diameter) with a low level of suspicion are often best investigated by doing a 3- to 4-mm punch biopsy in the area of highest suspicion (i.e., the blackest area or the area of greatest elevation).

### Lentigo maligna (melanoma in situ)

Flat, macular lesions suspected of being lentigo maligna (Fig. 5-3) present another problem because many of these lesions are very large (often over 2 cm in diameter) and frequently are present on the face. Excisional biopsy is preferred for small lesions, but this method is impractical for large lesions. Punch biopsy, preferably 3 to 4 mm, of one or two of the areas of highest suspicion is the diagnostic method of choice. These lesions can also be difficult for the pathologist to interpret because the characteristic pathology is often limited to a single line of

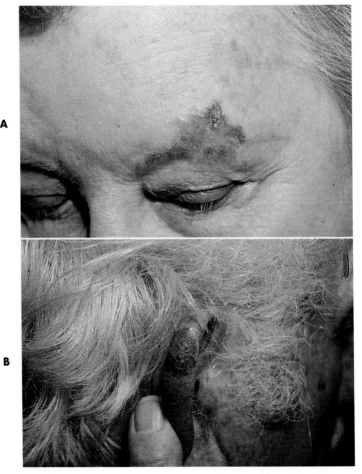

**FIG 5-3**
Lentigo maligna (melanoma in situ) (**A**) on the forehead and (**B**) on the ear.

atypical cells at the dermal-epidermal junction. To alert the pathologist, specimens should be labeled as "probable lentigo maligna." If you suspect that you are dealing with a benign lentigo, a single 2-mm punch biopsy or shave biopsy may be adequate.

Many benign lesions are so characteristic that biopsy is not necessary. On the other hand, early melanoma can be exceedingly difficult to diagnose (some lesions are not even pigmented). Considering this, and also taking into consideration that the morphology of benign pigmented lesions can be remarkably varied, it is best to be cautious when dealing with unusual pigmented lesions.

Biopsies should be performed on all questionable pigmented lesions. For lesions with a low level of suspicion for malignancy, shave biopsy is adequate. Lesions more suggestive of melanoma should be excised in toto; if this is not possible, a punch biopsy should be performed.

Benign pigmented lesions are much more common than melanoma. Unusual pigmented lesions are most often uncommon variants of benign lesions rather than melanomas. To help physicians diagnose melanoma, the American Cancer Society developed the ABCD guidelines (Box 5-1). These guidelines have been expanded to include **E** for **elevation** and/or **enlarging** lesions. Very little has been written to validate the efficacy of these guidelines, but some information can be found in a study done by McGovern and Litaker.[1] See Chapter 16 for photographic examples of the ABCDE criteria and further information on the use of these guidelines.

Any nevi that the patient reports have changed should be considered for biopsy.[2] For a summary of signs that suggest malignancy in pigmented lesions, see Table 5-1.

### Atypical moles (dysplastic nevi)

In 1978 Dr. Wallace Clark et al[3] published their finding of an exceedingly high risk of melanoma in certain families with atypical moles. Although these atypical moles, sometimes called *dysplastic nevi*,[4] are benign, they have clinical, histologic, and biologic behavior distinct from common nevocellular nevi. It was subsequently found that from 2% to 8% of the population have nevi that fit the clinical and histologic definition of atypical moles. Clinically, these nevi are large (5 to 12 mm in diameter), are characteristically multicolored (with shades of brown, tan, or pink),

---

**BOX 5-1    ABCDE Guidelines for Diagnosis of Melanoma**

**Asymmetry:** Benign nevi are symmetric; melanomas tend to have pronounced asymmetry.

**Border:** Benign lesions usually have smooth borders; melanomas tend to have notched, irregular outlines.

**Color:** Benign lesions usually contain only one color; melanomas frequently have a variety of colors.

**Diameter:** Melanoma is usually larger than 6 mm in diameter.

**Elevation:** Malignant melanoma is almost always elevated, at least in part, so that it is palpable.

OR

**Enlarging:** A pigmented lesion that is enlarging is more suspicious for melanoma.

---

**TABLE 5-1    Signs Suggesting Malignancy in Pigmented Lesions**

| Signs | Implication |
|---|---|
| **Change in Color** | |
| Sudden darkening; brown black | Increased number of tumor cells, the density of which varies within the lesion, creating irregular pigmentation |
| Spread of color into previously normal skin | Tumor cells migrating through epidermis at various speeds and in different directions (horizontal growth phase) |
| Red | Vasodilation and inflammation |
| White | Areas of regression or inflammation |
| Blue | Pigment deep in dermis, sign of increasing depth or tumor |
| **Change in Characteristics of Border** | |
| Irregular outline | Malignant cells migrating horizontally at different rates |
| Satellite pigmentation | Cells migrating beyond confines of primary tumor |
| Development of depigmented halo | Destruction of melanocytes by possible immunologic reaction and inflammation |
| **Changes in Surface Characteristics** | |
| Scaliness | |
| Erosion | |
| Oozing | |
| Crusting | |
| Bleeding | |
| Ulceration | |
| Elevation | |
| Loss of normal skin lines | |
| **Development of Symptoms** | |
| Pruritus | |
| Tenderness | |
| Pain | |

From Habif T: *Clinical dermatology: a color guide to diagnosis and therapy*, ed 3, St. Louis, 1996, Mosby.

and have irregular borders that tend to be indistinct (Fig. 5-4). They usually have a flat macular component, are frequently multiple, and are most common on the trunk. In contrast to common nevi, these atypical moles usually begin to appear during adolescence and continue to appear during young adult life.

The clinical approach to atypical moles has evolved since their first description. There still remains a difference of opinion as to their proper management. Characteristic atypical moles do not all require biopsy, especially if the patient has over 100 of these atypical moles. One must add to this statement the proviso that any pigmented lesion that the physician is uncertain about or that has changed should undergo biopsy. One of the most common reasons for which dermatologists are sued is failure to diagnose melanoma. Physicians who may be confronted with these lesions in practice should peruse several dermatology textbooks to familiarize themselves with the characteristic clinical features of atypical moles versus melanoma. When examining a patient who at first glance might appear to have multiple melanomas, one will almost always find that these are multiple dysplastic nevi.

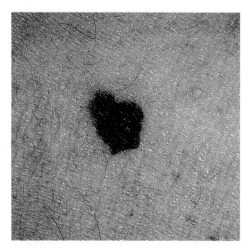

**FIG 5-4**
Atypical mole (dysplastic nevus) that is 6 mm in diameter. An elliptical excision was performed to rule out melanoma. Pathology showed dysplastic nevus only.

Patients with atypical moles should be divided into two groups: those with a personal history or a first-degree relative with a history of melanoma and those without such a history (sporadic atypical moles). Patients with sporadic atypical moles are probably not at great risk for developing melanoma and therefore require only routine follow-up.

Dysplastic nevus syndrome, defined as patients with first-degree relatives with melanoma and atypical moles, is now called *atypical mole syndrome*.[2] The NIH Consensus Panel refers to this syndrome as the *familial atypical mole and melanoma syndrome*. This syndrome is defined by (1) occurrence of melanoma in one or more first- or second-degree relatives; (2) large numbers of moles (often more than 50), some of which are atypical and often variable in size; and (3) moles that demonstrate certain distinct histologic features. These patients appear to have a greatly increased risk of developing melanoma.[5,6] These new melanomas may develop de novo, may arise in other common nevi, or may develop within existing atypical moles. Therefore these patients require careful follow-up. Whole-body photographs,[7] periodic skin self-examination, and careful cutaneous examinations every 3 to 6 months by a dermatologist are recommended for these high-risk patients.

A study published by Tucker et al[8] in 1997 suggests that persons with increased numbers of dysplastic nevi and/or large nevi have a greater risk of having melanoma even if they do not have a family history of melanoma. In their study, a nevus was considered to be dysplastic on physical examination if it met the following three criteria:

- 5 mm or larger
- Entirely flat or with flat component
- Having *at least* two of the following features:
    Asymmetric outline
    Irregular border
    Variable color
    Indistinct borders

### Nevi

Shave biopsy is the treatment of choice for most benign-appearing nevi. In Fig. 5-5, the raised lesion could be a benign nevus or a BCC. Therefore a shave biopsy would be the biopsy of choice. Removal of some nevi on the face will yield a better cosmetic result when accomplished by punch or meticulous excision. This is particularly true for nevi with a deeper intradermal component, which tend to recur or deeply pigment after shave removal, and for nevi with hair, for which shave biopsy is often too superficial to remove the deeper root of the hair follicle.

### Congenital nevi

Congenital nevi are frequently large (Fig. 5-6) and can meet all five ABCDE criteria. The diagnosis is made on history because congenital nevi have been present since birth. Biopsy is indicated if a congenital nevus changes in color, there is a new growth within the nevus, or bleeding without trauma occurs within the nevus.

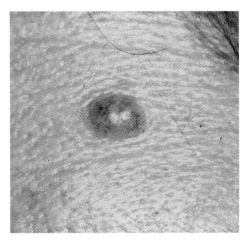

**FIG 5-5**
Benign nevus on the forehead. Because it has telangiectasias and is pearly, a shave biopsy was performed. Pathology revealed a nevus only.

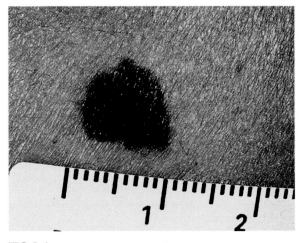

**FIG 5-6**
Congenital nevus that is not growing or changing (1 cm). The management plan is observation.

### Seborrheic keratoses

Most seborrheic keratoses will not need a biopsy (Fig. 5-7). However, because some of these lesions mimic malignant tumors such as melanomas, biopsy should be performed if any doubt exists. When performing a biopsy on seborrheic keratoses, care should be taken to avoid unnecessarily deep or destructive techniques. Seborrheic keratoses are epidermal lesions; if removed superficially, they will usually not recur or scar. Shave biopsy is the biopsy technique of choice unless the suspicion of melanoma is high. Treatment with cryotherapy, but without biopsy, is very acceptable for lesions in which the diagnosis is certain.

## Nonpigmented Lesions Suspicious for Cancer

### Basal cell carcinoma

The majority of BCCs are relatively small, raised tumors on the face, head, neck, or exposed parts of the trunk and extremities. Shave biopsy is preferred for most of these tumors and has the great advantage of not producing a full-thickness wound. Subsequent curettage and desiccation are therefore not hindered, such as they would be if a punch biopsy were performed.

Sclerosing (morpheaform) BCCs are flat and more difficult to diagnose clinically and histopathologically. Therefore a punch specimen is usually preferred, although a deeper shave often will be adequate to make the diagnosis. However, as seen in Fig. 5-8, these lesions are flat and difficult to biopsy with the shave technique.

When doing a shave biopsy on a suspected BCC, the physician should carefully record the site of the biopsy in the chart. In our office, we take Polaroid pictures of the biopsy site and place them in the chart. If this is not possible, physicians should write a description of the biopsy site and draw a picture in the chart. It can be helpful to record measurements from fixed landmarks (e.g., 3.2 cm inferior to the right pupil). Biopsy sites may heal quickly and can be difficult to find later when definitive treatment is necessary.

### Squamous cell carcinoma

Squamous cell carcinoma (SCC) can be difficult to diagnose by histopathology. It can easily be mistaken by the pathologist for actinic keratosis, especially if the

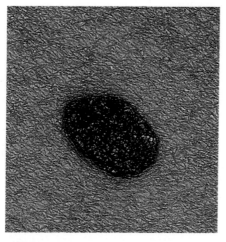

**FIG 5-7**
Classic seborrheic keratosis not suspicious for malignancy.

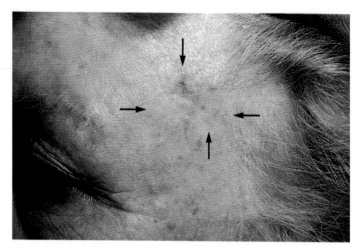

**FIG 5-8**
Sclerosing basal bell carcinoma, 3 cm in diameter, on the temple.

biopsy was made along the periphery of the lesion. Punch biopsies of these lesions will be easier for the pathologist to interpret, but can be difficult to perform when dealing with friable lesions. When performing a shave biopsy, care must be taken to get a specimen with adequate depth to enable the pathologist to render an accurate opinion. As with BCC, the physician should carefully record the site of biopsy. For large lesions, particularly those in or around the oral cavity and ears, it is important to check for lymphadenopathy before performing the biopsy. Prompt treatment after diagnosis of SCC is essential because some of these lesions have the potential for metastasis (See Chapter 16).

## UNKNOWN SKIN LESIONS

If skin lesions appear inflammatory or infiltrative, a punch biopsy is in order. If not, the physician should consider whether the lesion is raised. If it is, and melanoma is not likely to be the diagnosis, a shave biopsy may be adequate to give the diagnosis.

### Inflammatory Disorders

Some rashes and eruptions may require biopsy for diagnostic purposes (e.g., unusual lichen planus and discoid lupus erythematosus [DLE]). These lesions require punch biopsy to give the dermatopathologist an adequate specimen. The typical malar rash of systemic lupus erythematosus (SLE) in a patient with a strongly positive ANA does not require a biopsy for diagnosis (Fig. 5-9). However, an unusual case of DLE may need a biopsy for diagnosis. A 3-mm punch biopsy is usually preferred, but even 2-mm punch biopsy specimens can sometimes yield enough information for diagnosis.

Almost all inflammatory dermatoses have a dermal component. Punch biopsy is necessary to preserve the dermal architecture so the dermatopathologist can evaluate the cellular infiltrate, both as to its nature and its pattern. In most cases in which a punch biopsy is indicated, the biopsy need only go through the dermis, and the specimen is cut off at the top of the subcutaneous fat. However, to diagnose erythema nodosum (Fig. 5-10), the punch specimen should include as

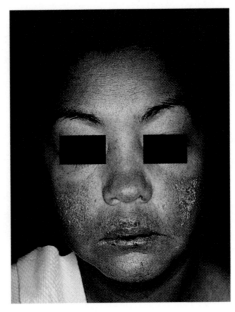

**FIG 5-9**
Typical malar rash of SLE that does not require
a biopsy.

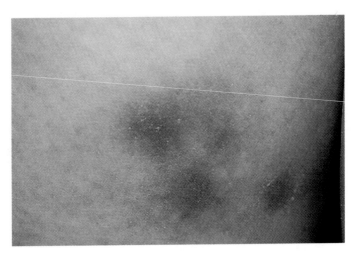

**FIG 5-10**
Erythema nodosum.

much of the subcutaneous fat as possible. This is because erythema nodosum is really a panniculitis, with the overlying dermis secondarily involved.

## Infiltrative Disorders

Infiltrative disorders, such as granulomas, also require punch rather than shave biopsy to deliver a suitable specimen for dermatopathologic examination. Examples of infiltrative disorders include granuloma annulare (Fig. 5-11), swimming-pool granuloma (Fig. 5-12), and sarcoidosis. A swimming-pool granuloma is an atypical mycobacterial infection.

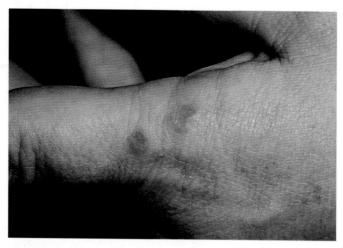

**FIG 5-11**
Granuloma annulare on the hand.

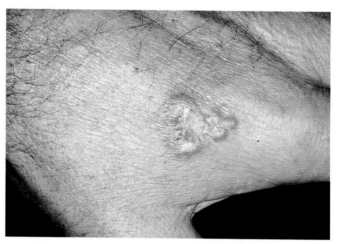

**FIG 5-12**
Swimming-pool granuloma (atypical mycobacterial infection).

## CONSIDERATIONS FOR SPECIFIC ANATOMIC AREAS

### Back and Anterior Shin

The thickness of the dermis on the back, which can exceed 1 cm, and the tightness of the skin on the shin make both excision and punch biopsy more hazardous in these locations. Possible consequences in these procedures include hematoma, dehiscence, infection, hypertrophic scarring, and keloid formation. For these reasons, shave biopsy is preferred when it is a reasonable alternative.

### Hands and Feet

Care must be taken when performing punch biopsies on the hands and feet because of proximity to vessels, tendons, bone, and nerves. The sensory nerves along the lateral sides of the fingers lie within reach of a biopsy punch. On the dorsum of the hand, tendons are vulnerable. Punch biopsies are difficult on the palmar and plantar surfaces because of skin thickness.

### Chest and Buttocks

The chest and buttocks may be considered cosmetic areas and may require particular care to avoid scarring. Keloidal or hypertrophic scarring is common in both of these areas. Large, deep shave biopsies should be avoided if possible.

### Scalp

The tautness, thickness, and vascularity of the scalp combine to make punch biopsies more difficult in this area. Shave biopsies are much more manageable and preferred. There is little or no risk of alopecia from shave biopsies on the scalp because the base of a hair follicle is deeper than the biopsy field.

### Ears, Eyelids, Nose, and Lips

Shave biopsies are easily done on the ears, eyelids, nose, and lips. If a punch biopsy is indicated, use of a 2-mm punch will avoid most problems with dog ears (See Chapter 10). On the eyelids, care must be taken to avoid the conjunctival margin; on the lips, care must be taken to align the vermilion border.

## HOW TO SUBMIT A SPECIMEN TO THE LAB

To obtain the most accurate diagnosis from the pathologist, it is important to provide all the relevant information on the submission form that accompanies the specimen. Drs. Boyd and Neldner[9] have come up with the following five D's mnemonic to remember what essential information should be included on the form:

- Description
- Demographics
- Duration
- Diameter
- Diagnosis

### Description

The physician should write a description of the appearance of the lesion. Examples of common descriptive terms include erythema, scale, pearly, raised, pigmented, ulcerating, crusted, nodular, papular, macular, vesicular, and bullous.

### Demographics

The age and sex of the patient should be noted. If a drug eruption is suspected, a list of the patient's medications should be included.

### Duration

How long a lesion has been present will help define the possible diagnoses.

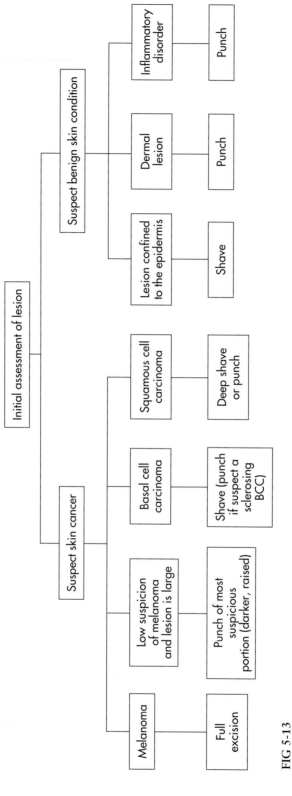

**FIG 5-13**
Algorithm for choice of biopsy based on initial assessment of lesion.

## Diameter

Recording the size of the lesion is especially important if the physician has not excised the entire lesion. Pigmented lesions larger than 6 mm are more likely to be melanoma. Unless recorded, the pathologist will not know the size of an incompletely excised lesion. For eruptions, one can record the distribution of the eruption.

## Diagnosis

A physician should write down the most likely diagnosis and the most likely alternative diagnoses. It is not expected that the diagnoses recorded will be correct all of the time; if they were, the pathologist would not be needed. However, submitting your best guess of the differential diagnosis may be helpful to the pathologist.

Following the five D's approach to submitting a specimen will improve communication with the pathologist and maximize the accuracy of the final histologic diagnosis.

## CONCLUSION

The choice of biopsy technique can substantially effect the cosmetic result, the diagnostic information obtained, and the time required to perform the procedure. Shave, punch, and excisional biopsies each have advantages and disadvantages. (See Chapters 6, 9, and 10 for further information on these procedures.) In Fig. 5-13, we summarize the recommendations in this chapter according to the initial assessment of the diagnosis of the lesion in question. This is merely a rough guideline because choosing among these techniques requires consideration of the size and morphology of the lesion in question, its anatomic location, the experience and skill of the physician, and the initial assessment of the diagnosis.

## REFERENCES

1. McGovern TW, Litaker MS: Clinical predictors of malignant pigmented lesions: a comparison of the Glasgow seven-point checklist and the American Cancer Society's ABCDs of pigmented lesions, *J Dermatol Surg Oncol* 18:22-26, 1992.
2. Habif T: *Clinical dermatology: a color guide to diagnosis and therapy*, ed 3, St. Louis, 1996, Mosby.
3. Clark WH et al: Origin of familial malignant melanomas from heritable melanocytic lesions: the B-K mole syndrome, *Arch Dermatol* 114:732-738, 1978.
4. Clark WH Jr: The dysplastic nevus syndrome, *Arch Dermatol* 124:1207-1210, 1988.
5. NIH Consensus Conference: Diagnosis and treatment of early melanoma, *JAMA* 268:10, 1314-1319, 1992.
6. Greene MH et al: High risk of malignant melanoma in melanoma-prone families with dysplastic nevi, *Ann Intern Med* 102:458-465, 1985.
7. Slue W, Kopf AW, Rivers JK: Total-body photographs of dysplastic nevi, *Arch Dermatol* 124:1239-1243, 1988.
8. Tucker MA et al: Clinically recognized dysplastic nevi: central risk factor for cutaneous melanoma, *JAMA* (5)277:18, 1439-1444, 1997.
9. Boyd A, Neldner K: How to submit a specimen for cutaneous pathology analysis, *Arch Fam Med* (6):64-66, 1997.

## SUGGESTED READINGS

Fewkes JL, Cheney ML, Pollack SV: The biopsy. In *Illustrated atlas of cutaneous surgery*, Philadelphia, 1992, Lippincott-Gower.

Robinson JK, LeBoit PE: Biopsy techniques. In Robinson JK et al: *Atlas of cutaneous surgery*, Philadelphia, 1996, WB Saunders.

Salopek TG et al: Management of cutaneous malignant melanoma by dermatologists of the American Academy of Dermatology. I. Survey of biopsy practices of pigmented lesions suspected as melanoma, *J Am Acad Dermatol* 33:441-450, 1995.

Winkelmann RK: Skin biopsy. In Epstein E, Epstein E Jr, editors: *Skin surgery*, ed 6, Philadelphia, 1987, WB Saunders.

# CHAPTER 6

# The Shave Biopsy

*Daniel Mark Siegel    Richard P. Usatine*

The shave biopsy is one of the more useful approaches for both obtaining tissue for diagnostic purposes and for the removal of benign surface neoplasms. It is especially fast, easy, and effective when the lesion is raised above the skin surface. The shave biopsy is also valuable for diagnosing many cutaneous malignancies, including basal cell carcinomas (BCCs) and squamous cell carcinomas (SCCs). It is also an effective tool for removing benign lesions such as seborrheic keratoses and benign melanocytic nevi. After a shave biopsy, hemostasis is easily obtained with a topical hemostatic agent. The raw surface is allowed to heal naturally, and no sutures are used. Because the raw surface is of an insignificant depth below the epidermis, the wound usually heals with a good cosmetic result.

## INDICATIONS

The following lesions are among those that can be diagnosed by shave biopsy:

- Actinic keratosis
- BCC
- SCC
- Keratoacanthoma
- Kaposi's sarcoma

Shave biopsy can also be used to remove the following lesions:

- Seborrheic keratosis
- Benign melanocytic nevus
- Sebaceous hyperplasia
- Pyogenic granuloma
- Skin tag with a large base
- Neurofibroma
- Porokeratosis

An example of a benign raised nevus that will do well with a shave excision is seen in Fig. 6-1. In Fig. 6-2, the lesion was easily diagnosed as a BCC after a shave biopsy specimen was sent for pathologic examination.

When a pigmented lesion appears to be benign and its removal is for cosmetic reasons, it is acceptable to use a shave excision. However, it is essential to send biopsies of all pigmented lesions for review by a pathologist.

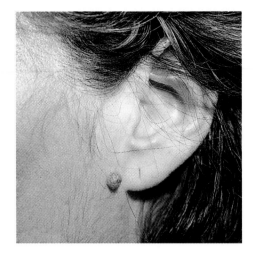

**FIG 6-1**
Benign raised nevus.

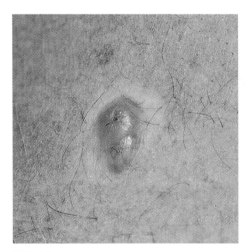

**FIG 6-2**
Nodular basal cell carcinoma. Shave biopsy is
preferred.

---

**BOX 6-1    Clark's Levels of Invasion of Primary Malignant Melanoma
From the Epidermis\***

Level I: Into the underlying papillary dermis
    II: To the junction of the papillary and reticular dermis
   III: Into the reticular dermis
   IV: Into the subcutaneous fat

---

\*The prognosis is worse as the level of the invasion deepens.

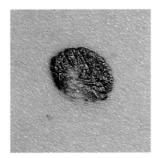

**FIG 6-3**
Melanoma. Excision rather than
shave biopsy is preferred.

## CONTRAINDICATIONS

Contraindications to shave biopsy include melanoma and any pigmented lesion highly suspicious for melanoma. There are no contraindications for shave biopsy based on location of the lesion.

When a lesion is suspicious for melanoma, the shave technique should not be used because it does not produce a full-thickness biopsy. If the lesion turns out to be a melanoma, the pathologist may be unable to give a depth or Clark's level (Box 6-1) because the shave biopsy may have removed only the superficial aspect of the melanoma. In Fig. 6-3, the lesion has the classic features of a melanoma, making excision rather than shave biopsy the method of choice. For further discussion on the diagnosis and treatment of melanoma, see Chapter 16.

## ADVANTAGES OF SHAVE BIOPSY

The advantages of shave biopsy can be broken down into two categories: those that are related to the physician and those that are related to the patient. Advantages of shave biopsy for the physician include the following:

- Can be performed rapidly
- Sutures are not needed
- Procedure is relatively easy to learn
- Multiple lesions can be excised at one time
- An assistant is not required
- Strict sterile procedure is not required
- Localization of the site after biopsy is facilitated by the healing wound

The following advantages of shave biopsy benefit the patient:

- There are no sutures that need to be removed
- Wound care is usually simple
- Restriction of activities is not needed during wound healing

## DISADVANTAGES OF SHAVE BIOPSY

As with the advantages of shave biopsy, the disadvantages can also be categorized into those that are related to the physician and those that are related to the patient. Disadvantages for the physician include the following:

- If the lesion turns out to be a melanoma, the shave will interfere with determining the depth of the lesion
- There is an art to mastering the technique of shave biopsy

For the patient, the disadvantages of shave biopsy include the following:

- Hypopigmentation may result
- Scarring may occur over the whole biopsy site
- A divot may remain if the shave was too deep

## EQUIPMENT

The minimum equipment necessary for a shave biopsy is a No. 15 scalpel, a 3-ml syringe and needle for local anesthesia, and cotton-tipped applicators for hemostasis (Fig. 6-4). Scalpel blades can be used alone or on a handle. Although all blades are disposable, a physician can choose between nondisposable scalpel handles or the ease of a totally disposable scalpel and blade combination. A No. 10 scalpel is useful for larger lesions (e.g., those greater than 1 cm). Some physicians also use a forceps to hold the lesion during the shave procedure.

As an alternative to the scalpel, a razor blade can be substituted. Razor blades such as Gillette Super Blues or Gillette Blue are optimal. However, many other brands of razor blades are available. There are also new devices in which the razor blade is incorporated into a handle; however, the cost is significantly higher than for plain razor blades. Razor blades are available presnapped in half and should be kept in a sterile urine specimen container. As they are needed, the blades can be sprinkled onto a piece of gauze. Autoclaving of blades is not recommended because it can dull the blade. The Gillette blades have a lubricant placed on them by the manufacturer that is antibacterial, and we have never had an infection from a Gillette razor blade used to obtain a biopsy.

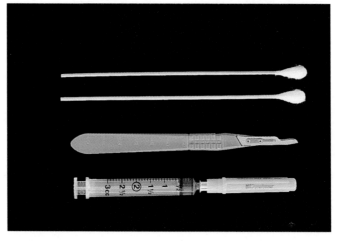

**FIG 6-4**
Equipment for shave biopsy. From top, cotton-tipped applicators for hemostasis, No. 15 blade with scalpel handle, and 3-ml syringe and needle for local anesthesia.

## SHAVE BIOPSY: STEPS AND PRINCIPLES

The primary focus of this discussion will be to help physicians perfect the shave excision with a scalpel. The razor blade shave excision technique and snip excisions are discussed later in the chapter.

The most important steps in the shave biopsy include the following:

- Using anesthetic to raise and stabilize the lesion
- Keeping the scalpel flat against the skin and using the middle of the blade to get the best control of the excision
- Stabilizing the lesion through various techniques to allow for complete removal of the lesion
- Dealing with any residual tissue after the initial shave

### Technique When Using a Scalpel

#### Preoperative measures

1. After determining that the shave technique is the best method for the patient, obtain informed consent for the procedure from the patient or patient's guardian (See Appendix A for sample consent form).
2. (Optional) Lightly prep the area with an alcohol swab or another antiseptic. There is no evidence that this preparation decreases the already extremely low infection rate.
3. Consider marking the margins of the lesion with a surgical marker if anesthetic will blur the margins. This is especially important if the lesion is sebaceous hyperplasia, because after injection the margins of the lesion may not be visible.

#### Local anesthesia

1. Draw up 1% lidocaine with epinephrine in a 3-ml syringe. Use a 30-gauge needle to inject the local anesthetic.
2. Inserting the needle into the dermis below the lesion, inject the anesthetic slowly until the tissue is distended (a wheal is raised) and blanching is seen. This distention helps to immobilize the lesion and facilitates smooth removal of the lesion using a shave technique.

#### Blade handling

1. Hold a No. 15 scalpel blade parallel to the surface of the skin.
2. Use the middle of the blade while cutting. Notice in Fig. 6-5, *A* that the tip of the scalpel was used to do the cutting. This does not give the physician maximal control and can lead to shaves that are uneven or too deep or leave residual tissue on one side. In Fig. 6-5, *B*, the middle of the scalpel blade is being properly used to produce an evenly controlled biopsy specimen. It requires some skill to adjust the scalpel blade on both sides of the lesion so as to remove the lesion in its entirety without affecting normal skin around the lesion.
3. Move the blade through the tissue using a minimal sawing movement. Ideally the motion would be straight—without sawing—but this is difficult to do. The slight sawing motion helps the blade move through the tissue, but too much sawing will produce scalloped edges. Note in Fig. 6-5, *A* and *B* how the fingers of the opposing hand are kept in the biopsy area to provide gentle countertraction and to stabilize the tissue. On certain areas of thin skin near vital structures such as the eye or hand, it may be necessary to pinch and elevate the surrounding skin with one hand while doing the biopsy with the other.

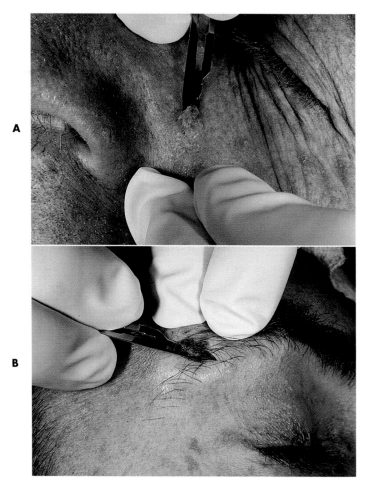

**FIG 6-5**
Performing a shave biopsy with the tip of the blade (**A**) is not optimal.
Using the middle of the scalpel blade (**B**) provides maximal control and
produces an even biopsy.

### Stabilization techniques

Lesions must be stabilized during shave biopsy; otherwise, they have a tendency to flip over at the end of the biopsy, making it difficult to cut the final portion of the excision. Fig. 6-6 shows four examples of methods used to keep the
lesion from moving during the shave biopsy. In Fig. 6-6, *A*, the lesion is stabilized with the tip of the same needle used to administer local anesthesia. In Fig.
6-6, *B*, the needle used to administer local anesthesia is inserted through the
lesion before starting the shave. In Fig. 6-6, *C*, forceps are used, and in Fig. 6-
6, *D*, the skin is pinched because the lesion is very flat. Regardless of which
method is used, it is important to not pull up on the lesion too much to avoid
producing an indentation.

### Hemostasis

If enough time has elapsed between the administration of anesthesia and the start
of the biopsy (10 to 15 minutes), the procedure can be virtually bloodless. After
this waiting period, however, it may help to recreate the wheal just before the
procedure to firm the tissue and raise a flat lesion.

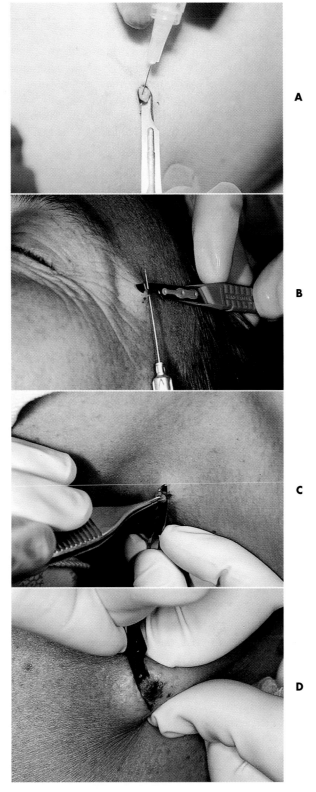

**FIG 6-6**
Stabilization techniques. **A,** The lesion is stabilized with the tip of the same needle used to administer local anesthesia. **B,** The needle from the local anesthetic is inserted through the lesion before starting the shave. **C,** Forceps are used for stabilization. **D,** The skin is pinched because the lesion is very flat.

After the biopsy, blot the site with a dry cotton-tipped swab or gauze to remove any pooled blood. Then roll an additional cotton-tipped swab that has been dipped in aluminum chloride back and forth over the site. Sometimes it helps to actually twist the swab over the site using significant pressure. It is important to not leave wet blood in the field because this will dilute the aluminum chloride and minimize its efficacy. Monsel's solution (ferric subsulfate) may also be used for hemostasis; it has a slight risk of tattooing but is slightly more effective than aluminum chloride for hemostasis. See Chapter 4 for further information on hemostasis.

### Remaining tissue after shave biopsy

If part of the lesion remains after the shave, options include doing a second shave, scraping with the side of the blade, using a curette, or electrodesiccating the remaining tissue (See Chapter 12 on electrosurgery). This remaining tissue is often found at the edge of the lesion where the scalpel or razor blade finished the shave biopsy. If using electrodesiccation, the charred tissue may be wiped away with a gauze or a curette. Our preferred method for finishing the shave removal of a seborrheic keratosis or other benign lesion is to lightly electrodesiccate any remaining tissue. This alone may be adequate treatment if only a small amount of tissue remains. For larger amounts of tissue, we use a small curette to lightly remove the electrodesiccated tissue and to ascertain whether any residual lesion remains. If tissue from the lesion remains, we repeat the electrodesiccation and curettage. Finally, we apply a hemostatic agent such as aluminum chloride or Monsel's solution to achieve the final hemostasis, rather than electrodesiccating the entire base. We suggest this approach because electrodesiccation to the base may increase the risk of scarring more than the chemical agents.

### Aftercare

After the procedure is complete, place a small amount of antibiotic ointment and a Band-Aid over the biopsy site and give the patient wound care instructions. See Appendix E for a sample patient handout entitled *Wound Care Instructions for Naturally Healing Wounds*.

### Pathology

Send all pigmented lesions and any lesion suspicious for cancer to the pathologist. Skin tags may not need to be sent if they are typical and benign in their appearance. Although the shave biopsy is easy for the physician and patient and often produces a good cosmetic result, it is not a technique meant to produce a complete excisional biopsy in all cases. If the pathologist reports that the lesion appears benign, does not have atypical features, but is incompletely excised, there is usually no need to do a further or deeper excision. However, if the pathologist recommends further excision because of a suspicion of malignancy, this recommendation must be followed.

If the lesion turns out to be malignant, definitive treatment will be necessary. If the lesion is premalignant (such as an actinic keratosis), it should be reexamined after it fully heals. If there is remaining scaling or evidence of the original lesion, it may be treated with cryotherapy instead of doing another excision.

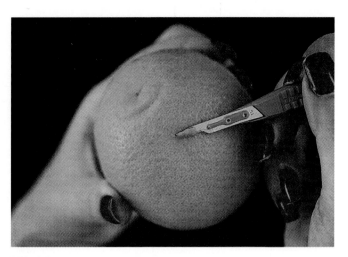

**FIG 6-7**
Practicing the shave biopsy on an orange helps develop technique.

## Suggestions for Learning Shave Biopsy Technique

When learning shave biopsy technique, it may be helpful to practice on an orange. Use a No. 15 blade and attempt to remove the outer layer without encroaching on the underlying pulp (Fig. 6-7). As skill levels improve, practice removing small hair follicles from the skin of a turkey or chicken to refine technique even further. The most difficult technique for the beginner to master is the ability to keep the blade parallel to the skin surface, creating a tendency to cut too deeply.

## Complications

Complications that may arise from shave biopsy include the following:

- Producing a divot, or indentation, in the skin
- Erythema
- Hypopigmentation
- Regrowth of incompletely excised lesion
- Infection (rare)

Serious complications are extremely infrequent with shave biopsy. However, caution must be taken to keep the blade parallel to the skin surface or an unintentional divot can be created, which can be cosmetically unappealing (especially on the central face).

After shave biopsy, erythema may persist for a few weeks, and hypopigmentation may be permanent in some individuals. In the case of melanocytic nevi, approximately 1 in 20 will regrow after removal by this technique. In nevi with hair, the hair is likely to regrow if the nevus is excised with a shave biopsy alone. This type of nevus may be best removed with a deeper elliptical excision. Alternatively, the hair follicles remaining after a shave biopsy may be destroyed with electrosurgery.

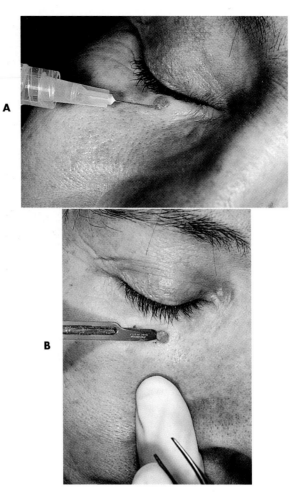

**FIG 6-8**
Shave biopsy of a suspected nevus on the face. **A,** Local anesthetic is injected into a raised, pigmented lesion on lower eyelid. **B,** Beginning of shave excision using a No. 15 blade. Note stabilization of eyelid skin with finger.

## TREATMENT OPTIONS BY SPECIFIC LESION

### Suspected Benign Nevus on Face (Raised)

Fig. 6-8 shows a shave biopsy of a suspected benign pigmented lesion on the lower eyelid. Because the lesion appeared completely benign and the patient wanted it removed for cosmetic reasons, it was acceptable to do a shave excision. By appearance, the lesion is probably an intradermal nevus, compound nevus, or seborrheic keratosis. The patient received local anesthesia with 1% lidocaine with epinephrine through a 30-gauge needle (Fig. 6-8, *A*). The shave excision was performed with a No. 15 blade on a scalpel handle.

In Fig. 6-8, *B*, note how the eyelid skin is stabilized by the physician's finger with gentle downward traction. This figure also shows the tip of the blade advancing into the lesion, which usually is less preferable than using the body of the blade. However, because the lesion was so close to the eye, the physician used the tip of

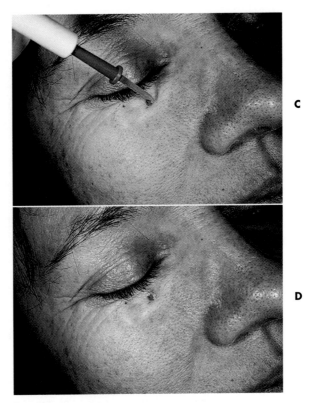

**FIG 6-8, cont'd**
Shave biopsy of a suspected nevus on the face. C, Light
electrodesiccation of the base of the lesion to achieve hemostasis and to eliminate any residual nevus. D, Final appearance. Electrodesiccation was not used over the entire surface of the lesion. Aluminum chloride was applied first to
achieve hemostasis.

the blade to avoid getting too close to the globe. Although an excellent result is
achieved here, we prefer to use the middle of the scalpel blade whenever possible.

In Fig. 6-8, C, light electrodesiccation is applied to the edge of the lesion to
destroy residual nevus tissue that was left on the edge of the lesion (probably secondary to using the tip of the blade).

Fig. 6-8, D shows the final appearance after the shave excision. Notice that
electrodesiccation was not used over the entire surface of the lesion. Instead, aluminum chloride in an aqueous solution was applied first to achieve hemostasis.
The use of a topical hemostatic agent in addition to electrodesiccation is the preferred method to minimize scarring. If aluminum chloride in an alcohol solution
is applied first, the site should be dried before applying electrosurgery.

The pathology report on the lesion in Fig. 6-8 indicated it was a seborrheic keratosis with some inflammation. For a true nevus, it is helpful to let the patient know
that it may recur even though initially no pigment is apparent after the surgery.

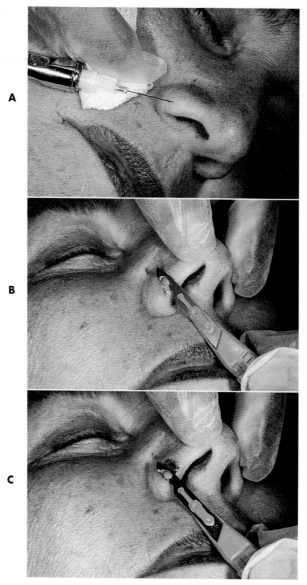

**FIG 6-9**
Biopsy to rule out basal cell carcinoma on the nose.
A, 1% lidocaine with epinephrine is injected into an elevated, pearly nodule. Notice how the epinephrine causes vasoconstriction. B, The scalpel blade is advanced so that the lesion is placed in the center of the blade. C, The top of the lesion is completely removed, revealing the residual cyst of a large milia.

## Possible Basal Cell Carcinoma on the Nose

The patient in Fig. 6-9, A to E, had a history of a pearly bump on the nose for 6 months. To remove the lesion, 1% lidocaine with epinephrine is injected with a 30-gauge needle beneath the lesion to raise it before beginning the shave biopsy (Fig. 6-9, A). Notice that the epinephrine causes vasoconstriction, which minimizes bleeding during the procedure. As stated in Chapter 3, epinephrine can safely be used for local anesthesia on the nose.

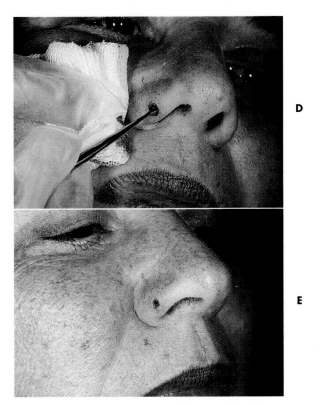

**FIG 6-9, cont'd**
Biopsy to rule out basal cell carcinoma on the nose.
**D,** The residual cyst is removed with a 2-mm curette to
prevent recurrence. **E,** Hemostasis is achieved after light
electrodesiccation and application of Monsel's solution.

In Fig. 6-9, *B*, the No. 15 blade is advanced so that the lesion is placed in the center of the body of the blade, where it is the easiest to control. The blade is advanced into the lesion using the fingers to stabilize the nose and to provide countertraction. In Fig. 6-9, *C*, the top of the lesion is completely removed, revealing the residual cyst beneath the surface. The lesion can now be identified as a large milia and not a BCC. The residual lesion is then removed with a 2-mm curette to prevent recurrence (Fig. 6-9, *D*). Hemostasis is achieved (Fig. 6-9, *E*) after light electrodesiccation, which also removes any residual lesion. Monsel's solution is also applied.

## Pigmented Lesions

If a physician is considering the diagnosis of a melanoma, a shave biopsy should not be performed. It is important to know the entire depth of a melanoma because measuring the Clark's level of melanoma invasion is necessary for determining treatment and prognosis. A shave biopsy will rarely be deep enough to determine the entire depth of the lesion. If clinical suspicion is very low for melanoma, a pigmented lesion can be excised with a shave biopsy that removes the entire base. Because the shave biopsy is fast and easy to perform, it is acceptable and common for physicians to use this technique with nevi and seborrheic keratoses that are unlikely to be melanoma.

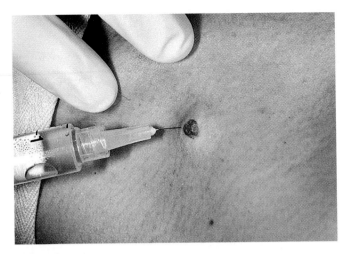

**FIG 6-10**
Benign raised nevus on the back being elevated with anesthetic before
shave with a No. 15 blade.

## Benign Nevus

A young woman requested the removal of a nevus on her back (it was catching
on her clothes). This nevus was perfect for a shave excision because it was raised
and had only benign features. Local anesthesia was used to numb the area and
raise the lesion further (Fig. 6-10). The nevus was easily shaved off using a No.
15 blade and forceps. The pathology revealed a benign nevus. The cosmetic result
was excellent.

## Sebaceous Hyperplasia

A middle-aged man had what appeared to be sebaceous hyperplasia on his forehead. He wanted it removed for cosmetic purposes. The lesion was marked with
a surgical marker before local anesthesia was administered. The physician
pinched the skin slightly and followed the marking while removing this lesion
with a No. 15 blade (Fig. 6-11). Pathology showed sebaceous hyperplasia only.

## Pyogenic Granuloma

A 54-year-old man noted a growth on his nose for 4 months. It appeared vascular, and the differential diagnoses were angioma, pyogenic granuloma, and BCC.
The lesion was shaved off with a No. 15 blade (Fig. 6-12). Hemostasis was
obtained with aluminum chloride (aqueous solution) and electrosurgery. The
pathology revealed a pyogenic granuloma, which has not recurred.

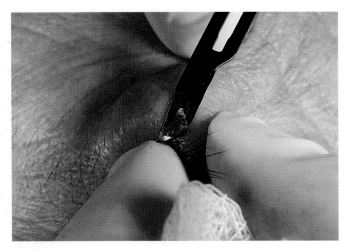

**FIG 6-11**
Shave biopsy of sebaceous hyperplasia on the forehead after the lesion
was marked with gentian violet.

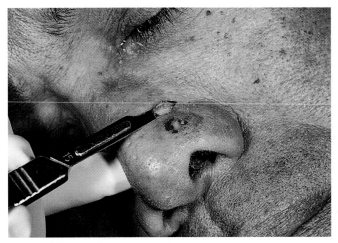

**FIG 6-12**
Shave biopsy of a pyogenic granuloma on the nose with a No. 15 blade
on a reusable handle.

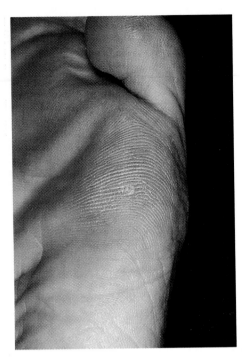

**FIG 6-13**
Porokeratosis.

## Porokeratosis

The hyperkeratotic spot on the sole of the foot in Fig. 6-13 appeared to be a porokeratosis, a benign hyperkeratotic lesion caused by hypertrophy of the stratum corneum about the duct of a sweat gland. It is usually seen on the sole of the foot and can cause pain with ambulation (as it did in this case). A porokeratosis can be mistaken for a plantar wart. In this case, the simple but complete removal of the lesion with a No. 15 blade was both therapeutic and diagnostic. A plantar wart would have shown pinpoint bleeding spots and disrupted the skin lines further.

## Actinic Keratosis

A 62-year-old woman had a number of actinic keratoses on the back of her hand that were treated with cryotherapy. The keratotic lesion in Fig. 6-14 did not respond to therapy. Because of its thickness, it was decided to do a biopsy to rule out SCC. On the back of the hand, a shave biopsy is safer and easier to perform than punch or deep excision biopsies. However, because the lesion was so flat, the skin needed to be pinched to facilitate the shave biopsy. When pinching the skin in this manner, the physician must be very careful not to cut his or her fingers.

The pathology of this lesion showed actinic keratosis only.

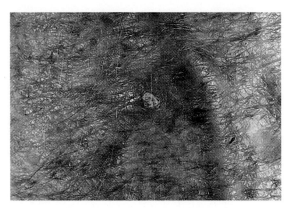

**FIG 6-14**
Actinic keratosis on the dorsum of the hand before shave
with a No. 15 blade.

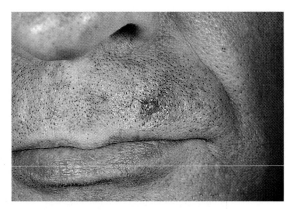

**FIG 6-15**
Basal cell carcinoma on the face.

## Basal Cell Carcinoma

A middle-aged man developed a new lesion over his lip that he repeatedly nicked
while shaving. The lesion, as seen in Fig. 6-15, was nodular with telangiectasias.
A shave biopsy confirmed the diagnosis of a BCC. Further treatment was provided. Curettage and desiccation or excision are adequate treatment modalities.

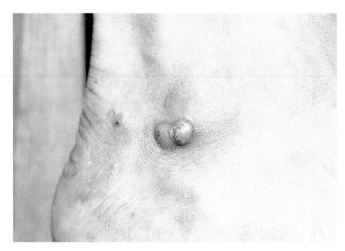

**FIG 6-16**
Kaposi's sarcoma in a man with AIDS.

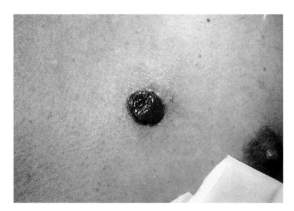

**FIG 6-17**
Cutaneous bacillary angiomatosis in a man with AIDS.
(Courtesy Frances Dann, MD.)

## Kaposi's Sarcoma vs. Bacillary Angiomatosis

Fig. 6-16 shows an example of Kaposi's sarcoma (KS). The lesion is raised, and a shave biopsy will provide adequate tissue for diagnosis. Because cutaneous bacillary angiomatosis (BA) (Fig. 6-17) can mimic nodular KS, it is important to biopsy all suspected cases of KS.[1,2] When a suspicious lesion is flatter than shown in Fig. 6-16, a punch biopsy is the better method for making the diagnosis. See Fig. 9-4 for an example of a flat KS lesion and a discussion of the punch technique.

Both BA and KS occur in patients that are HIV positive. BA is caused by two organisms, *Bartonella (Rochalimaea) henselae* and *Bartonella quintana*. Clinically, the BA skin lesions vary from a single lesion to thousands. The cutaneous lesion appears as a bright-red, round papule; a subcutaneous nodule; or a cellulitic plaque.[3] The patient with BA might present with nonspecific signs and symptoms of chills, headaches, fever, malaise, and anorexia. BA can produce

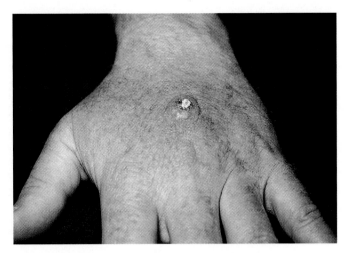

**FIG 6-18**
Keratoacanthoma that has grown rapidly on the back of the hand.

extracutaneous lesions involving the liver, spleen, lymph nodes, and bone. Oral and anal mucosal lesions can also occur with BA.[3]

The reason that it is so important to distinguish between KS and BA is that BA is a potentially fatal opportunistic infection that usually responds rapidly to appropriate antimicrobial therapy.[4] In fact, therapy for BA can be as easy as erythromycin 500 mg 4 times a day for 2 to 8 weeks.[3] There are treatments for KS as well, so knowing the proper diagnosis is essential. When sending a biopsy of a potential KS or BA lesion to the laboratory, it is important to alert the pathologist to the differential diagnosis so the proper studies will be done to achieve a correct diagnosis.

## Keratoacanthoma

Keratoacanthomas can usually be distinguished by their clinical history of rapid growth (Fig. 6-18). Patients will frequently say that these lesions have doubled or quadrupled in size within the preceding 3 or 4 weeks before their visit. Skin cancers such as BCC and SCC don't grow this rapidly.

A superficial shave biopsy is not an adequate technique when dealing with a keratoacanthoma because these lesions are invariably much deeper and will recur if treated only with a superficial shave biopsy. In addition, keratoacanthomas can be difficult to diagnose by superficial shave biopsy because without their full architecture visible to the pathologist, they may be misdiagnosed as squamous cell carcinoma.

When a shave biopsy is performed on a keratoacanthoma, an attempt should be make to perform a deep shave biopsy. In the deep shave technique, the blade goes deeply under the lesion, leaving a dish- or bowl-type defect. Yet even when this is accomplished, there frequently is residual lesion going deeper into the dermis. After the deep shave, we recommend performing a superficial curettage and desiccation to prevent recurrence.

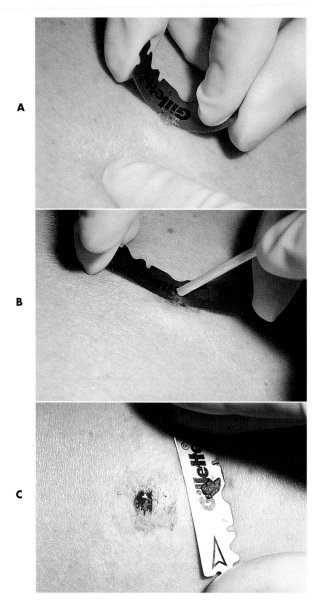

**FIG 6-19**
Shave biopsy using a razor blade. **A,** One end of the razor blade is grasped between the thumb and forefinger while pressure is placed on the other end of the blade by the middle finger. The blade is gently advanced into the lesion while moving the blade in a side-to-side fashion. The other hand performs traction of the tissue for stabilization. **B,** The stick end of a cotton-tipped swab that will be used for hemostasis is used to prevent the specimen from rolling or curling. **C,** The specimen lies flat on the blade.

## SHAVE BIOPSY USING A RAZOR

The following technique describes the steps needed to perform a shave biopsy using a razor:

1. Raise a wheal with local anesthesia.
2. Grasp one end of the razor blade between the thumb and forefinger and push on the other end with the middle finger, creating a half circle with the blade (Fig. 6-19, *A*). Place the blade on the skin surface and gently advance it into the lesion while moving the blade in a side-to-side fashion along the arc of what would be the imaginary circle that would be created by the curvature of the blade. Apply gentle pressure during this process and allow the blade to move through the lesion without excess pressure. Use the other hand to perform traction of the tissue to facilitate stabilization (Fig. 6-19, *A*).
3. On some thin specimens, there is a tendency for the specimen to roll or curl. This can be minimized by using the stick end of the cotton-tipped swab that will be used for hemostasis or by using the needle from the syringe that was used for anesthesia to stabilize the lesion on top of the blade as the biopsy proceeds (Fig. 6-19, *B*).
4. At the completion of the procedure, the specimen lies flat on the blade and a small bit of blood is frequently seen at the base of the biopsy (Fig. 6-19, *C*).

## SNIP EXCISION (SIMPLE SCISSOR EXCISION)

Another variation of the shave excision for small raised lesions is the snip excision performed with sharp scissors (Fig. 6-20). Anesthesia and hemostasis are executed in the same manner as for the scalpel shave excision. The only difference is that the lesion is snipped off with sharp scissors rather than shaved with a blade. Lesions particularly amenable to snip excision are skin tags, small warts, and polypoid nevi. We recommend using a good pair of sharp iris scissors (straight or curved).

After the lesion is anesthetized with 1% lidocaine and epinephrine, it is grasped with forceps and cut at the base with the scissors. Any remaining tissue can be handled the same as described for shave excisions. Hemostasis can be achieved with aluminum chloride, Monsel's solution, or electrosurgery.

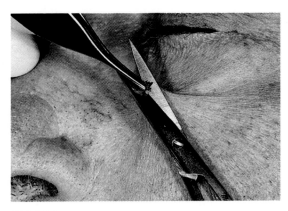

FIG 6-20
A snip excision is performed with a straight iris scissor. The lesion was marked before the biopsy with gentian violet.

## CONCLUSION

The shave biopsy is one of the most useful techniques in dermatologic surgery. It is widely applicable to many skin lesions and can be performed rapidly in the office setting with minimal equipment. Every primary care physician that performs skin surgery should learn to master this technique.

## REFERENCES

1. Caldwell BD, Kushner D, Young B: Kaposi's sarcoma versus bacillary angiomatosis, *J Am Podiatr Med Assoc* 86(6):260-262, 1996.
2. Tappero JW et al: Cutaneous manifestations of opportunistic infections in patients infected with human immunodeficiency virus, *Clin Microbiol Rev* 8(3):440-450, 1995.
3. Ramirez Ramirez CR, Saavedra S, Ramirez Ronda C: Bacillary angiomatosis: microbiology, histopathology, clinical presentation, diagnosis and management, *Bol Asoc Med P R*, 87(7-9):140-146, 1995.
4. Schwartzman W: *Bartonella (Rochalimaea)* infections: beyond cat scratch, *Ann Rev Med* 47:355-364, 1996.

## SUGGESTED READING

Shelly WB: The razor blade in dermatologic practice, *Cutis* 15:843-845, 1975.
Shelly WB: Epidermal surgery, *J Dermatol Surg* 2:125-128, 1976.

# CHAPTER 7

# Suture Material*

*Ronald L. Moy*

There are many suture types available. Absorbable sutures are used for removing tension across the wound; nonabsorbable sutures are used to closely approximate skin edges. The ideal suture is strong, handles easily, and forms secure knots. It causes minimal tissue inflammation and does not promote infection. It stretches to accommodate wound edema and recoils to its original length with wound contraction. Ideally, it is also inexpensive. Although no single suture material possesses all of these features, proper selection of sutures helps achieve better results in skin surgery. Among the absorbable sutures are catgut and treated catgut (both are used infrequently) and the synthetic sutures, which are designed for good tensile strength, easy handling, and low tissue reactivity. Nonabsorbable sutures include silk (now infrequently used) and several synthetic materials designed for elasticity, easy handling, good knot security, and minimal tissue irritation.

## HISTORY

The search for new and improved suture materials started with the Egyptians, who as early as 2000 BC used linen to close wounds.[1] Around AD 75, Galen experimented with catgut, and in 1869 Listeria introduced the practices of impregnating catgut with chromic acid and sterilizing suture material. In the early part of this century, Halsted promulgated the advantages of silk over catgut, and silk soon became the most common suture material in surgical practice.[2] Within the past two decades, a variety of synthetic products have entered the market. With a wide array of suture materials to choose from, it is increasingly important to understand the basic properties of suture materials to make the most appropriate suture selection for wound closure.

## PROPERTIES OF SUTURE MATERIAL

Because no single suture possesses all of the features of an ideal suture, it is the physician's task to weigh the advantages and disadvantages of the available suture materials. A number of standardized terms describe the properties of suture materials.[2]

**Tensile strength** is defined as the amount of weight required to break a suture, divided by its cross-sectional area. The *U.S. Pharmacopeia* provides a standard

*Modified from Moy R, Lee A, Zalka A: *Am Fam Phys* 44(6):2123-2128, 1991.

for identifying tensile strength in a digit-hyphen-zero form, where increasing digits correspond to decreasing suture diameter. Thus 3-0 nylon suture has a greater diameter than 5-0 nylon and possesses greater tensile strength.

**Knot strength** is a measure of the amount of force necessary to cause a knot to slip and is directly related to the coefficient of friction of a given material.[3]

**Physical configuration** refers to monofilamentous or multifilamentous sutures. Multifilamentous sutures come in twisted and braided types. Braided sutures tend to be the easiest to handle and tie, but they also have the potential to sequester bacteria between the strands, resulting in increased risk of infection.

**Elasticity** refers to the intrinsic tension generated in a suture after stretching, which causes it to return to its original length. Elasticity is a desirable feature because it allows the suture to expand during wound edema (without causing strangulation or cutting of tissue) and to recoil during wound retraction (thereby maintaining wound edge apposition).

**Memory** refers to the inherent tendency of a suture material to return to its original shape after being manipulated and is a reflection of its stiffness. A suture with a high degree of memory is stiffer, more difficult to handle, and more likely to become untied compared with suture material that has less memory.

**Tissue reactivity** refers to the inflammatory response generated by the presence of suture material in the wound. This response peaks within 2 to 7 days[2,4] and is a function of the quantity of material present as well as its type and configuration. Sutures of superior tensile strength and knot security not only minimize the risk of suture line disruption but also reduce the amount of foreign material left in the wound by allowing the use of finer sutures and fewer knots. This, in turn, reduces tissue reaction and infectious complication.[3] Postlethwaite, Willigan, and Ulin[5] found that multifilamentous natural fibers such as catgut and silk, which possess relatively low tensile strength, cause the most intense inflammatory reactions, whereas monofilamentous synthetic materials with increased tensile strength, such as nylon and polypropylene, generate less reaction.

**Fluid absorption** and **capillarity** are suture characteristics that have a relationship to the risk of infectious complications. Fluid absorption refers to the amount of fluid that a material soaks up when immersed, and capillarity measures the extent to which the fluid is transmitted along the strand. In general, braided sutures have higher capillary action than monofilamentous sutures, and for this reason have additional potential for infectious complications.

The choice of suture material for any given wound closure should not be made arbitrarily, but rather with careful attention to the physical and handling properties of the suture, as well as its propensity for eliciting tissue reaction and promoting infection.

## ABSORBABLE SUTURE MATERIALS

An absorbable suture material is loosely defined as one that loses most of its tensile strength within 60 days after being placed below the skin surface. The term *absorbable suture* does not imply complete absorption, however; catgut may persist in the tissue for years.[2] Currently, the most commonly used absorbable sutures are synthetic substances: polyglycolic acid, polyglactic acid, polydioxanone, and polyglyconate.

Catgut is discussed primarily as a basis for comparison; its use is steadily declining, except for chromic gut used in episiotomy repairs and fast-absorbing forms used in cosmetic facial procedures. To decrease the tension on wound edges, absorbable sutures are generally used as buried sutures. The ideal

**TABLE 7-1    Absorbable Sutures and Their Features**

| Product | Features | Advantages | Disadvantages |
|---|---|---|---|
| Gut (plain) | Natural product, absorbed by proteolysis | Inexpensive, maintains tensile strength for 4-5 days | Poor tensile strength, poor knot security, high tissue reactivity, quickly absorbed |
| Gut (chromic) | Natural product, absorbed by proteolysis | Less tissue reactivity than untreated catgut, prolonged tensile strength | Moderate tissue reactivity, poor knot security |
| Polyglycolic acid (Dexon) | Synthetic product, monofilament, absorbed by hydrolysis | Delayed absorption, greater tensile and knot strength, diminished tissue reactivity | Stiff, difficult to handle (braided version easier to handle) |
| Polyglactic acid (Vicryl) | Synthetic product, coated with lubricant, absorbed by hydrolysis | Easy to handle, tensile strength approximately equal to polyglycolic acid, diminished tissue reactivity | Dyed form may be visible through skin |
| Polyglactic acid (PDS) | Synthetic product, monofilament, hydrolyzes slowly | Extended duration of tensile strength (about 74% at 2 weeks), minimal foreign body reaction | Quite stiff, difficult to handle |
| Polyglyconate (Maxon) | Synthetic product, monofilament, hydrolyzes slowly | Extended duration of tensile strength (about 81% at 2 weeks); supple, easy to handle | Expensive; new product, limited experience |

Modified from Moy R, Lee A, Zalka A: *Am Fam Phys* 44(6):2123-2128, 1991.

absorbable suture has high tensile strength, low reactivity, good knot security, and delayed absorption time. The advantages and disadvantages of each absorbable suture type are described in Table 7-1. Characteristics of absorbable suture materials are described in Table 7-2.

## Gut

Catgut is derived from sheep intestinal intima. After being used for centuries, catgut is gradually being phased out because of its relatively poor tensile strength, poor knot security in vivo, and high tissue reactivity. Catgut retains significant tensile strength for only 4 to 5 days, and wound security essentially disappears within 2 weeks.[6]

Compared with the untreated variety, catgut treated with chromic acid (mild chromic gut) has delayed absorption time and decreased tissue reactivity and can be used as the top layer of skin closure. A newer form of catgut (fast-absorbing gut) that is not treated with chromic acid can also be used as percutaneous suture

**TABLE 7-2    Characteristics of Absorbable Suture Materials**

| Material | Tensile strength half-life, days | Tissue reaction* | Configuration | Ease of handling* | Knot security* | Color† |
|---|---|---|---|---|---|---|
| Gut (fast absorbing) | 2‡ | 2 | Mono | 1 | 1 | N |
| Gut (plain) | 4‡ | 4 | Mono | 1 | 1 | N |
| Gut (chromic) | 7‡ | 4 | Mono | 1 | 2 | N |
| Dexon | 14 | 2 | Braided | 3 | 4 | G, W |
| Vicryl | 14 | 2 | Braided | 3 | 4 | V, G |
| PDS | 28 | 2 | Mono | 2 | 3 | C, V |
| Maxon | 21-28 | 2 | Mono | 3 | 3 | C, G |

From Lask G, Moy R, editors: *Principles and techniques of cutaneous surgery*, New York, 1996, McGraw-Hill.
*1 = lowest; 4 = highest.
†C, Clear; G, green; N, natural; V, violet; W, white.
‡Variable.

in split-thickness skin grafts or in wounds in children, in which suture removal may be difficult. In general, however, synthetic sutures may be more suitable for use than catgut because synthetic materials have more predictable absorption and substantially decreased tissue reaction.

## Dexon: a Polyglycolic Acid Suture

Introduced in 1970, polyglycolic acid (Dexon), a polymer of glycolic acid, was the first synthetic absorbable suture. It was hailed for its excellent tensile strength and knot strength, as well as delayed absorption and markedly diminished tissue reactivity compared with catgut. In animal studies, the absorption of polglycolic acid suture was found to be about 40% after 7 days.[7] By 15 days, it loses more than 80% of its original strength.[8,9] By 28 days, this material retains only 5% of its original tensile strength, and it is completely dissolved by 90 to 120 days.[10] Whereas catgut is absorbed by proteolytic degradation, polyglycolic acid is absorbed by hydrolysis, reducing the inflammatory response.

As a monofilament, Dexon is stiff and difficult to work with. However, it is available in braided form for easier handling. Dexon also comes with a synthetic coating (Dexon Plus) to facilitate knot tying and passage through tissue.

## Vicryl: Polyglactic Acid

Polyglactic acid (Vicryl), the second synthetic suture material to be marketed (in 1974), is a copolymer of lactide and glycolide and is manufactured with a coating composed of polyglactin 370 and calcium stearate. This lubricant coating gives Vicryl excellent handling and smooth tying properties.

Technical studies have shown Dexon to have slightly greater tensile and knot strength than Vicryl,[11] but the differences are clinically insignificant. As with Dexon, Vicryl suture material retains only 8% of its original tensile strength by 28 days. However, complete absorption of Vicryl is more rapid, occurring between 60 and 90 days.[10] Like all synthetic polyesters, Vicryl degrades by hydrolysis and causes minimal tissue reaction.

Vicryl is a braided suture and is available in violet-dyed and undyed forms. When used in skin surgery, the dyed form can sometimes be seen beneath the skin surface. A buried Vicryl or Dexon suture may occasionally (10% of the time) be extruded through the suture line.

### PDS: Polydioxanone

Also a polyester, polydioxanone (PDS) is described as having prolonged tensile strength in vivo compared with Dexon and Vicryl. PDS retains 74% of its original strength at 2 weeks, 58% at 4 weeks, and 41% at 6 weeks.[12] Thus PDS is a useful suture in situations where extended wound tensile support is needed. Although PDS is hydrolyzed much more slowly than the other synthetic absorbable sutures (complete absorption does not occur until 190 days after placement), foreign body reactions to this material are judged to be minimal. Unlike Dexon or Vicryl, PDS is monofilament and is less likely to harbor microorganisms. PDS is stiffer than the braided synthetics, is more difficult to handle, and costs about 14% more than Vicryl or Dexon.

### Maxon: Polyglyconate

Polyglyconate (Maxon) is the newest synthetic absorbable suture on the market. It is a monofilament that was designed to combine the excellent tensile-strength retention properties of PDS with improved handling characteristics. As with PDS, Maxon provides wound support over an extended period of time, with an average strength retention of 81% percent at 14 days, 59% at 28 days, and 30% at 42 days. Complete absorption occurs between 180 and 210 days, with minimal tissue reaction. Moreover, Maxon is much more supple and easier to handle than PDS, with 60% less rigidity.

## HOW TO CHOOSE ABSORBABLE SUTURES

Compared with Dexon or Vicryl, Maxon has a smoother knot rundown and an excellent first-throw holding capacity, thus simplifying tissue approximation and minimizing the need for knot repositioning.[13] Maxon costs approximately 7% more than Dexon or Vicryl. Its superior strength and handling qualities make it a very useful absorbable suture (Table 7-3).

See Fig. 7-1 for a graphical depiction of the loss of in vivo strength of absorbable sutures over time. Because the data for the graph comes from different sources, the graph does not exactly match Table 7-1 in exact numbers, but does show the same trends.

The type of suture selected depends on the costs and the personal preference of the physician. The most commonly used absorbable sutures include Vicryl and Dexon II. Because these sutures are braided and coated, they pass through tissue easily. These two brands of absorbable sutures also dissolve the quickest (60 to 120 days). The amount of time they actually retain tensile strength is usually adequate for most skin surgery.

There are newer suture types that retain their tensile strength in tissue for a greater period of time. These sutures (Maxon, PDS) usually are not braided but are monofilamentous, making it easier to tie the first knot. There are very few

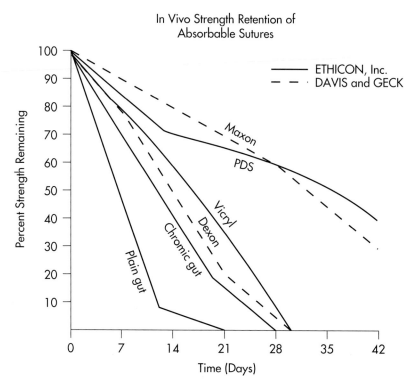

**FIG 7-1**

In vivo strength retention of absorbable sutures over time. (From Moy R, Lee A, Zalka A: *Am Fam Phys* 44(6): 2123-2128, 1991.)

**TABLE 7-3    Absorbable Sutures: Retained Tensile Strength Over Time**

| | Retained strength | | | Full absorption (days) |
|---|---|---|---|---|
| | 2 weeks | 4 weeks | 6 weeks | |
| Dexon | 55% | 5% | <5% | 90-120 |
| Vicryl | 55% | 8% | <8% | 60-90 |
| PDS | 74% | 58% | 41% | 180 |
| Maxon | 81% | 54% | 30% | 180-210 |

studies that show that these sutures produce a better cosmetic result even though they are retained in the tissue longer. Because these sutures are more expensive, it is probably unnecessary to use them in most cases. However, they may be helpful in closing a wound under excessive tension, which may be susceptible to dehiscence and stretching of the scar line over time. Additionally, these monofilamentous, absorbable sutures are nonreactive for a longer period and can be used for both deep and superficial placement, minimizing the number of suture packets used in a given procedure (Table 7-4).

**TABLE 7-4    Recommended Absorbable Suture Size**

| Wound location | Suture size |
| --- | --- |
| Under tension | 3-0 to 4-0 |
| Small and not under tension | 5-0 |
| Face | 5-0 |

# NONABSORBABLE SUTURE MATERIALS

Nonabsorbable sutures (Table 7-5) are defined by the *U.S. Pharmacopeia* as "strands of material that are suitably resistant to the action of living mammalian tissue." The most commonly used nonabsorbable suture are silk, nylon polypropylene, braided polyesters, and polybutester. The characteristics of nonabsorbable suture materials can be seen in Table 7-6.

## Silk

Silk is a naturally occurring proteinaceous filament. It is made into a braided suture and has perhaps the best handling and tying characteristics of any suture material. Unfortunately, it has the lowest tensile strength of any material tested[3] and elicits considerable tissue reaction, second only to catgut.[5] Silk also has a high degree of capillarity because of its braiding and should not be used in wounds where there is much potential for infection (e.g., distal extremities).

## Nylon

As a monofilament, nylon (Ethilon, Dermalon) is the most widely used nonabsorbable suture in skin surgery. It has high tensile strength, minimal tissue reactivity, excellent elastic properties, and low cost. The major drawback to nylon is its high degree of memory. A greater number of knot throws (three or four) are required to hold a given stitch in place. Pliabilized Ethilon can be ordered presoaked in alcohol to increase pliability and decrease memory.

Nylon hydrolyzes at a slow rate. Studies in rabbits have shown that buried nylon retains 89% of its tensile strength at 1 year and 72% by 2 years.[14] At this point, degradation apparently stabilizes; Moloney[15] has found that nylon sutures retain approximately two thirds their original strength after 11 years.

## Polypropylene

Polypropylene (Prolene, Surgilene) is an extremely inert suture with tensile strength and tissue reactivity comparable to that of nylon. A slippery material with low adherence to tissue, this suture can be withdrawn easily from wounds,[16] and is especially useful for subcuticular closures. On the other hand, this very characteristic compromises knot security, and extra throws are required. Polypropylene is noted for its plasticity.[2] Although it stretches to accommodate wound edema, it remains loose when wound edema recedes. Another disadvantage is that it costs 13% more than monofilament nylon suture.

**TABLE 7-5    Nonabsorbable Sutures and Their Features**

| Product | Features | Advantages | Disadvantages |
|---|---|---|---|
| Silk | Natural product, protein, braided | Best-handling suture, minimal skin irritation | Lowest tensile strength, high capillary (may increase risk of infection), high tissue reactivity |
| Nylon (Ethilon, Dermalon) | Synthetic product, monofilament, hydrolyzes slowly | Excellent elasticity, inexpensive, high tensile strength, minimal tissue reactivity | High degree of memory (stiffer, harder to handle), requires many knot throws |
| Polypropylene (Prolene, Surgilene) | Synthetic product | Low tissue adherence, stretches to accommodate wound edema | Poor knot security, requires many knot throws, remains loose when wound edema resolves, expensive |
| Braided Polyester (Ethibond, Ethiflex, Mersilene, Dacron) | Synthetic product, braided, monofilament | Easy handling, good knot security | Uncoated version causes friction and tissue drag, expensive |
| Polybutester (Novafil) | Synthetic product, monofilament | Excellent elasticity, accommodates increasing and decreasing wound edema, less stiff, less drag | Moderately expensive |

Modified from Moy R, Lee A, Zalka A: *Am Fam Phys* 44(6):2127, 1991.

**TABLE 7-6    Characteristics of Nonabsorbable Suture Materials**

| Material | Tissue reaction* | Configuration | Ease of handling* | Knot security* | Color† |
|---|---|---|---|---|---|
| Silk | 4 | Braided | 4 | 4 | B, W |
| Nylon (mono) | 1 | Mono | 2 | 2 | B, C, G, K |
| Nylon (braided) | 2 | Braided | 3 | 4 | B, W |
| Polypropylene | 1 | Mono | 1 | 1 | B, C |
| Polybutester | 1 | Mono | 2 | 3 | B |
| Polyester (uncoated) | 1 | Braided | 3 | 3 | G, W |
| Polyester (coated) | 2 | Braided | 4 | 2 | B, C, W |

From Lask G, Moy R, editors: *Principles and techniques of cutaneous surgery*, New York, 1996, McGraw-Hill.
*1 = lowest; 4 = highest.
†C, Clear; G, green; N, natural; V, violet; W, white.

**TABLE 7-7    Recommended Nonabsorbable Suture Size (Nylon)**

| Wound location | Suture size |
|---|---|
| Face | 5-0 to 6-0 |
| Extremities | 4-0 to 5-0 |
| Under tension | 4-0 |
| Trunk | 4-0 |

## HOW TO CHOOSE NONABSORBABLE SUTURES

There is a strong element of personal preference involved in the choice of sutures. With regard to size, the smallest suture that will allow proper closure of the wound should be used to minimize excess suture material in the wound and reduce the risk of suture tracks and tissue necrosis from overtight tying of large-gauge sutures (Table 7-7).

## CHOOSING NEEDLE TYPES FOR USE WITH SUTURES

Because there are so many possible needle types associated with sutures, it can be difficult to decide which needle should be used for the different types of sutures available. To add to the confusion, there is no standard needle nomenclature among the different suture companies. Each physician may develop a personal preference that makes standard recommendations difficult. The best general advice is to use smaller needles for facial closures and larger needles for closures on the trunk or extremities. Although smaller needles may work better for finer work on thinner skin, these needles may have a tendency to bend more easily.

There is minimal difference between a reverse cutting needle (sharp edge on the outside curve of the needle) and a conventional cutting needle (sharp edge on the inside curve of the needle) (Fig. 7-2). Therefore this classification scheme does not apply when choosing the needle type.

The major manufacturers of sutures in the United States are Ethicon and Davis & Geck. The Ethicon nomenclature uses the *FS* abbreviation as "for skin," whereas the Davis & Geck equivalent is the *CE* needle. See Box 7-1 for needle recommendations for nylon suture. The 4-0 and 5-0 sutures and needle combinations are for thicker skin areas on the trunk or extremities, and the 6-0 nylon will be adequate for most facial closures. Box 7-2 lists needle recommendations for absorbable sutures.

One advantage of the FS or CE needle-suture combinations is that they are half the cost of the precision (P, PS, or Pre) needles. The PS needles are basically FS needles that are sharper and made of better steel. The P series needles are even sharper and smaller than the PS or FS. PC denotes "precision cosmetic" needles. These are the sharpest needles and are intended for fine cosmetic work. The actual difference in clinical results may be small if the sutures and needles are of the same approximate size. However, we do recommend the precision needles when using 6-0 suture on the face.

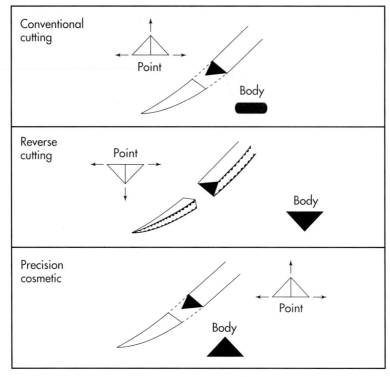

**FIG 7-2**
Needle point and body shape. (From Moy R, Lee A, Zalka A: *Am Fam Phys* 44(6): 2123-2128, 1991.)

| BOX 7-1   Needle Choice for Nylon Sutures | | |
|---|---|---|
| **Nylon** | **Ethicon** | **Davis & Geck** |
| 4-0 | FS-2 | CE-4 |
| 5-0 | FS-3 | CE-4 |
| 6-0 | P-3 | Pre-2 |

| BOX 7-2   Needle Choice for Absorbable Sutures | | |
|---|---|---|
| **Absorbable** | **Vicryl (Ethicon)** | **Dexon (David & Geck)** |
| 4-0 | FS-2 | CE-4 |
| 5-0 | FS-3 | Pre-2 |

## CONCLUSION

Qualities of the ideal suture include the following:

- Strong
- Handles easily
- Forms secure knots
- Causes minimal tissue inflammation
- Does not promote infection
- Able to stretch to accommodate wound edema
- Can recoil to its original length with wound contraction
- Inexpensive

In this chapter we have provided information to help physicians become familiar with the types of sutures available and the rationale for their use. There is nothing like experience to help you get to know these materials. If you are in a practice situation in which someone else chooses the sutures, we encourage you to become familiar with the sutures available to you. If you have the opportunity to choose your own sutures, start with at least one type from the absorbable and nonabsorbable categories and experiment until you find the suture materials that meet your needs. In Chapter 8, we apply what you have learned about suture materials to the actual techniques needed to use sutures in skin surgery.

## REFERENCES

1. Goldenberg I: Catgut, silk, and silver: the story of surgical sutures, *Surgery* 46:908-912, 1959.
2. Bennett RG: Selection of wound closure materials, *J Am Acad Dermatol* 18(4 Pt 1):619-637, 1988.
3. Herrmann JB: Tensile strength and knot security of surgical suture materials, *Am Surg* 37:209-217, 1971.
4. Macht SD, Krizek TJ: Sutures and suturing: current concepts, *J Oral Surg* 36:710-712, 1978.
5. Postlethwaite RW, Willigan DA, Ulin AW: Human tissue reaction to sutures, *Ann Surg* 181:144-150, 1975.
6. Swanson NA, Tromovitch TZ: Suture materials, 1980's: properties, uses, and abuses, *Int J Dermatol* 21:373-378, 1982.
7. Morgan MN: New synthetic absorbable suture material, *Br Med J* 2:203, 1969.
8. Herrmann JB, Kelly RJ, Higgins GA: Polyglycolic acid sutures: laboratory and clinical evaluation of a new absorbable suture material, *Arch Surg* 100:486-490, 1971.
9. Postlethwaite RW: Polyglycolic acid surgical suture, *Arch Surg* 101:489-494, 1970.
10. Craig PH et al: A biologic comparison of polyglactin 910 and polyglycolic acid synthetic absorbable sutures, *Surg Gynecol Obstet* 141:489-494, 1975.
11. Bloomstedt B, Jacobson S: Experience with polyglactin 910 in general surgery, *Acta Chir Scand* 143:259, 1977.
12. Ray JA et al: Polydioxanone (PDS): a novel monofilament synthetic absorbable suture, *Surg Gynecol Obstet* 153:497-507, 1981.
13. Moy RL, Kaufman AJ: Clinical comparison of polyglactic acid (Vicryl) and polytrimethylene carbonate (Maxon) suture material, *J Derm Surg Oncol* 17:667-669, 1991.
14. Postlethwaite RW: Long term comparison study of non-absorbable sutures, *Ann Surg* 271:892, 1970.
15. Moloney GE: The effect of human tissue on the tensile strength of implanted nylon sutures, *Br J Surg* 48:528, 1961.
16. Freeman BS et al: An analysis of suture withdrawal stress, *Surg Gynecol Obstet* 131:441-448, 1970.

# CHAPTER 8

# Suturing Techniques[*]

*Ronald L. Moy*

Proper suturing technique is essential for achieving good cosmetic results and avoiding infection, scarring, and poor wound healing. Techniques that must be mastered include good eversion and precise approximation of skin edges while maintaining uniform tensile strength along the skin edges. The goal of these techniques is to minimize scar formation while avoiding suture marks. Vertical mattress sutures have the advantage of good wound eversion and closure of dead space. Running continuous sutures can be quickly placed and divide tension equally along the skin edge. Interrupted sutures are more time-consuming but allow more precise wound edge approximation, whereas subcuticular sutures are useful for avoiding suture marks in conspicuous areas.

## WOUND HEALING

The primary function of a suture is to maintain wound closure and promote wound healing when the integrity of the wound is most vulnerable. The type and amount of suture used, the suturing technique, and the degree of tension on the suture all influence wound healing. The process of wound healing has been divided into three phases: (1) the initial lag phase (days 0 to 5), in which there is no gain in wound strength; (2) the fibroplasia phase (days 5 to 14), when a rapid increase in wound strength occurs; and (3) the final maturation phase (day 14 until final healing), which is characterized by further connective tissue remodeling[1,2] (Box 8-1).

Wounds never gain more than 80% of the strength of intact skin. Only 7% of the final tensile strength of the repair is achieved after 2 weeks. Thus nonabsorbable skin sutures, which are typically removed between days 5 and 10, and buried absorbable sutures play a crucial role during the initial 5-day lag phase.[3] Absorbable sutures play a very important role in the two final phases.

Table 8-1 summarizes the advantages and disadvantages of different suturing techniques. The ideal wound closure technique is one that produces maximal wound eversion, is technically simple to perform, maintains tensile strength throughout the healing process, allows for precise wound-edge approximation, and does not leave suture marks. These are also factors that should be considered before choosing a method for wound closure.

Sutures that are too tight or left in place too long can lead to permanent suture marks, or "railroad tracks." The greatest strength of the skin, and ultimately of

[*]Modified from Moy R, Lee A, Zalka A: *Am Fam Phys* 44(5):1625-1634, 1991.

---

**BOX 8-1    The Three Phases Of Wound Healing**

**Phase 1** (initial lag phase, days 0 to 5)
  No gain in wound strength
**Phase 2** (fibroplasia phase, days 5 to 14)
  Rapid increase in wound strength occurs
  At 2 weeks, the wound has achieved only 7% of its final strength
**Phase 3** (final maturation phase, day 14 until healing is complete)
  Further connective tissue remodeling
  Up to 80% of normal skin strength

---

**TABLE 8-1    Suturing Techniques: Advantages and Disadvantages**

| Technique | Advantages | Disadvantages |
| --- | --- | --- |
| Simple interrupted suture | Allows precise adjustments between stitches, allows removal of only selected (e.g., every other) stitches | More likely to cause uneven tension along wound edges, more prone to cause "railroad track" scars |
| Vertical mattress suture | Increased wound eversion, good dead-space closure, increased wound strength | Time consuming, prone to prominent suture marks if removal is delayed, edge approximation may be difficult |
| Shorthand vertical mattress suture | Has the advantages of vertical mattress suture, but can be placed much faster | As with vertical mattress suture, edge approximation may be difficult |
| Buried suture | Approximation of wound edges | Minimal eversion |
| Buried vertical mattress suture | Prolonged eversion, permitting early removal of top layer of sutures | If placed too superficially, suture may "spit" through |
| Running continuous suture | Speed, even tension, additional wound eversion | Suture must be removed entirely |
| Corner suture | Minimizes blockage of blood supply when suturing skin flaps | Edge approximation difficult, risk of trauma to skin flap |
| Subcuticular suture | Low incidence of suture scars, best for edge approximation without tension | Time consuming, poor strength under tension, poor wound eversion |
| Horizontal mattress suture | Good dead-space closure, some hemostasis, good wound eversion | Risk of epidermal necrosis, prone to suture scars |
| Wound closure tapes | Minimal wound trauma, no suture marks; more resistant to infection | Poor wound eversion, edge approximation difficult |

Modified from Moy R, Lee A, Zalka A: *Am Fam Phys* 44(5):1625-1634, 1991.

the repaired wound, lies in the dermal layer. The epidermis is a superficial covering that gives a polished effect to the wound but does not contribute to the strength of the repair.

## WOUND EVERSION

Eversion is important because the natural tendency of sutured wound edges is to become inverted after wound contraction has occurred. Thus everted wounds heal as flat scars after wound contraction. Wounds that are sutured so that the skin surface is flat are likely to leave a more visibly indented scar after wound contraction has occurred.

Wound eversion is accomplished by pushing down on the wound edges as the needle enters the skin at a 90-degree angle to the skin surface and pushing up on the wound edges as the needle exits the skin (Fig. 8-1). Pushing up or down on the wound edges can be done with a finger or an instrument, such as a forceps or skin hook. Eversion can also be accomplished by everting the skin with the skin hook as the needle enters or exits the skin. Furthermore, eversion occurs if the path of the needle is wider at the deepest part of the wound so that the entire path of the needle is flask-shaped (Fig. 8-2, A).

## SPECIFIC SUTURING TECHNIQUES

### Simple Interrupted Suture

The interrupted suture is one of the most commonly used suture techniques. It is easy for beginners to learn and perform. It may allow more careful wound approximation when small adjustments must be made. It is also a good technique to use in conjunction with buried sutures that have not completely approximated the wound edges.

The interrupted suture is more time-consuming to perform than a running suture and is more likely to leave "railroad track" scars on the skin surface. However, it is a better technique to use if the wound is not well approximated or has more than a little tension. Interrupted and running sutures can even out height differences between wound edges. Fig. 8-2, B, shows how this can be done with the interrupted suture. The needle should exit or enter the skin on the high side superficially and exit or enter the skin deeply on the low side ("high on the high side, low on the low side"). Interrupted sutures allow the removal of every other suture (an uncommon need).

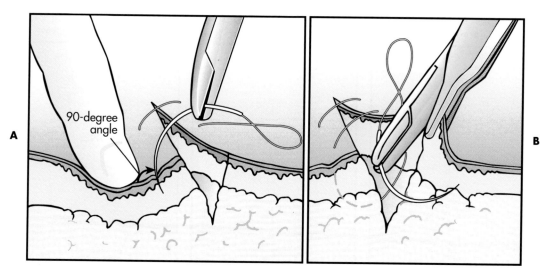

**FIG 8-1**
Additional wound eversion is created (**A**) by pushing down on the wound edges as the needle enters the skin at a 90-degree angle to the skin surface and (**B**) by pulling up on the wound edges as the needle exits the skin.

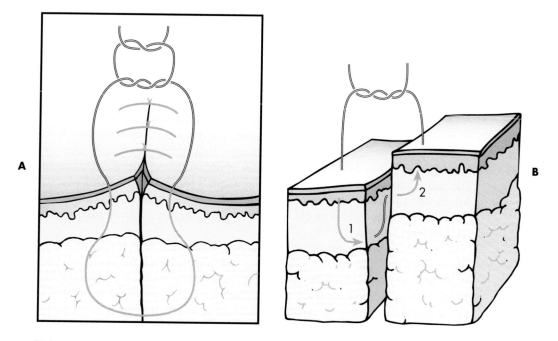

**FIG 8-2**
**A,** Wound eversion with interrupted sutures can be created by pushing down on the skin as the needle enters and pushing up on the skin as it exits and by creating a flask-shaped path with the needle. **B,** To even out height differences in wound edges, *(1)* suture low on the low side (low in the dermis) and *(2)* high on the high side (higher in the dermis).

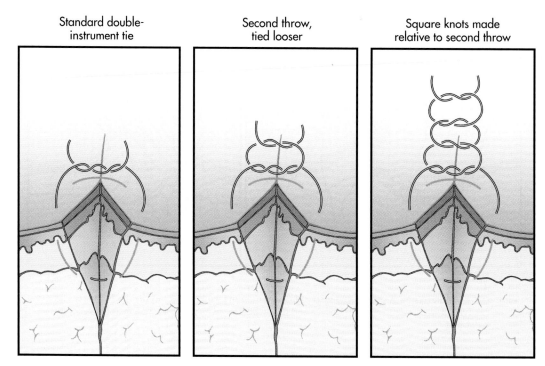

| Standard double-<br>instrument tie | Second throw,<br>tied looser | Square knots made<br>relative to second throw |

**FIG 8-3**
Loop throw used with interrupted suture.

A common mistake encountered with the simple interrupted suture is that if it is tied too tightly, it causes suture marks after postoperative edema.[4] Suture marks can be prevented by using a loop throw instead of the normal square knot[5] (Fig. 8-3). The first throw is the standard double-instrument tie; the second throw is tied looser, leaving a small loop; and the third and fourth knots are squared. The loop stitch allows expansion of the stitch if edema occurs. Squaring the knots allows them to lie flat and ensures adequate holding power.

Three throws may be minimally sufficient with a nylon suture, but Prolene (polypropylene) sutures usually require four throws because of their increased memory (the inherent tendency to return to original shape after manipulation). Furthermore, compared with nylon, Prolene and Novafil (polybutester) are more elastic (the intrinsic tension generated after stretching, which causes the suture to return to its original length). Thus if edema occurs, these sutures stretch slightly.

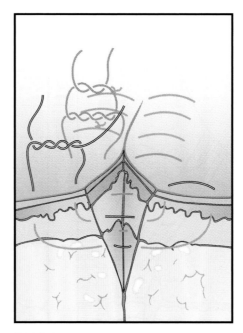

**FIG 8-4**
Vertical mattress suture.

## Vertical Mattress Suture

The main reason for using a vertical mattress suture is to produce greater wound eversion (Fig. 8-4). Vertical mattress sutures also close dead space and provide increased strength across the wound. To use a vertical mattress suture, begin by taking a slightly wider bite than that taken in a simple interrupted suture. Then reverse the direction of the needle and start closer to the wound edge on the same side that the suture just exited. Enter the skin superficially closer to the wound edge, taking a narrower bite. Finally, tie the suture on the same side of the wound as the suture originally pierced the skin.

Disadvantages of the vertical mattress suture include difficulty in closely approximating wound edges and prominent suture marks if the sutures are not removed sooner than other techniques require. This is a somewhat time-consuming technique that can take twice as long as a simple interrupted suture. Some physicians alternate between vertical mattress sutures and simple interrupted sutures along the length of the wound. The more accomplished the physician becomes in everting wound edges, the less often the vertical mattress suture is used.

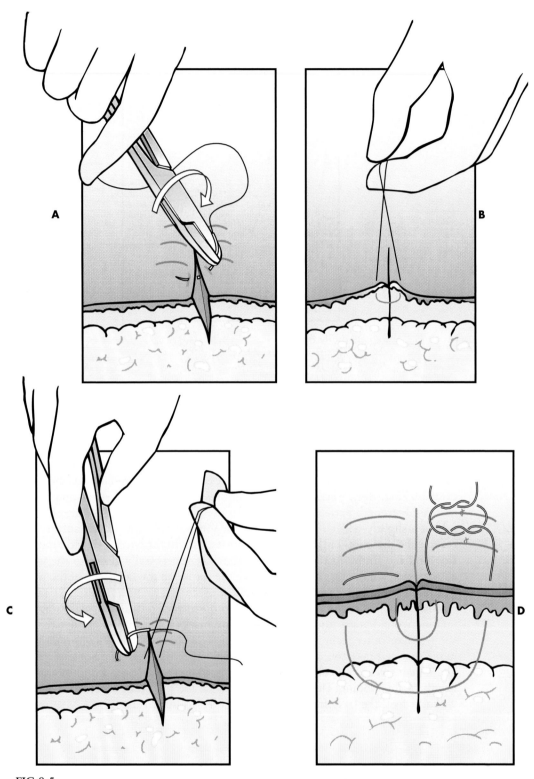

**FIG 8-5**
Shorthand vertical mattress suture. **A,** Superficial loop created using backhand rotation. **B,** Free end and proximal portion of superficial loop lifted upward to elevate opposite skin margins. **C,** Deep loop created by reversing the direction of the needle and using forehand rotation. **D,** Shorthand vertical mattress suture completed with a double knot.

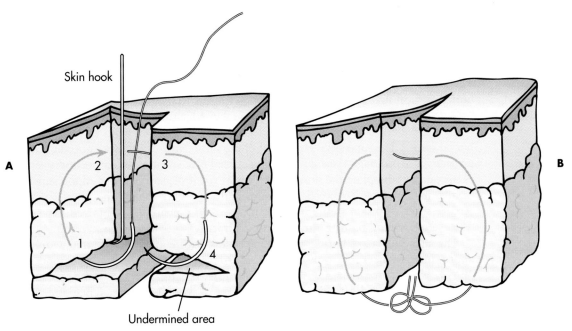

**Skin hook**

**Undermined area**

**FIG 8-6**

Buried vertical mattress suture (deep stitch with absorbable suture material). **A,** The needle should enter deep in the skin below the dermis where the undermining was accomplished *(1)* and exit in the upper dermis *(2)*. The needle enters in the upper dermis *(3)* and exits below the dermis where the undermining was accomplished *(4)*. **B,** The buried vertical mattress suture is tied at the bottom of the wound to avoid having the knot stick out of the incision.

### Shorthand Vertical Mattress Suture

The shorthand vertical mattress suture was described by Snow, Goodman, and Lemke.[6] When properly performed, this technique accomplishes the same degree of tissue eversion as the classic vertical mattress suture, but in half the time. Using backhand rotation, the needle is inserted superficially close to the wound edge and removed at a point equidistant on the opposite wound edge (Fig. 8-5). This step approximates the epidermal edges. The opposite skin margins are gently lifted upward by grasping the free end and proximal portion of the suture between the thumb and index finger. Then, using forehand rotation, the needle is reversed and deeply inserted far from the wound edge and passed through the deep dermis to an equidistant point on the opposite edge.

### Buried Sutures: Deep Absorbable Sutures

Buried sutures are important for obtaining wound eversion, providing prolonged wound tensile support, and closing dead space. The width of a resultant scar may be estimated by the distance between the skin edges only after buried sutures are placed. The most common suture materials used in this technique are Vicryl (polyglactic acid), Dexon (polyglycolic acid), PDS (polydioxanone), and Maxon (polyglyconate). (See Chapter 7 for descriptions of these materials.) The buried suture technique is shown in Fig. 8-6. In the classic description of this technique, the knot is buried downward[7] (Fig. 8-6, *B*). What is often not emphasized is that eversion can be obtained with the buried suture without leaving noticeable suture marks.

Buried sutures need not be placed as close together as external sutures. Often only 1 to 3 deep sutures are needed to close the dead space and bring the wound margins together. Of course, this varies based on the length of the incision and the skin tension.

### Buried Vertical Mattress Suture

The buried vertical mattress suture everts the wound in a fashion similar to the non-buried vertical mattress suture (Fig. 8-6). With this technique, the suture is buried with a slightly different path than the classic buried suture. The path of the needle is slightly wider and closer to the epidermal surface than the path in a common buried suture. The superficial placement of the suture and slightly wider needle path provide more prolonged eversion. The superficial placement of the suture approaches the point of dimpling the skin surface. However, if the suture is placed too superficially, it may "spit." A vertical buried mattress suture allows the physician to remove superficial skin sutures earlier, since wound eversion is maintained longer.[8] The everted wound flattens after wound contraction, providing a good result.

The ideally placed buried vertical mattress suture provides everted wound approximation itself, so only a loose final layer is necessary. If the wound is already well approximated with a buried suture, this final surface layer provides additional support during the first 3 to 6 days of wound healing. When approximation of wound edges is already completed with the buried suture, a running continuous suture is a good technique to approximate the skin surface.

## Running Continuous Suture

The running continuous suture can be performed quickly and distributes tension evenly along the length of the wound so that the suture is less likely to be too tight (Fig. 8-7). A running stitch is used primarily for wounds that are well

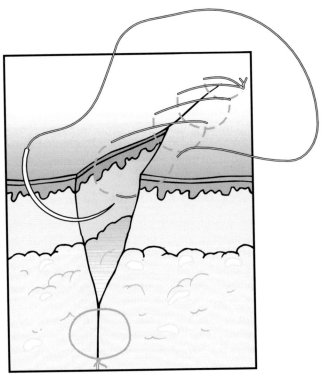

**FIG 8-7**
Running continuous suture.

approximated and have little tension. These two conditions are usually present when buried sutures are well placed. Small adjustments in the height of the wound edge can be made by exiting the needle superficially in the dermis on the higher wound edge and deeper in the dermis on the lower wound edge.

A running continuous suture is a disadvantage if subsequent removal of only a few sutures at a time is desired. In this situation, the end of the suture can be tied to a remaining loop so that the suture will not unravel. Theoretic concerns about increased wound infection or decreased final tensile strength with this type of suture have not been proved in clinical situations or animal studies.[9,10] A running continuous suture is useful in many situations because it is quick and shows good results.

## Corner Suture

The corner suture, or half-buried mattress suture, has been considered necessary for suturing of star wounds from trauma without compromising blood supply. This complication is highly unlikely under suturing flaps because a simple superficial interrupted suture through a flap tip has not been shown to cause flap tip necrosis in pigs or in clinical experience with human patients.[11-13]

When a corner suture is used, it is started on the opposite wound edge from the tip (Fig. 8-8). The nonabsorbable suture enters this wound edge across from the tip and then enters the tip at the same depth as it exited the opposite wound edge. The suture then goes through the dermis of the flap tip and enters the opposite wound edge. It exits the surface of the wound edge opposite to the flap tip and adjacent to the initial entry point. It is thus tied on the side opposite to the flap tip.

The main disadvantage of this suturing technique is that close approximation of the wound edges without trauma to the flap tip can be difficult.

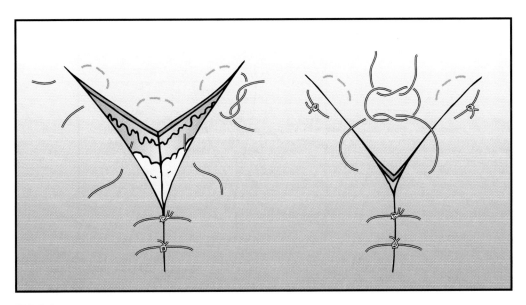

**FIG 8-8**
Corner suture, or half-buried mattress suture, consisting of a superficial interrupted suture through the flap tip and a horizontal mattress suture.

## Subcuticular Suture

An elegant but difficult suturing technique is the subcuticular suture, or running intradermal suture, which was first described by Halsted.[14] This technique is valuable when sutures need to be in place for more than 1 week but suture marks must be avoided. For example, subcuticular closure can be useful on the extremities, on the forehead of a patient with telangiectatic erythematous skin, or on sebaceous skin, where prominent suture marks can occur.

Subcuticular sutures are placed totally within the dermis, so that the only possibility of suture marks is at the ends of the wound, where the suture enters and exits (Fig. 8-9). The path of the needle crosses back and forth horizontally across the wound within the dermis. The needle holder can be held like a pencil, with the needle moving across the wound in a horizontal direction and the loops backtracking slightly. Usually, the more loops that are placed across the wound edges, the closer the approximation.

Securing the suture ends requires multiple knots at the end of the suture and the use of surgical tape. Buried sutures and simple interrupted sutures are often necessary to approximate the wound edges because the subcuticular closure cannot always provide close wound approximation under tension. A running subcuticular closure is time-consuming and does not evert wound edges. However, a well-placed subcuticular suture can be the ideal technique in certain locations of the body. It is often used as the final suturing technique in the standard episiotomy repair. For skin surgery, a long run of subcuticular suture should have an occasional loop above the surface to facilitate removal of the suture.

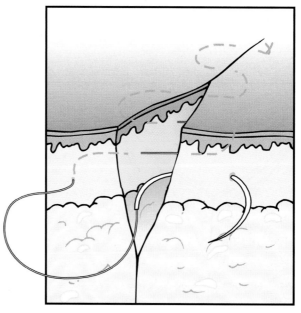

**FIG 8-9**
Subcuticular suture.

## WOUND-CLOSURE TAPES

Wound-closure tapes offer distinct advantages over both sutures and staples. They minimize iatrogenically induced trauma and apply less tension to the wound. Wounds closed with tape are more resistant to infection than sutured wounds.[15] On the other hand, tape cannot provide adequate skin-edge eversion or deep-tissue approximation when used alone. Thus tape is most commonly used as an adjunct to sutures or staples. However, tape may be used alone for small, superficial wounds (especially in young children.) For instance, tape helps reinforce wounds closed subcuticularly or with conventional suturing techniques; sutures or staples can be removed sooner if tape is applied to healing, sutured wounds. In areas where contamination is suspected, foreign material within the wound may be reduced by alternating tape with sutures or staples to close the wound.

The performance of surgical tape is characterized by its tensile strength, porosity, and adhesion.[15] Tensile strength is required for maintenance of wound-edge apposition, and adequate porosity is necessary to prevent buildup of gas and water vapor, which can cause the tapes to separate from the skin. A good adhesive ensures firm tape-to-skin attachment.

Adhesion is enhanced by the application of a tacky substance to the skin surface. Traditionally, tincture of benzoin has been used for this purpose, but a preparation containing gum mastic (Mastisol) has been shown to provide stronger adhesion.[16] Although some tape manufacturers indicate that Mastisol is not required, in our experience all wound-closure tapes have significantly enhanced adhesion when Mastisol is used. Wound-closure tape combined with the application of Mastisol is necessary after suture removal to prevent dehiscence. In addition, wound-closure tape may be used at the time of surgery. We typically apply wound-closure tapes, such as Steri-Strips, at the time of surgery and keep them in place until the sutures are removed. When placed over the suture, wound-closure tape can take tension off the wound edge, provide a semi-occlusive environment, and prevent the patient from looking at or handling the wound until days after suture removal.[17]

## WHEN TO REMOVE SUTURES

Guidelines for number of days required before removal of external sutures are provided in Table 8-2.

**TABLE 8-2    Guidelines for the Number of Days Before Removal of External Sutures**

|  | Span (days) | Average number of days |
|---|---|---|
| Face | 3-7* | 5 |
| Neck | 5-7 | 7 |
| Trunk (and genitalia) | 7-14† | 10 |
| Extremities (hands) | 7-14 | 10 |
| Scalp | 7-14 | 10 |

*Leave sutures in longer when the wound is under greater tension.
†Take external vertical mattress sutures out sooner.

## CONCLUSION

In summary, the ideal wound-closure technique accomplishes the following:

- Produces maximal wound eversion
- Allows for precise wound-edge approximation
- Maintains tensile strength throughout the healing process
- Does not leave suture marks
- Is technically simple to perform

These factors, combined with suturing time and the suturing materials available, should be considered before choosing a method for wound closure.

## REFERENCES

1. Lober CW, Fenske NA: Suture materials for closing the skin and subcutaneous tissues, *Aesthetic Plast Surg* 10:245-248, 1986.
2. Swanson NA, Tromovitch TA: Suture materials, 1980s: properties, uses, and abuses, *Int J Dermatol* 21:373-378, 1982.
3. Harris DR: Healing of the surgical wound. I. Basic considerations, *J Am Acad Dermatol* 1:197-207, 1979.
4. Crikelair GF: Skin suture marks, *Am J Surg* 96:631-639, 1958.
5. Bernstein G: The loop stitch, *J Dermatol Surg Oncol* 10:587, 1984.
6. Snow SN, Goodman MM, Lemke BN: The shorthand vertical mattress stitch: a rapid skin everting suture technique, *J Dermatol Surg Oncol* 15:379-381, 1989.
7. Stegman SJ, Tromovitch TA, Glogau RG: *Basics of dermatologic surgery,* St. Louis, 1982, Mosby.
8. Zitelli JA, Moy RL: Buried vertical mattress suture, *J Dermatol Surg Oncol* 15:17-19, 1989.
9. Borgstrom S, Sandblom P: Suture technique and wound healings: an investigation based on animal experiments, *Ann Surg* 144:982-990, 1956.
10. McLean NR et al: Comparison of skin closure using continuous and interrupted nylon sutures, *Br J Surg* 67:633-635, 1980.
11. McQuown SA et al: Gillies' corner stitch revisited, *Arch Otolaryngol* 110:450-453, 1984.
12. Tromovitch TA, Stegman SJ, Glogau RG: *Flaps and grafts in dermatologic surgery,* St. Louis, 1989, Mosby.
13. Swanson NA: *Atlas of cutaneous surgery,* Boston, 1987, Little, Brown Co.
14. Fisher GT, Fisher JB, Stark RB: Origin of the use of subcuticular sutures, *Ann Plast Surg* 4:144-148, 1980.
15. Edlich RF et al: Wound healing and wound infection. In: Hunt TK, editor: *Wound healing and wound infection: theory and surgical practice,* New York, 1980, Appleton-Century-Crofts.
16. Mikhail GR, Selak L, Salo S: Reinforcement of surgical adhesive strips, *J Dermatol Surg Oncol* 12:904-905, 908, 1986.
17. Taube M, Porter RJ, Lord PH: A combination of subcuticular suture and sterile Micropore tape compared with conventional interrupted sutures for skin closure: a controlled trial, *Ann R Coll Surg* 65:164-167, 1983.

# CHAPTER 9

# The Punch Biopsy

*Daniel Mark Siegel    Richard P. Usatine*

The punch biopsy is a fast and easy procedure to perform to obtain a small, full-thickness specimen for pathologic diagnosis of lesions that may be malignant or that have an unknown etiology. Punch biopsy is the method of choice for flat lesions and is especially useful in flat lesions in which a shave biopsy would leave a divot. The main advantage of the punch biopsy over the shave technique is that it yields deeper tissue with preserved architecture for pathologic evaluation. If the punch defect would need to be sutured, however, the shave biopsy is faster and easier to perform.

Flat lesions that are amenable to punch biopsy include inflammatory skin conditions such as drug eruptions, dermatosis, psoriasis, fungal infections, and lupus vasculitis. Also, a punch biopsy works well for flat neoplastic lesions such as Bowen's disease (superficial squamous cell carcinoma [SCC]), superficial or sclerosing basal cell carcinoma (BCC), and T-cell lymphomas.

Punch excisions may be useful to remove small, flat nevi while obtaining tissue for pathology. Because most punch biopsies are sutured, the cosmetic results are usually very good. Therefore the punch technique can be used to remove small, flat nevi for cosmetic purposes even when the nevi are not suspicious for malignancy.

The main disadvantage of doing a punch biopsy applies only to BCC or superficial SCC in that it may obligate the physician to use an excision instead of curettage and desiccation to treat the lesion. If curettage and desiccation are performed after a punch biopsy, the curette will sink into the deeper hole caused by the punch technique, making the procedure technically more difficult and possibly reducing the cure rate. See Chapter 12 for further information on curettage and desiccation.

Punch biopsy is frequently used to obtain specimens in which undistorted cores of tissue encompassing epidermis, dermis, and subcutaneous tissue are desired. A punch biopsy is of great value in evaluating inflammatory skin disease and can also be used to assess malignancies such as BCC, SCC, and melanoma. It is of particular value in the diagnosis of melanoma if the entire lesion is large, making it too difficult to remove the whole lesion at the time of biopsy. In this case, the diagnostic yield will generally be best if a biopsy is performed on the darkest, most elevated, and/or most suspicious areas.

If the suspicion for melanoma is high, excising the entire lesion is preferred to improve the diagnostic yield. If the suspicion is low, such as in a large solar lentigo, it is best to do a small punch biopsy rather than a large excision. In the solar lentigo in Fig. 9-1, a small punch biopsy would be sufficient. In Fig. 9-2, the lesion is darker and more suspicious. Because it might have been a solar lentigo only, a punch biopsy was done at the darkest portion of the lesion rather than doing an initial large excision. The biopsy results showed melanoma in situ (lentigo maligna), and the lesion was fully excised with Mohs' surgery.

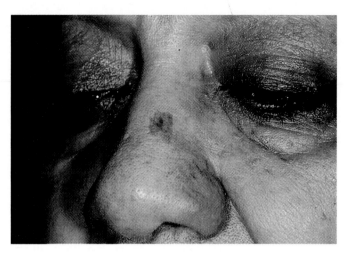

**FIG 9-1**
Benign solar lentigo. This is an appropriate lesion for a 2-mm punch biopsy at the darkest portion.

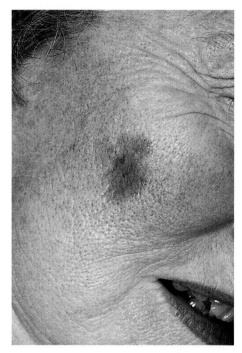

**FIG 9-2**
This seemingly benign-appearing lesion turned out to be a lentigo maligna (melanoma in situ).

# INDICATIONS

### Diagnosis

Punch biopsy can be used to diagnose the following lesions:

- Inflammatory skin disease such as dermatosis, psoriasis, vasculitis
- Granulomas: sarcoid, atypical mycobacteria
- Erythema nodosum
- Keratoacanthoma
- Kaposi's sarcoma
- BCC
- SCC
- Melanoma
- Cutaneous T-cell lymphoma

### Removal

Punch biopsy can be used to remove the following lesions:

- Small nevus
- Neurofibroma
- Dermatofibroma

# CONTRAINDICATIONS

Punch biopsy can be a less optimal biopsy technique for SCC or BCC because the biopsy may breach deeper planes than the tumor, necessitating a more aggressive approach to the removal of the tumor at the time of definitive treatment.

A punch biopsy does have certain risks that are greater than those of a shave biopsy, including the possible disturbance of deeper underlying structures such as nerves or arteries. Therefore physicians must be familiar with the underlying anatomy. For example, care must be taken to avoid cutting the temporal branch of the facial nerve or the supraorbital branch of the trigeminal nerve while doing a biopsy (See Fig. 19-6). Punch biopsies in critical areas, such as the digits or the eyelid overlying the globe, are generally to be avoided. When possible, it is also prudent to avoid doing a punch biopsy over superficial arteries such as digital or temporal arteries. Caution should also be exercised over areas where there is little soft tissue between the skin and the bone (over the tibia, digits, and ulna) because the punch can cut through the underlying bone.

## ASKING A QUESTION

Any biopsy, including a punch or shave biopsy, asks a question. All biopsies should be done selectively where indicated. It helps to have a good idea of the differential diagnosis before choosing the biopsy type and location. For most punch biopsies, a physician should excise the whole lesion or the portion of the lesion that appears to have the worst pathology. However, for bullous disorders such as pemphigus vulgaris or pemphigoid, it is best to punch the edge of the bulla to include the perilesional skin. When performing a biopsy on a lesion of unknown origin that has no morphologic form other than an ulcer, it is helpful to remove tissue from the edge of the ulcer rather than the center portion. For example, if pyoderma gangrenosum is suspected, the biopsy should include the edge of the lesion, with some perilesional skin. However, if the ulcerated lesion is a suspected SCC, perilesional skin does not need to be included.

Additionally, before starting the biopsy the physician should also have in mind whether this is to be a standard formalin-fixed hematoxylin and eosin (H & E)–stained specimen or whether it will be sent off for immunofluorescence or split for some combination of these procedures along with possible culture for various organisms. For example, to diagnose bullous disorders it helps to send the specimen for both H & E and immunofluorescent analysis. The biopsy for immunofluorescence is best performed on perilesional skin rather than on the middle of the blister. Suspected conditions for which a biopsy should be sent for immunofluorescence include the following:

- Dermatitis herpetiformis
- Discoid lupus erythematosus
- Pemphigus vulgaris
- Pemphigoid
- Systemic lupus erythematosus

Firm dermal nodules may represent a granulomatous process such as sarcoid. A punch biopsy of sarcoid will not grow organisms on culture. However, sporotrichosis, atypical mycobacterial infections (Fig. 9-3), and some deep fungal infections will grow organisms even if the pathology is a nonspecific granuloma. If a fungal infection is suspected, processing of the specimen should be discussed with the laboratory.

If a patient is HIV positive and has the typical lesions of Kaposi's sarcoma (KS), a biopsy is still needed to prove the diagnosis of KS because cutaneous bacillary angiomatosis can mimic KS (See Chapter 6). If the lesion is flat, a small punch biopsy should be sufficient to make a diagnosis. Fig. 9-4 shows an example of Kaposi's sarcoma. The lesion is flat, and a 2-mm punch biopsy will provide a sufficient specimen for diagnosis. A 2-mm punch defect in this case does not require suturing and therefore minimizes the risk of a needlestick to the physician. A larger punch could also be used to excise an isolated whole lesion if desired, but the defect will require suturing.

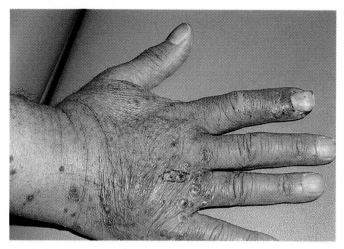

**FIG 9-3**
Atypical mycobacterium infection of the hand.

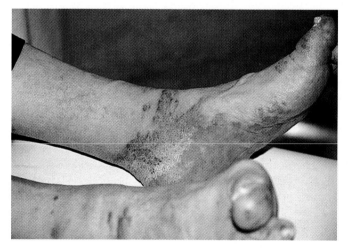

**FIG 9-4**
Kaposi's sarcoma. A 2-mm punch would work well for diagnosis.

## EQUIPMENT

- Punches (2 to 8 mm)
- Fine, sharp scissors
- Forceps
- Needle holder and sutures or hemostatic solution

Punches come in various sizes ranging from 2 mm to 8 mm and are available as reusable steel punches and disposable punches (Fig. 9-5). Disposable punches have the advantage of being presterilized and requiring no maintenance. Reusable punches are more expensive, require sterilization between procedures, and must be maintained by proper, skilled sharpening. We use disposable punches for the majority of procedures because of convenience.

Occasionally, a specimen removed with the punch will retract into the punch itself. When this happens, the specimen can be removed by using a cotton-tipped swab stick from above to push it out of a hollow punch. If a nonhollow punch is used, impaling the specimen from below or injecting a bit of local anesthetic around it may dislodge it. A nonhollow disposable punch may be pulled apart with a mosquito forceps, and the specimen can then be pushed through from above.

Basic punch instrumentation is quite simple. A basic setup consists of the punch; a pair of fine, sharp scissors; and a pair of pickups (Fig. 9-6). A syringe and needle for administering local anesthetic are also shown in Fig. 9-6. In a punch biopsy, the pickups could be used for placement of the suture as an alternative needle driver. However, it is easier to have a needle driver also available.

## CHOOSING PUNCH SIZE

A 2- to 3-mm punch is usually adequate to obtain sufficient tissue for pathology. When the lesion is smaller than 6 mm, the punch size may be determined by the diameter required to completely excise the tissue. Punch biopsies done with 7 and 8 mm punches may produce "dog ears" when closure is attempted (See Chapter 10). If the lesion requires a punch of larger than 6 mm, it is best to do an elliptical excision. Punch biopsies between 2 and 6 mm should produce adequate tissue and be easy to close with a good cosmetic result. A 3-mm punch is a good standard, and a 2-mm punch has the advantage of not always requiring sutures to close.

## TECHNIQUE

In contrast to shave biopsy, punch biopsy often results in a wound that needs to be closed; therefore a more rigorous approach to sterile technique is necessary. There is wide variation in the manner of prepping the biopsy site, but generally acceptable techniques include preparation with alcohol, Betadine, or Hibiclens. Using a sterile drape provides a larger working area, but its use is optional for solitary punches.

After selecting the biopsy site, a punch must be chosen. In most cases, a punch that will remove the lesion with a minimal margin of normal skin is adequate. In some cases, such as with a suspected melanoma, a larger margin around the specimen is preferred.

Before performing the punch biopsy, the area is infiltrated with local anesthetic. Usually, 1% lidocaine with epinephrine is used. Lidocaine without epinephrine should be used for digital blocks and for local anesthesia if there is any

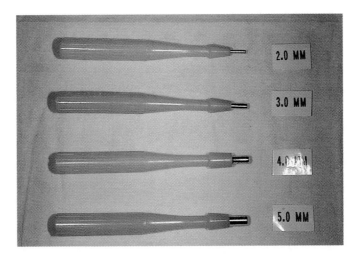

**FIG 9-5**
Disposable punches.

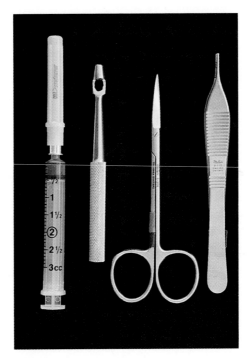

**FIG 9-6**
Basic instrumentation for a punch biopsy.

question of vascular compromise on distal fingers or toes (See Chapter 3). It is important to infiltrate the skin surface and the dermis to the full depth of the planned punch. Allowing the anesthetic to settle in for 10 to 15 minutes minimizes distortion of the tissue and enhances hemostasis by allowing maximum vasoconstriction. In most cases, waiting this long is not necessary.

If the lesion is on a surface with prominent relaxed skin tension lines or areas where skin folds are important, the physician's nondominant hand should be used to hold tension perpendicular to those lines (Fig. 9-7). This tension should be maintained throughout the punch procedure until the dermis is fully breached. This stretching perpendicular to relaxed skin tension lines will allow the resultant wound, circular under tension, to revert to an oval or fusiform shape when the retention is relaxed. The oval defect will be aligned with the relaxed skin tension line to facilitate closure and optimize cosmesis.

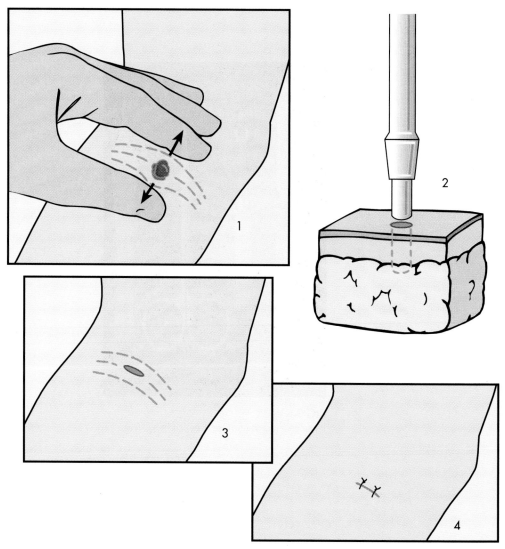

**FIG 9-7**
Line drawing showing how to stretch the skin during a punch biopsy. *1,* Skin stretched perpendicular to skin lines. *2,* Punch to subcutaneous fat. *3,* Oval defect. *4,* Closed defect is now linear.

The intradermal nevus shown in Fig. 9-8, *A* is about to be removed by punch technique; the nondominant hand is creating tension around the area. The punch is held above the area and is brought down over the specimen so that the specimen is centered under the punch. The punch is then held between the thumb and forefinger of the dominant hand (Fig. 9-8, *B*). With gentle downward pressure, the punch is rapidly rotated back and forth between the fingers, allowing it to drill a corelike sample around the specimen. The punch should penetrate completely through the dermis, exposing the subcutaneous fat. This provides a better specimen and facilitates closure. The punch is then removed, and the specimen remains in the center of the site. If the process is inflammatory, with involvement of underlying fat, or if the fat is fragile for various physiologic reasons, the specimen may shear off and pull away with the punch. If this happens, it can be removed from the punch with the same needle used for administering anesthesia.

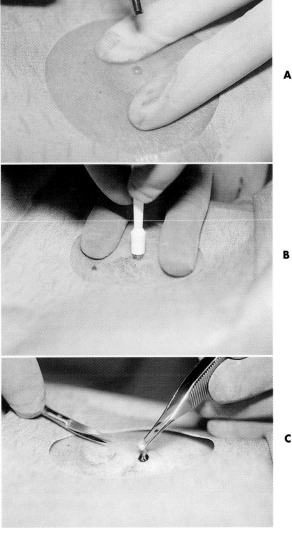

**FIG 9-8**
**A,** Intradermal nevus about to undergo biopsy. **B,** Punch is held between thumb and forefinger and lowered directly over lesion. **C,** Specimen is gently raised with forceps.

*Continued*

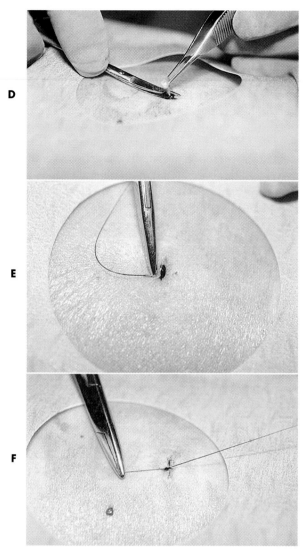

**FIG 9-8, cont'd**
D, Specimen is snipped with sharp scissors just below the dermis. E, Needle driving suture. F, Suture tied with instrument tie.

This may also occur when the punch is rotated slowly instead of rapidly, resulting in shearing and twisting of the specimen.

A gentle, downward compression of the area around the specimen often results in elevation of the specimen. The specimen can then be further elevated gently with a forceps (being careful not to crush the specimen) (Fig. 9-8, C) and amputated from its base with a sharp scissor (Fig. 9-8, D). Variations on this method include putting a skin hook or small needle into one side of the specimen and elevating it. Personal preference determines the actual approach chosen, regardless of what technique is used for removal of the specimen. It is important to remember that every effort needs to be made to handle the specimen lightly and to resist the tendency to compress or crush the specimen with the teeth of the forceps. The forceps should be used not as a grasping item, but rather as a shelf on which the specimen must lie with almost no compression around it. To demonstrate this utilization of forceps, be it with or without teeth, consider grasping your own eyelid or ear and gently moving the tissue around with the forceps. You will be amazed at how easily this can be done with gentle nudging and no compression, squeezing, or crushing of the tissue.

Two-millimeter punch defects can be left to heal by secondary intention or they can be sutured to promote more rapid and comfortable healing. When not suturing the punch defect, some physicians place a small amount of gel foam in the defect to aid in hemostasis. However, using aluminum chloride or Monsel's solution for hemostasis is equally effective and much less expensive. After placing the gel foam, the physician should then cover the punch site with a dressing. Allowing a punch defect to heal by secondary intention will minimize the risk of a needlestick to the physician when dealing with a patient that is known to have hepatitis, AIDS, or syphilis.

On areas where the round punch flattens to an almost straight line along relaxed skin tension lines, cosmesis can be excellent. Defects caused by the 3-mm to 4-mm punches are gently closed with one simple stitch; larger punch defects may require two or more sutures to close them. Punch defects are closed by inserting the suture needle perpendicular to the skin at the edge of the defect and rotating the needle directly through the tissue into the opposite side of the wound (Fig. 9-8, *E*). Alternatively, the needle can be passed into the hole and then reinserted into the other side of the intact skin. Then a hand knot or instrument tie can be performed (Fig. 9-8, *F*). The site can then be dressed with a small amount of antibiotic ointment and a simple dressing.

The suture placed after a punch biopsy is frequently a nonabsorbable suture such as nylon. There is rarely a need for subcutaneous sutures after a punch biopsy. Subcutaneous sutures, such as 5-0 PDS or Maxon, may be considered when a very large punch is used (8 mm). These dissolvable sutures can be used both below the surface and at the surface, minimizing the number of suture packets necessary for the procedure. Sutures are generally left in place for 5 to 7 days on the face and 7 to 14 days elsewhere on the body. See Chapter 18 for further details of postoperative wound care.

Patients should be informed that a punch biopsy obtained on mobile areas such as the back, which is stretched each time we bend or breathe, or the arms, which are stretched each time the muscles are flexed or pumped, may well result in some stretching of the wound. The ultimate scar, while frequently flat and flesh-colored, may well approximate the size of the area that was removed via punch technique. Hypertrophic or keloidal scarring may rarely occur, particularly with patients predisposed to their occurence.

If a biopsy is being performed on an inflammatory lesion in which there may be a secondary bacterial infectious component, it is better not to suture the wound, but rather to allow it to heal by secondary intention. Although the worsening or induction of an infection in a punch biopsy is extremely rare, it is even more rare to see an infection if the site has been left open.

## SPECIFIC EXAMPLES

### Solar Lentigo

Some solar lentigines have features suspicious enough to warrant punch biopsies. The patient in Fig. 9-9 sought treatment because the spot on his face was growing. He is fair-skinned and had a history of many sunburns as a child. A biopsy was done to rule out melanoma because of the growth in size (Fig. 9-9, *A* to *F*). However, because the suspicion was low, a punch biopsy was done in the darkest area only. The pathology result showed a solar lentigo.

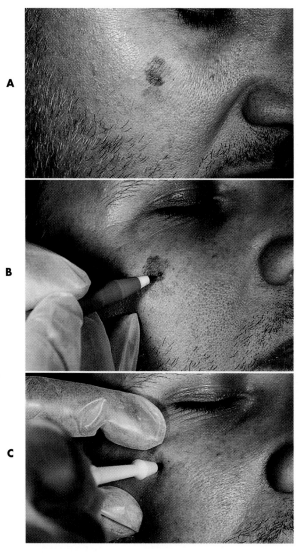

**FIG 9-9**
**A,** Probable solar lentigo on the face. Biopsy should be done to rule out melanoma based on growth and size of the lesion. **B,** The darkest area of the lesion is marked. **C,** A 2-mm disposable punch is used to perform the biopsy.

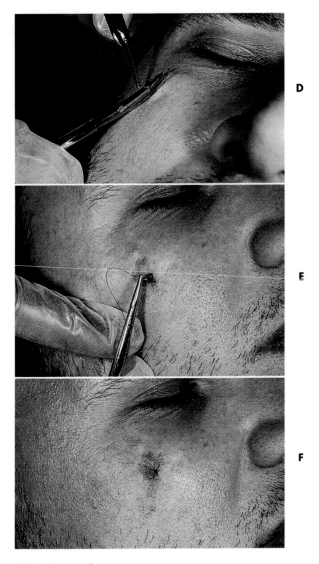

**FIG 9-9, cont'd**
D, The specimen is snipped at its base. E, The wound is sutured with a single simple interrupted suture. F, The final result.

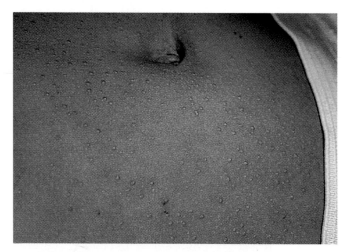

**FIG 9-10**
Inflammatory dermatosis, later diagnosed as lichen nitidus, was not responding to empiric treatment and diagnosis was uncertain.

## Inflammatory Dermatoses

Fig. 9-10 shows a child who developed an extensive eruption on his trunk that was not responding to empiric treatment; the diagnosis was uncertain but was suspected to be lichen nitidus. A punch biopsy was done and the diagnosis was confirmed.

## Psoriasis

The diagnosis of psoriasis can be made based on the clinical presentation in almost all cases, using clues such as the distribution, appearance, and chronicity of the lesions. In Fig. 9-11, *A*, the appearance and distribution of psoriatic plaques are so typical that a biopsy is not needed. A punch biopsy can be used to confirm the diagnosis in an atypical presentation when there is a great deal of uncertainty. In Fig. 9-11, *B*, a darkly pigmented person has thick, scaling plaques that do not show the same amount of erythema. Because the lack of erythema is not unusual in darker-pigmented skin, the lesions are still classic enough that a biopsy is not needed; even in this case, the diagnosis is a clinical one.

## Vasculitis

In Fig. 9-12, this leukocytoclastic vasculitis secondary to clindamycin use was difficult to diagnose. The punch biopsy enabled the physician to make the diagnosis. If lesions are polymorphous, as is often the case in inflammatory vascular processes, proper lesion selection is important. Lesions that are too new may not show a fully evolved pathologic process, and lesions that are too old may show nonspecific changes associated with resolution or necrosis. Therefore lesions in an intermediate stage may provide the best histologic information.

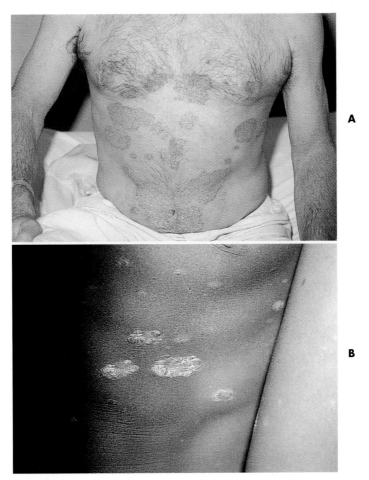

**FIG 9-11**
A, Classic psoriasis. There is no need for a biopsy to make a diagnosis.
B, Psoriasis in a darkly pigmented person does not show the same amount
of erythema. However, it is classic enough to not warrant a biopsy, and
the diagnosis is a clinical one.

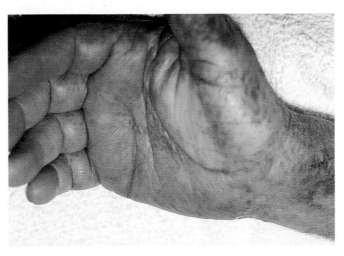

**FIG 9-12**
Leukocytoclastic vasculitis secondary to clindamycin use.

## Nevi

In Fig. 9-13, the patient had a small, very dark nevus that was itching. Although the most likely diagnosis was a blue nevus, the history of itching and the darkness of the pigment called for a biopsy. Because the lesion was small and round, it was possible to excise the whole lesion with a full-depth biopsy using a 3-mm punch. The pathology result was blue nevus (a benign nevus). The punch technique is also a good method for removing a small, flat nevus (less than 6 mm) that appears benign when the patient is requesting removal for cosmetic reasons.

## Malignancies

In Fig. 9-14, the lesion was suspected to be a keratoacanthoma because of its appearance with the central volcano-like ulceration and a history of fast growth. The diagnosis was confirmed with a punch biopsy, and the lesion was treated with full excision.

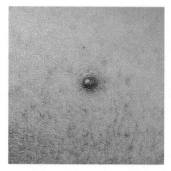

**FIG 9-13**
Small blue nevus.

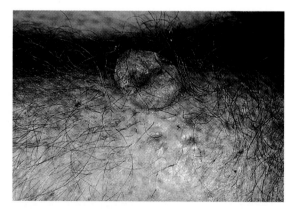

**FIG 9-14**
Keratoacanthoma.

In Fig. 9-15, the patient has what appears to be a flat morpheaform BCC on his face. This is one example of a BCC in which a punch biopsy is better than a shave biopsy. The punch biopsy confirmed that the lesion was a morpheaform (sclerosing) BCC.

Fig. 9-16 is a 1-cm raised lesion on the back of a young woman. The lesion has the classic features of a nodular BCC. Because it is raised and a probable BCC, a shave biopsy would be the method of choice. However, the figure shows that the physician performed a punch biopsy instead. The pathology report confirmed that the lesion was a nodular BCC. After a punch biopsy, a simple curettage and desiccation treatment is technically more difficult to perform and this may reduce the cure rate. Therefore the options for treatment include an elliptical excision and cryotherapy.

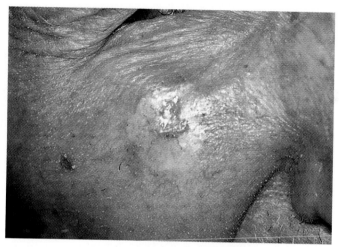

**FIG 9-15**
Morpheaform basal cell carcinoma.

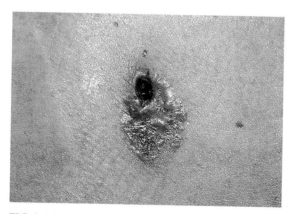

**FIG 9-16**
Nodular basal cell carcinoma with punch biopsy on the back of a young woman. Because punch biopsy was done, the definitive treatment should involve full excision (not curettage and desiccation). The better choice for biopsy of this lesion would have been a shave technique.

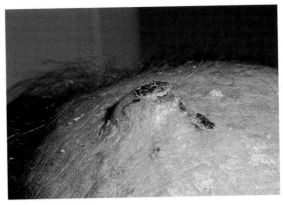

**FIG 9-17**
Squamous cell carcinoma on scalp. A shave or punch biopsy could be used.

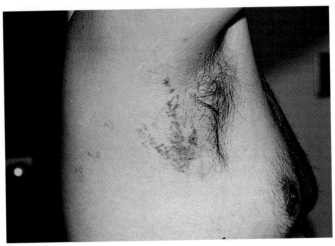

**FIG 9-18**
Punch biopsy was performed in the darkest area of this lesion below the axilla. Biopsy confirmed melanoma and acanthosis nigricans.

Fig. 9-17 shows an SCC on the scalp, a condition best suited to a shave biopsy. A punch biopsy is an alternative.

Fig. 9-18 shows a very large, dark spot that appeared under the patient's axilla in the previous few months. The differential diagnosis included acanthosis nigricans and melanoma. Full excision of a lesion this size could not be done in most offices. Therefore a punch biopsy was performed on the darkest portion of the lesion. The biopsy showed melanoma (Clark's Level I), and the lesion was fully excised in the operating room by a surgeon who specializes in surgical treatment of melanoma. The remainder of the lesion showed only acanthosis nigricans. The original pathology on the punch was rechecked by a number of dermatopathologists who also confirmed the diagnosis of melanoma.

## COMPLICATIONS

Complications from a punch biopsy include the following:

- Producing a divot or indentation
- Infection (rare)
- Erythema
- Hypertrophic scar
- Dog ears

Complications are extremely infrequent with the punch biopsy. Informed consent should be obtained so that the patient will understand the purpose of the biopsy (to help make a diagnosis) and the risks associated with it, including infection, scarring, and the need for further procedures. A complete consent form is included in Appendix A.

## CONCLUSION

The punch is a relatively easy and convenient procedure for getting a full-thickness biopsy. It is much easier to perform than an elliptical excision, but neither as easy nor as fast as the shave biopsy. It is preferentially used when a shave biopsy is too superficial, and a small 2- to 6-mm biopsy will provide adequate tissue sampling. Usually, a physician should not be doing more punch biopsies than shave biopsies.

## SUGGESTED READING

Devereux DF: Diagnosis and management of dysplastic nevus syndrome and early melanoma, *Oncology* 4:73-81, 1990.

Fewkes JL, Cheney ML, Pollack SV: The biopsy. In *Illustrated atlas of cutaneous surgery*, Philadelphia, 1992, Lippincott-Gower.

Koh HK: Cutaneous melanoma, *N Engl J Med* 325:171-182, 1991.

Robinson J, LeBoit PE: Biopsy techniques. In Robinson J et al: *Atlas of cutaneous surgery*, Philadelphia, 1996, WB Saunders.

# CHAPTER 10

# Elliptical Excision

*Ronald L. Moy    Richard P. Usatine*

The elliptical excision is used to excise a lesion or subcutaneous mass that is too large for a punch biopsy. As with the punch biopsy, the elliptical excision removes the full thickness of the skin and is sutured for closure. The major steps involved in the elliptical excision involve the following:

- Planning and designing the excision
- Anesthesia
- Incision
- Undermining
- Hemostasis
- Wound closure

## PLANNING AND DESIGNING THE EXCISION

Important factors to consider when planning an excision include the following:

- Avoiding vital structures
- Placement of incision lines
- Size of the surgical margin
- Whether the closure can be accomplished with a side-to-side closure
- Whether anatomic distortion will occur

### Avoiding Vital Structures

When planning an elliptical excision, it is crucial to avoid damage to any vital structures, including nerves, arteries, bones, tendons, ligaments, cartilage, sensory organs, and internal organs. For example, a deep elliptical excision over the medial antecubital fossa may result in cutting the brachial artery. When possible, a shave technique can be used to perform a biopsy without the risk of cutting deep structures.

In planning the surgical excision, it is important to avoid cutting the temporal branch of the facial nerve or the spinal accessory nerve. Both of these nerves are superficial; if they are cut, it will result in permanent limitations in movement. For a superficial skin cancer, the physician may choose to perform a superficial curettage and desiccation instead of an elliptical excision. Mohs' micrographic surgery is an alternative technique for skin cancer in these areas because the tissue is removed layer by layer.

The temporal branch of the facial nerve can be damaged by any surgery of the temple area. The nerve lies very superficially with the fat layer; it can be impossible to see, and there is enough anatomic variation that its location can be unpredictable. The best way to locate the nerve is to draw an imaginary line from the tragus to the eyebrow and another imaginary line from the tragus to the upper forehead wrinkle area. The area between these two lines within the temple area is where the temporal branch of the facial nerve is most superficial. If this nerve is cut, the patient will not be able to wrinkle the forehead because the innervation to the frontalis muscle is lost. The patient will also likely have permanent drooping of the upper eyelid (See Fig. 19-6, *B*). If any surgery is to be performed in this area, it is important that this risk is discussed with the patient.

The spinal accessory nerve lies within the posterior triangle posterior to the sternocleidomastoid muscle (See Fig. 19-7). The nerve can lie very superficially posterior to the sternocleidomastoid muscle. If this nerve is cut, the patient cannot raise the trapezius muscle. Fine hand-arm coordination can also be impaired.

## Placement of the Incision Line

Major factors to be considered when determining the placement of the incision line are wrinkle lines and relaxed skin tension lines. The physician may also want to perform a circular excision first and observe the direction in which the circle becomes elongated.

The design of the ellipse is usually done so that any incision line is placed within a wrinkle line. This method works on any older individual who has wrinkles (Fig. 10-1). If there are no wrinkles, the next best method is to use the relaxed

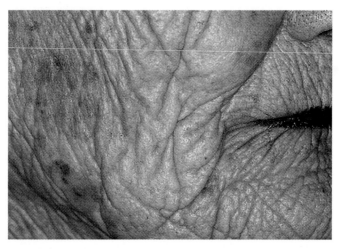

**FIG 10-1**
Wrinkle lines may be used to plan an incision line.

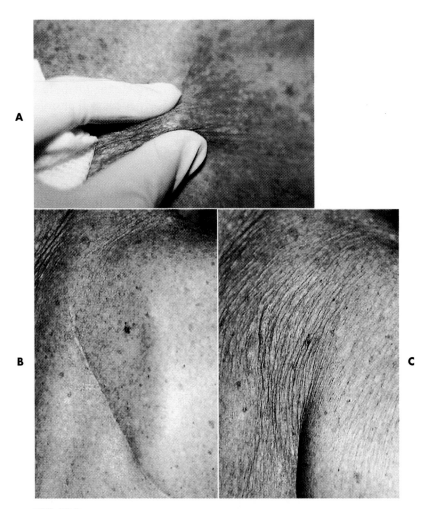

**FIG 10-2**
A, Relaxed skin tissue lines demonstrated by pinching the skin on the upper chest. B, The skin on the back is smooth near the darkly pigmented lesion (disregard old scar). C, By asking the patient to swing his arm back, skin tension lines are visible running vertically in the area of the lesion to be excised. (From Fewkes JL, Cheney ML, Pollack SV: *Illustrated atlas of cutaneous surgery,* Philadelphia, 1991, Lippincott-Gower.)

skin tension lines. These lines are the parallel skin lines that are seen when the skin is pinched together (Fig. 10-2). For example, when the skin is pinched together on the wrist, the relaxed skin tension lines run horizontally from the lateral wrist to the medial wrist. The relaxed skin tension lines are used to plan the ellipse on the trunk, extremities, and on facial areas where wrinkle lines are not apparent (Fig. 10-3).

The wrinkle lines and the relaxed skin tension lines usually are the same except in certain areas such as the side of the nose, the lateral canthal area, and the peri-

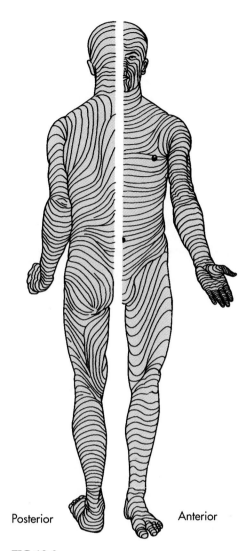

Posterior                          Anterior

**FIG 10-3**
Relaxed skin tension lines on the body. (From
Fewkes JL, Cheney ML, Pollack SV: *Illustrated
atlas of cutaneous surgery,* Philadelphia, 1992, Lippincott-Gower.)

oral area. Wrinkle lines should be used in these areas. If neither the wrinkle lines
nor the relaxed skin tension lines are obvious, it is sometimes necessary to use the
circular excision method of line placement. In this method, the lesion is excised
in a circular fashion, and the surgical defect is undermined in all directions. The
line of closure is chosen by looking at the direction in which the circle becomes
elongated. The sides that are closer together or that can be pushed together most
easily are sutured. Alternatively, the sides can be pulled together with skin hooks
to determine the best direction of closure.

**TABLE 10-1   Choosing Surgical Margins**

| Lesion | Margin during excision (mm) |
|---|---|
| **Melanoma** | |
| Melanoma in situ (lentigo maligna) | 5* |
| Confirmed level <1 mm | 10* |
| Confirmed level 1-2 mm | 20 |
| Confirmed level >2 mm | At least 20 |
| Moderate to high suspicion | 1 |
| Low suspicion | 1 or shave |
| **Basal Cell Carcinoma** | |
| Diagnosis confirmed | 3-5 |
| Moderate to high suspicion | Shave |
| Low suspicion | Shave |
| **Squamous Cell Carcinoma** | |
| Diagnosis confirmed | 4-6 |
| Moderate to high suspicion | Shave |
| Low suspicion | Shave |

*Data from NIH Consensus Conference: *JAMA* 268:1314-1319, 1992.

## Surgical Margin

The ellipse is designed so that the lesion is cleared with a margin. The surgical margin will be at least 3 to 5 mm for basal cell carcinomas, 4 to 6 mm for squamous cell carcinomas, and 1 to 2 cm for melanomas (Table 10-1). When the suspicion for malignancy is low, a shave biopsy or an excision with smaller margins of 1 to 2 mm is usually adequate.

It is very helpful to mark the biopsy margins with a sterile surgical marking pen. To orient the ellipse properly, determine the wrinkle line or relaxed skin tension line that will define the axis of the ellipse. The lesion should first be prepped and scrubbed with an antiseptic. A clean and nonsterile surgical marking pen is acceptable if you prep the skin again after marking the lesion. The usual ellipse is drawn so that the length of the ellipse is at least three times the width of the ellipse (Fig. 10-4). Conditions in which a 3:1 or greater ratio should be used for an elliptical incision include looser skin (3:1) and tighter skin, skin over the extremities, and curved surfaces (>3:1).

The ends of the ellipse should be approximately 30-degree angles so that potential dog ears are minimized. Dog ears consist of bulging skin at the ends of a sutured wound. Looser skin areas sometimes allow slightly larger angles at the

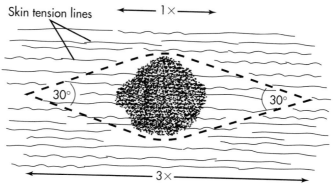

**FIG 10-4**
3:1 ratio for marking an elliptical incision.

end of the ellipse because the dog ears flatten slightly. Undermining the end of the ellipse also helps minimize these potential dog ears. A physician should explain to patients before the surgery that the length of the incision needs to be about three times the diameter of the lesion. It is helpful to draw this for patients so they can see how large their incision will be.

Once the ellipse has been drawn with a surgical marking pen, it is advisable to pinch the skin again to make sure that the ellipse can be closed and that minimal anatomic distortion occurs. A final wash with an antiseptic may be necessary.

## Is Side-to-Side Closure Possible?

The way to decide whether side-to-side closure can be accomplished is to pinch the skin to determine whether there is loose enough skin within the area. The physician has to predict from pinching the skin whether the two sides of the ellipse can be brought together. Areas such as the cheek, trunk, and arms are areas where an elliptical excision can be easily accomplished. Areas that are most difficult are over the sternum and tibia.

## Avoiding Distortion of Tissue

Elliptical excisions on the forehead, upper lip, and around the eye require careful planning because they can distort the eyebrow, lip, or eyelid. If there is doubt about whether the ellipse can be closed or if there is potential for anatomic distortion, it is possible that a flap or graft will be necessary. These procedures are beyond the scope of this book. There may be instances when the closure can be very tight. Wider undermining or thicker sutures may be required to accomplish the closure.

## ANESTHESIA

Local anesthesia can be performed using 1% lidocaine with epinephrine after the ellipse has been designed. The area of anesthesia must be wide enough to cover the whole ellipse and to anesthetize the skin that will hold the sutures. This can often be done with one or two injections. Adequate or tumescent anesthesia will promote hemostasis. Tumescent anesthesia involves the use of a large volume of anesthesia to distend the tissue for greater hemostasis.

It is best to wait at least 10 minutes before making the incision so that the epinephrine can take effect and any bleeding will be minimized (See Chapter 3).

## INCISION

The incision is performed with a No. 15 blade. The scalpel should be held like a pencil, with the hand holding the scalpel resting comfortably on the patient. The corner of the ellipse is incised with the tip of the blade. The belly of the blade is used to cut the majority of the ellipse. Care should be taken to make the incision perpendicular to the skin surface (Fig. 10-5). If the incision is made so that the skin is beveled outward, it can be difficult to obtain a fine-line closure.

The incision should be made through the dermis, keeping the scalpel perpendicular to the cutting axis. While making the incision, it should be spread open and checked to ensure that the cut is perpendicular and the ends are vertical. When making a curved incision, there is a natural tendency to lean the scalpel to the outside of a curve. This is poor technique. The physician should excise the ellipse, remembering to keep the blade vertical or leaning 10 degrees to the inside curve, which may help evert the skin edges.

The incision should be carried down to subcutaneous fat. It helps to have a surgical assistant stretch the skin perpendicular to the axis of the incision so that the incised skin will separate easily. The entire ellipse should be excised at the same level in the subcutaneous tissue to allow for a good closure (Fig. 10-6).

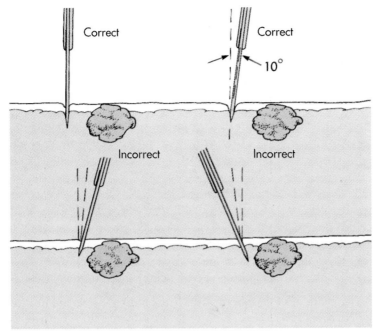

**FIG 10-5**
Scalpel handling. (From Fewkes JL, Cheney ML, Pollack SV: *Illustrated atlas of cutaneous surgery*, Philadelphia, 1992, Lippincott-Gower.)

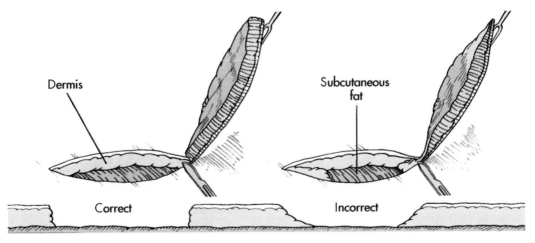

**FIG 10-6**
Incision carried down to the subcutaneous fat. (From Fewkes JL, Cheney ML, Pollack SV: *Illustrated atlas of cutaneous surgery*, Philadelphia, 1992, Lippincott-Gower.)

## UNDERMINING

Undermining may be performed by spreading blunt tenotomy scissors under the edges of the incision (Fig. 10-7). Undermining allows one to mobilize the tissue so that it can be advanced to close the defect.[1] Alternatively, sharp iris scissors or the No. 15 scalpel may be used. The sharper the instrument, the greater the chance that bleeding will occur because vessels are more likely to be cut using this approach, whereas blunt dissection can push the vessels out of the way atraumatically. Most areas of the body are undermined within the subcutaneous fat. Some areas of the body, such as the scalp, are better undermined in a deeper plane. The scalp should be undermined in a subgaleal plane (right above the skull) because it is a bloodless, easy plane in which to widely separate the tissue. Appropriate levels of undermining include the following:

- Scalp: deep to the galea aponeurotica, above the skull
- Face: high fat
- Nose: deeper fascia or connective tissue plane
- Trunk and extremities: deep subcutaneous fat above the muscle

The width of undermining is determined by the size and location of the defect. Undermining is useful to loosen the surrounding skin, but should not be excessive. Undermining should allow the skin edges to come together without too much tension and allow eversion of the wound edges with suturing.

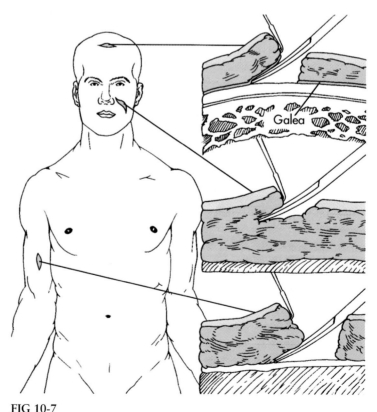

**FIG 10-7**
Levels of undermining. Blunt tenotomy scissors are inserted at the appropriate level and are then opened to push aside the surrounding tissue. (From Fewkes JL, Cheney ML, Pollack SV: *Illustrated atlas of cutaneous surgery*, Philadelphia, 1992, Lippincott-Gower.)

## HEMOSTASIS

Hemostasis is achieved by electrocoagulation during and after the undermining. Creating a dry surgical field is essential for good viewing of the tissues at the time of the final repair. Suturing with a dry field helps prevent hematoma formation, wound infection, and dehiscence. Minimal use of the Hyfrecator (or other electrosurgical unit) should be attempted so that tissue injury is minimized. The use of firm pressure by the surgical assistant and rolling cotton-tipped applicators across the surgical field will help locate the bleeding points. It helps to have an assistant retract the skin edges with skin hooks to locate bleeding around the undermined skin. The whole hemostasis process should be done systematically so that every area of the surgical wound is examined. The surgical site should be dry before initiating wound closure (See Chapter 4).

## WOUND CLOSURE

The first suture usually is a buried absorbable vertical mattress suture used to bring the skin edges together. Sometime a thick, interrupted, nonabsorbable suture will be used to decrease tension before placing the buried absorbable suture. The buried suture should be pulled lengthwise along the wound. The goal is to have the wound edges closely approximated using only buried sutures. If the ellipse is small and narrow and not under much tension, a buried suture is not needed (See Chapter 8).

### Dog Ear Repair

Repair of the elevated cone of tissue at either end of an elliptical excision is easily accomplished by extending the length of the excision (Fig. 10-8). This is usually accomplished by extending the excision through the center of the elevated cone of tissue. This results in two overhanging edges of tissue that need to be trimmed to flatten out the elevated cone of tissue. This trimming is done with a No. 15 blade to neatly trim the tissue to the very end of the excision. The No. 15 blade is used rather than iris or tenotomy scissors because it results in a sharper and more perpendicular cut than most scissors. When trimming this tissue, it is important to trim only a small amount at a time so that not too much tissue is removed from the end of the ellipse.

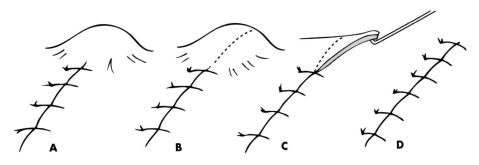

FIG 10-8
Dog ear repair. **A**, Bulging dog ear. **B**, The tissue is cut along the dotted line with a No. 15 blade. **C**, The extra tissue is brought across with a skin hook, and a cut is made along the new dotted line. **D**, Two new sutures are placed, and the dog ear is flattened.

It may be tempting to leave a dog ear or an elevated bulge of tissue at the end of an excision. However, this only works on an area where the skin is loose, such as on an elderly person, so that the elevated tissue may flatten with time. The usual recommendation is to excise any dog ear so that the skin surface is flat. Dog ears usually do not flatten out with time and are best avoided by careful planning, such as marking the ellipse as described.

## LABELING TISSUE FOR THE PATHOLOGIST

Labeling one end of an elliptical excision is important. If the pathology report comes back with a report of tumor remaining, it may be possible to go back and excise the appropriate skin edge if it was marked. If this orientation is not maintained, the entire scar line may need to be reexcised. It may be better to refer the patient to a surgeon for Mohs' micrographic surgery if it is not clear from where the remaining tumor should be excised.

The usual way to label tissue is to suture the superior pole of the tissue specimen. Tissue dye, such as bluing ink or commercially available tissue dyes, can also be used. It is important to communicate the labeling to the pathologist so the pathology report can reflect the labeling orientation.

## PUTTING IT ALL TOGETHER

Fig. 10-9 shows a full elliptical excision of an atypical nevus to rule out melanoma. All of the steps described above are illustrated in this series of photographs. The lesion was determined by pathology to be a benign atypical nevus with clear margins.

## FLAPS

There are a number of flaps that can be useful in excising benign and malignant lesions. Performing flaps well takes considerable training and experience. It is important to master the more basic techniques in this book before progressing to flaps. Flaps have a higher risk of complications such as bleeding, dehiscence, infection, and necrosis. A poorly performed flap with a complication can be a cosmetic disaster (especially for a cosmetic lesion). When using a flap to treat a malignancy, there is an additional risk of uncertainty or inability to determine tumor origin if the malignancy recurs. That is, did the cancer come from the site from which the flap was cut or from the site where the flap was placed? For these reasons, we recommend flaps be used only by the most experienced skin surgeons.

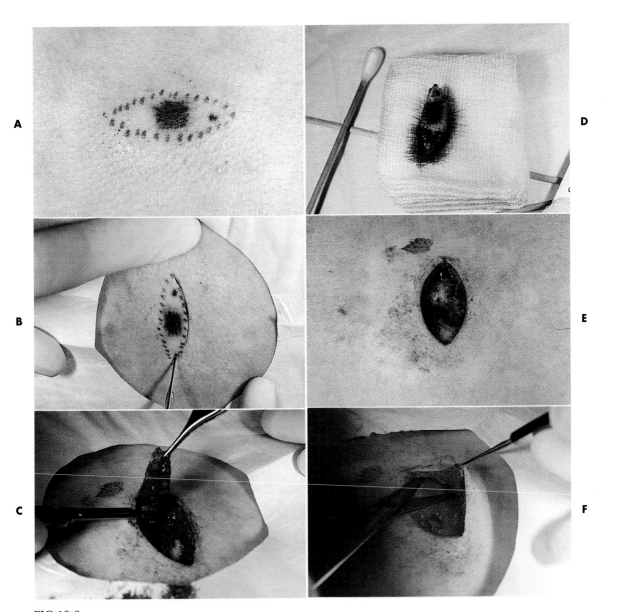

**FIG 10-9**

Excision of atypical nevus. **A,** Atypical nevus, including small satellite lesion, with ellipse marked with surgical marking pen. Epinephrine effect is noted by the blanching of the skin. **B,** Incision is made with a No. 15 blade so that the blade is perpendicular to the skin. The incision should be made down to subcutaneous fat. **C,** The ellipse is removed at the level of the subcutaneous fat. **D,** The specimen will be sent to the pathology laboratory. **E,** The ellipse has been removed. **F,** Undermining is performed with tenotomy scissors about 5 to 10 mm within the fat layer. Hemostasis is achieved with electrocoagulation after undermining.

*Continued*

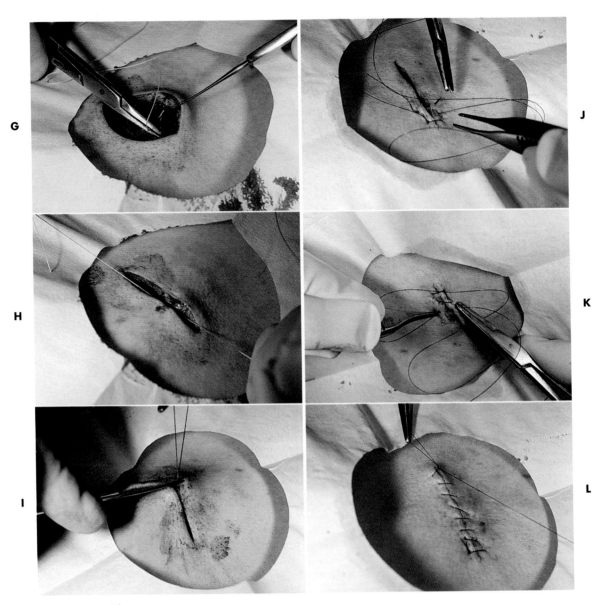

**FIG 10-9, cont'd**
Excision of atypical nevus. **G,** An absorbable buried suture is placed. **H,** The buried suture is tightened by pulling along the length of the ellipse. **I,** The buried sutures are cut short right above the knot. **J,** The tension across the wound is lessened with the buried sutures so that the running continuous sutures can be placed with minimal wound tension. **K,** The wound is everted with a forceps. **L,** Final closure. Running continuous sutures should be reserved for experienced skin surgeons. Simple, interrupted sutures are otherwise preferred, even though they take longer to place.

## EQUIPMENT

See Chapter 1 for in-depth discussion of the following lists of equipment.

- Skin marking pen
- Sterile gauze pads
- Surgical wash: povidone/iodine (Betadine) or chlorhexidine gluconate (Hibiclens)
- 5-ml syringe with needles (20-gauge for drawing up local anesthetic and 30-gauge for injection)
- Injectable local anesthetic: 1% lidocaine with epinephrine for most areas
- Sterile drape
- Sterile gloves
- Specimen jar with formalin solution and label
- Nylon suture for skin closure (4-0, 5-0, or 6-0, depending on the location of the lesion)
- 4-0 Vicryl or Dexon suture if deep sutures are anticipated

### Small Elliptical Excision Set

- Adson forceps
- Iris scissors
- Webster needle-holder (smooth)
- No. 15 scalpel blade with handle
- Designated suture scissor (optional)

### Large Elliptical Excision Set

- Adson forceps
- Iris scissor
- Webster needle holder
- Blunt tenotomy scissor
- Mosquito hemostat
- Two skin hooks (single, sharp prong)
- No. 15 scalpel blade with handle
- Designated suture scissor (optional)

Consider adding cotton-tipped swabs and a metal basin to this setup as needed.

## SPECIAL CONCERNS

### Hair-Bearing Areas

To minimize hair loss in such hair-bearing areas as the scalp and eyebrows, it helps to orient the scalpel in the direction of the hair and hair follicle. This will cause less damage to hair follicles and decrease the chance for permanent hair loss.

## Epidermal Inclusion Cysts

Fig. 10-10 shows the elliptical excision of an epidermal inclusion cyst on the forehead of a 29-year-old woman. Further information on the excision of epidermal cysts and lipomas is provided in Chapter 15.

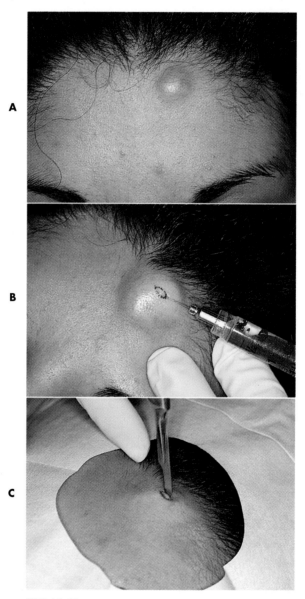

**FIG 10-10**
**A,** Epidermal inclusion cyst on the forehead of a 29-year-old woman. **B,** The ellipse is marked smaller than the cyst but large enough to remove the cyst. Anesthesia is placed around the cyst without puncturing it. Two injections were made, with one above the cyst and another aimed below it, without puncturing the cyst. **C,** The ellipse is incised, keeping the blade perpendicular to the skin.

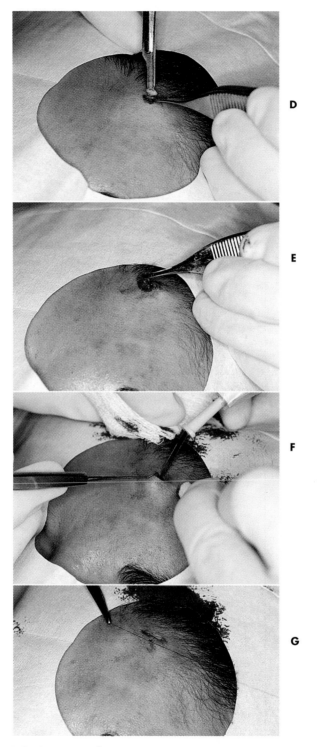

**FIG 10-10, cont'd**

**D,** A forceps is used to remove the excised skin. **E,** Cyst is separated from the subcutaneous tissue. **F,** A skin hook helps provide exposure while electrocoagulation is applied. **G,** Defect is closed with buried and nonabsorbable sutures.

## CONCLUSION

The elliptical excision is used commonly to excise benign and malignant skin lesions, epidermal cysts, and lipomas. It has the advantage of allowing the physician to produce a full-thickness excision that can be closed with minimal tension and good cosmetic results. The best results can be achieved when the physician pays close attention to the fine points of planning, designing, and executing the excision as described in this chapter. For a step-by-step outline of the elliptical excision procedure, see Appendix B.

## REFERENCE

1. Fewkes JL, Cheney ML, Pollack SV: Basic excisional technique. In *Illustrated atlas of cutaneous surgery*, Philadelphia, 1992, Lippincott-Gower.

## SUGGESTED READING

Devereux DF: Diagnosis and management of dysplastic nevus syndrome and early melanoma, *Oncology* 4:73-81, 1990.

Koh HK: Cutaneous melanoma, *N Engl J Med* 325:171-182, 1991.

NIH Consensus Conference: Diagnosis and treatment of early melanoma, *JAMA* 268:1314-1319, 1990.

Robinson J, LeBoit PE: Biopsy techniques. In Robinson J et al: *Atlas of cutaneous surgery*, Philadelphia, 1996, WB Saunders.

# CHAPTER 11

# Cryosurgical Techniques

*Richard P. Usatine    Edward L. Tobinick*

Cryosurgery (cryotherapy) of the skin involves the use of extreme cold to remove both benign and malignant lesions of the skin. The technique involves the application of liquid nitrogen, chemical refrigerants, or cold cryoprobes to the skin. Liquid nitrogen can be applied using cotton-tipped applicators or cryoguns. Cryoprobes with nitrous oxide cryoguns can also deliver the cold directly to the lesions to be frozen. Cryosurgery has wide applicability to a variety of skin lesions and has the advantages of ease of use, low cost, and acceptable cosmetic results. With these techniques, the physician is able to treat multiple lesions rapidly.

Cryotherapy selectively destroys cells, leaving the fibroblast tissue matrix intact. Because fibroblasts do not usually form extensive scar tissue during the healing process, healing occurs with little to no scar formation.

## METHODS AND TEMPERATURES

In this chapter we will focus on the use of liquid nitrogen as our preferred method of performing cryotherapy for skin lesions. It is the coldest cryogen available for cryotherapy (Table 11-1) and has the most data to support its efficacy in the treatment of benign and malignant skin lesions. Nitrous oxide is a reasonable alternative for those physicians who don't keep liquid nitrogen in their offices and who use nitrous oxide for cryotherapy of the cervix. Verruca-Freeze is associated with lower start-up and equipment maintenance costs, but it does not have the long track record of liquid nitrogen for the treatment of cutaneous lesions. Verruca-Freeze is not approved to treat malignancies. Nitrous oxide can be used to treat malignancies. Indications and contraindications to cryosurgery can be found in Tables 11-2 and 11-3. Box 11-1 lists the advantages and disadvantages of cryosurgery.

## EQUIPMENT

Liquid nitrogen
- Storage dewar (tank)
- Cryogun (Fig. 11-1)
- Cotton-tipped swabs
- Cotton balls
- Styrofoam cups

**TABLE 11-1    Methods and Temperatures of Cryosurgery**

| Methods | Temperatures |
|---|---|
| Liquid nitrogen | −196° C |
| Cotton-tipped applicator | |
| Cryogun | |
| Nitrous oxide (cryoguns with cryoprobes) | −90° C |
| Verruca-Freeze (chemical refrigerant) | −70° C to −94° C |

**TABLE 11-2    Indications for Cryosurgery**

| Indications | Estimates of cryotherapy efficacy[*] |
|---|---|
| **Benign Skin Lesion** | |
| Angioma | L |
| Condyloma acuminata | M-H |
| Dermatofibroma | M |
| Freckles (ephelides) | M |
| Granuloma annulare | L |
| Hypertrophic scar | L or M[†] |
| Keloid | M[*] |
| Lentigo | M |
| Molluscum contagiosum | M |
| Mucocele | M[‡] |
| Prurigo nodularis | M |
| Sebaceous hyperplasia | L-M |
| Seborrheic keratosis | M |
| Skin tag (acrochordon) | L |
| Verruca (wart and plantar wart) | M-H |
| Xanthelasma | L |
| **Premalignant Lesion** | |
| Actinic keratosis | H |
| **Malignant Lesion** | |
| Superficial basal cell carcinoma | H |
| Superficial squamous cell carcinoma (when diagnosis is known) | H |

*H*, High efficacy; *M*, moderate efficacy; *L*, low efficacy.
[*]Estimates based on authors' experience.
[†]Better results with use of concomitant intralesional steroid.
[‡]Better results with use of concomitant incision and drainage.

**TABLE 11-3   Contraindications for Cryosurgery**

| Contraindications | Category |
|---|---|
| **By Lesion** | |
| Nevus* | R |
| Recurrent basal cell carcinoma | A |
| Melanoma | A |
| Any undiagnosed lesion suspected of malignancy (you must send tissue for pathology first) | A |
| Morphea | A |
| Sclerosing basal cell carcinoma | A |
| Large vascular lesion (hemangioma) | R |
| | |
| **By Area** | |
| Eyelids and thin skin | R |
| Over superficial cutaneous nerves | R |
| Elbow or digit (because of superficial cutaneous nerves) | R |
| On eyebrow, eyelash, and scalp (may kill hair follicles) | R |
| Neoplasm of ala nasi and nasolabial fold | R |
| Neoplasm of anterior tragus | R |
| Neoplasm of upper lip near vermilion border | R |
| Neoplasm over the shins | R |
| | |
| **By Patient** | |
| Previously adverse reaction to cryotherapy (e.g., cold anaphylaxis) | A |
| Darkly pigmented skin (greater risk of hypopigmentation) | R |
| Cryoglobulinemia | R |
| Myeloma, lymphoma | R |
| Autoimmune disorders (including pyoderma gangrenosum) | R |
| Raynaud's disease, especially when lesion is on fingers, toes, nose, ears, penis | R |
| Chronic systemic corticosteroid therapy | R |
| Concurrent treatment with immunosuppressive drugs | R |
| Extremity with any vascular compromise | R |

*A*, Absolute; *R*, relative.
*We do not recommend freezing nevi. Nevi that recur after freezing can be confusing to manage because they can be difficult to interpret morphologically and histologically.

**BOX 11-1   Advantages and Disadvantages of Cryosurgery**

**Advantages**
*For the physician*
Procedure can be performed with little time
Technique is easy to learn
Multiple lesions can be treated at one time
An assistant is not needed

*For the patient*
No injections of local anesthetic needed
Pain is tolerable (less so for children)
No sutures to remove
Wound care is usually simple

**Disadvantages of Cryosurgery/Complications**
*For the physician*
Equipment cost
Arranging for delivery and storage of liquid nitrogen or nitrous oxide
(Verruca-Freeze has a small canister so delivery and storage are not problems)
There is an art to mastering these techniques

*For the patient*
Postoperative pain
Lesion recurrence
Hypopigmentation may result
Area may be more prone to sunburn
Multiple visits may be necessary
Blisters may be tense and painful
Numbness in area may last for months
Scarring may occur

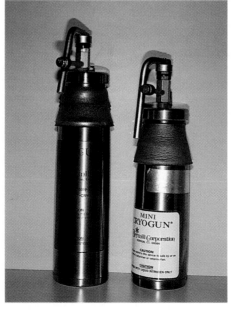

**FIG 11-1**
Cryogun for liquid nitrogen.

**Nitrous oxide**

- Tanks with cart
- Hand gun (Fig. 11-2)

**Verruca-Freeze**

- Canister and speculum (Fig. 11-3)

## Liquid Nitrogen

Use of liquid nitrogen in the office requires a storage dewar (tank). Storage dewars cost hundreds of dollars because they are made from high-strength aluminum and must have superb insulation to minimize the evaporation of the liquid nitrogen. The dewar uses a simple cap or a withdrawal device, including a nozzle, pressure valves, and a gauge. Standard storage dewar tanks for the office come in sizes that

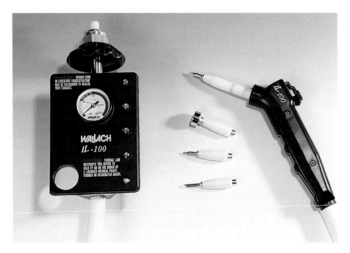

**FIG 11-2**
Hand gun and probes to use with nitrous oxide.

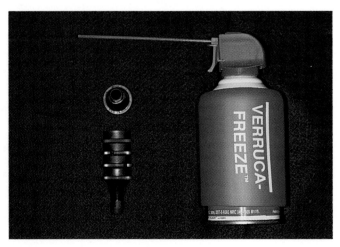

**FIG 11-3**
Verruca-Freeze with canister and speculum.

hold from 10 to 50 liters. Delivery is needed approximately every 1 to 4 weeks to replace the liquid nitrogen as it is used and evaporates. Approximately 20 liters every 4 weeks is probably an adequate amount for a small practice, whereas 35 liters every week may be needed for a large group practice.

Liquid nitrogen can be put in a Styrofoam cup and applied to the patient using cotton-tipped swabs. A cryogun provides a continuous spray to the skin for larger and deeper freezes and can also be controlled for light and superficial freezes. When using cotton-tipped swabs, the swab must be dipped repeatedly into the liquid nitrogen and applied to the skin. Deeper freezes can be achieved with large cotton-tipped swabs (Fig. 11-4) or with extra cotton added to the standard swab. This extra cotton provides a larger reservoir for the liquid nitrogen within the cotton tip and delivers more cryogen to the skin. Care should be taken not to create too large an applicator, which will create a resulting halo larger than desired. The physician should make or choose an applicator tip appropriate for the lesion size.

Liquid nitrogen cryoguns come with special applicator tips that have different size apertures. The "C" tip with the Brymill cryoguns is the best all-purpose aperture. It allows for a controlled spray diameter that will match most needs. The "B" tip may be used for larger-diameter lesions, but continuous spraying with the "C" tip will produce an expanding area of frozen tissue. When the lesion is small, it helps to spray intermittently for better control. With liquid nitrogen in the cryogun, the spray tip should be oriented perpendicular to the skin surface. When the halo gets to the desired size, the spraying should be stopped for a moment to allow the halo to recede, and then spraying should resume until an adequate freeze time is obtained.

Cryoguns come in varying sizes. The mini cryogun should be adequate for most offices and probably needs only to be filled once or twice a day, depending on the frequency of use. Larger practices that do a lot of cryotherapy may prefer the Cryogun II, which is larger and more expensive, but has twice the holding time as the mini cryogun.

## Nitrous Oxide

Use of nitrous oxide requires a gas cylinder, pressure gauge, a regulator, and a cryogun with an assortment of tips. (This is a different cryogun than is used with liquid nitrogen). We don't recommend purchasing this equipment for cryotherapy of the skin alone. For an office that already uses this equipment for cryotherapy

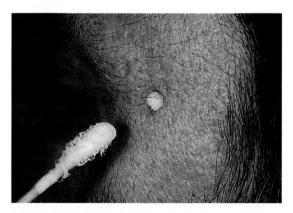

**FIG 11-4**
Application of liquid nitrogen to a seborrheic keratosis with cotton-tipped swab.

of the cervix, it is an alternative method for treating lesions. Even though nitrous oxide does not evaporate as quickly as liquid nitrogen, it is costly to refill the tank. Because the treatment temperature is not as cold as liquid nitrogen, nitrous oxide is not as good a therapy for malignant lesions. For more information about using this technique in your office, we recommend consulting the Cryotherapy chapter in Torre, Lubritz, and Kuflik's *Practical Cutaneous Surgery*.[1]

## Verruca-Freeze

Verruca-Freeze is the least expensive cryotherapy system to acquire. It does not require a storage tank, and the chemical refrigerant can be shipped directly from the manufacturer. It is very portable to off-site clinics, nursing homes, and hospitals. Unfortunately, its use is not indicated for malignant lesions, and it does not have the long track record of liquid nitrogen for use on benign lesions.

Verruca-Freeze equipment consists of a small canister with a nozzle spray tube and a series of cones to control the size of the area being treated. In Fig. 11-5, the cryogen is being sprayed into a cone that is surrounding a wart on the finger. The starter kit comes with a training video to help learn this technique. Although our preference is for liquid nitrogen, the Verruca-Freeze system is an alternative for physicians with limited start-up funds and storage space. In Fig. 11-6, the cryogen is cold enough to produce a blister around the wart that was frozen.

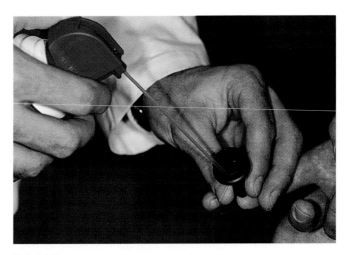

**FIG 11-5**
Verruca-Freeze being used to freeze a wart.

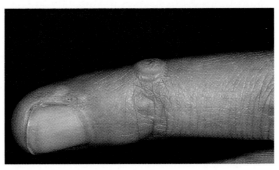

**FIG 11-6**
A blister around a wart after Verruca-Freeze treatment.

## ISSUES TO CONSIDER BEFORE THE PROCEDURE

Patients should be informed before the procedure that cryosurgery does produce discomfort. In general, cryosurgery is done without anesthesia. Although it is reassuring to patients that no injections are necessary, the technique can be rather painful if long freeze times are needed. Patients should be informed that they may have discomfort that will persist for several minutes and sometimes up to 20 minutes after the procedure. Physicians should be aware that in some cases the discomfort is of sufficient magnitude to cause vasovagal reactions. For this reason, patients should be positioned so that they can be put into the prone position or into a feet up, head down position after the procedure. Patients should also be advised of the nature of the healing process. Painful blisters can be popped sterilely with a needle and the fluid expressed. Patients may need analgesics for the pain.

Risks of cryosurgery include hypopigmentation, increased susceptibility to sunburn in the area treated, some numbness in the area that can last as long as months, and occasional scarring. Patients with dark skin have a greater risk of hypopigmentation or hyperpigmentation after cryotherapy. The patient should also be informed that more than a single treatment may be necessary. In particular, patients should be advised that there is a significant recurrence rate after cryosurgery for warts, and if this occurs the procedure may be repeated.

Part of providing informed consent is to describe the benefits of the procedure, which is intended to eradicate the skin lesion. Alternative treatments may be described, such as electrosurgery (See Chapter 12). It is not required to have the patient sign a consent form for this procedure because it is done routinely in many offices and is not a surgical procedure in which tissue is cut. For physicians who choose to have some patients sign a consent form, a sample form is included in Appendix C. Obtaining consent may be advisable before treatment of a malignant lesion with cryotherapy.

## MEASURING THE DEGREE OF FREEZE BY HALO SIZE

Because we cannot see the freezing that goes on below the surface, we have to use other methods to judge the depth of the tissue destruction. Thermocouples can be inserted into the skin to measure the freezing temperature, but few physicians have or use this equipment. The standard methods to judge the degree of a freeze are freezing times, halo size around the lesion, halo thaw time, and total thaw time. The halo is measured in millimeters from the edge of the lesion to the edge of the white freeze. Fig. 11-7 shows a 2-mm freeze around a wart. The larger the halo on the skin, the larger, deeper, and colder the freeze. With liquid nitrogen, freezing time is the amount of time the lesion turns white. The halo thaw time is the number of seconds it takes for the halo to recede to the border of the lesion. The total thaw time is the time it takes for the entire white area to disappear. All of these measurements are tools to estimate the degree of tissue destruction. Table 11-4 summarizes the recommended halo sizes for various lesions. These recommendations may need adjusting based on specific characteristics of the lesion, location, and patient.

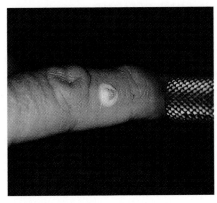

**FIG 11-7**
Halo. A 2-mm freeze around a wart.

**TABLE 11-4    Halo Size for Cryotherapy**

| Indications | Healthy tissue halo (mm) |
|---|---|
| **Benign Skin Lesions** | |
| Angiomas | 1-2 |
| Condylomata acuminata | 1-2 |
| Dermatofibromas | 0-1 |
| Freckles (ephelides) | 0-1 |
| Granuloma annulare | 0-1 |
| Hypertrophic scars | 0 |
| Keloids | 0 |
| Lentigines | 0-1 |
| Molluscum contagiosum | 1 |
| Mucoceles | 2 |
| Prurigo nodularis | 0-1 |
| Sebaceous hyperplasia | 0-1 |
| Seborrheic keratoses | 1 |
| Skin tags (acrochordons) | 1 |
| Verrucae vulgaris (warts) | 1-2 |
| Verrucae plana (plantar warts) | 1 |
| Xanthelasma | 0-1 |
| | |
| **Premalignant Lesions** | |
| Actinic keratoses | 1-2 |
| | |
| **Malignant Lesion** | |
| Superficial basal cell carcinomas | 5 |
| Superficial squamous cell carcinomas (when diagnosis is known) | 5 |

## TREATMENT OF BENIGN SKIN LESIONS

The primary concern in treating benign skin lesions is avoiding complications from the treatment. Cryosurgery can be a potent modality, and its power must be respected. In general, when treating benign tumors of the skin, the goal should be to achieve a total freeze of the entire mass of the lesion with a small halo of frozen tissue around the base of the lesion. In general, the halo should be about 1 to 2 mm surrounding the base of the lesion. We will discuss the treatment of specific lesions using liquid nitrogen with direct application of cotton-tipped swabs or with spray. This method will usually produce complete removal of the lesion with an excellent cosmetic result.

### Angiomas

Cryosurgery has limited use with angiomas. Treating angiomas by freezing the complete mass of the lesion with a 1-mm halo of frozen tissue will remove some small angiomas, including cherry angiomas (Fig. 11-8). However, shave excision and electrosurgery are more effective treatment modalities (See Chapter 12).

### Condyloma Acuminata

Cryosurgery is one of the treatment modalities of choice for treating sexually transmitted warts (Fig. 11-9). In general we attempt to treat a slightly larger area around the condyloma than with other benign lesions because it has been shown that human papilloma virus is present in normal-appearing tissue surrounding each of the visible lesions. Therefore we try to treat with about a 2-mm halo of frozen tissue around the visible extent of the lesion. Care must be taken when treating multiple lesions in sensitive areas. For patients with multiple lesions that make up a considerable extent of the surface area of the penis or the vulva, other methods of treatment are recommended, including electrosurgical techniques described in the Chapter 12. Cryosurgery is ideal for isolated lesions on the penile shaft or on the vulva.

### Dermatofibromas

Dermatofibromas are benign scarlike nodules that often have a hyperpigmented halo and are most commonly found on the legs of adults (Fig. 11-10). Because they have a tendency to recur, dermatofibromas may be difficult to "cure" with any modality. Punch excision may be used to remove small lesions. Larger lesions are more difficult to excise. Cryotherapy is a good method of treatment for those patients who insist on being treated. Before treatment, patients should be advised that these lesions are of cosmetic concern only and do not have malignant potential. A biopsy should be performed for pathologic confirmation on lesions of uncertain diagnosis. For those typical lesions for which surgical excision is not chosen, cryotherapy can produce reasonably good results. The technique involves freezing the entire lesion with either no halo or a very small halo of normal skin. Patients should be advised that lesions may recur and hyperpigmentation may persist despite treatment.

Another option is to do a shave excision of the central dermatofibroma and to follow that with cryotherapy of the remaining tissue.

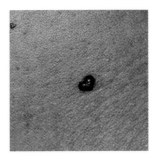

**FIG 11-8**
Cherry angioma.

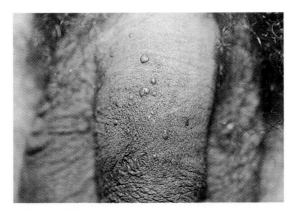

**FIG 11-9**
Condyloma acuminata on the shaft of the penis.

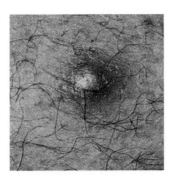

**FIG 11-10**
Dermatofibroma.

## Freckles

Freckles require very light treatment, particularly with use of one of the colder modalities such as liquid nitrogen. Freckles should be frozen without a margin of normal skin being treated, with only a 2- to 5-second freeze with liquid nitrogen. In general, we prefer not to treat multiple freckles on a patient because of the risk of hypopigmentation. The treatment technique of choice for freckles usually is application of a cryogen with a cotton-tipped swab, but the cryogun with a small aperture can also be used.

## Hypertrophic Scars and Keloids

Cryotherapy is an excellent adjunctive therapy for the treatment of hypertrophic scars and keloids when used before intralesional injection of steroid (Fig. 11-11). We freeze a keloid or hypertrophic scar to a moderate extent before steroid injection. We do not freeze a margin of normal tissue but attempt to confine the ice-ball to the very center of the lesion with a 3- to 5-second freeze. This minimizes pain and also will prevent the destruction of normal tissue around the lesion. After liquid nitrogen or another freezing modality is applied to the scars, they are

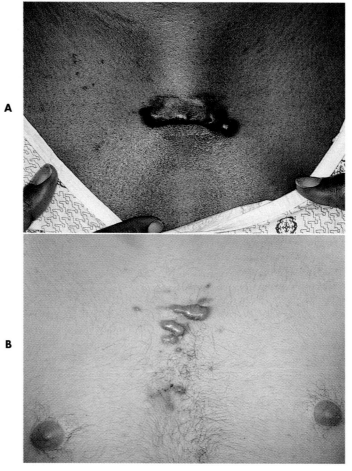

**FIG 11-11**
Keloids over the sternum in an African-American woman (**A**) and in a Caucasian man (**B**).

allowed to thaw and develop edema. This generally takes 1 to 2 minutes, allowing the easier introduction of intralesional corticosteroids into the center of the lesions. Multiple treatment sessions usually are required, but we attempt to space the time between treatments to at least 2 to 3 weeks. Spacing treatments too closely increases risk of atrophy from the intralesional corticosteroids.

## Lentigines

Lentigines (plural for *lentigo*) respond relatively well to cryotherapy. As with freckles, these lesions require very light treatment to avoid postinflammatory hypopigmentation. Generally a 2- to 5-second freeze with liquid nitrogen is all that is necessary. An attempt should be made to freeze lentigines to their borders but not beyond. Multiple treatment sessions for large lesions may be necessary. Accurate diagnosis before treatment is necessary. Any lentigines with variegation of pigmentation or other suspicious characteristics, such as extremely large size (See Fig. 9-2), require biopsy before treatment. These atypical lesions may be lentigo maligna (melanoma in situ), and histopathologic diagnosis is necessary.

## Molluscum Contagiosum

Cryotherapy is an acceptable treatment for molluscum contagiosum (Fig. 11-12). For lesions that cannot be curetted, we proceed with cryotherapy, attempting to freeze to the borders of the lesion but not beyond. Multiple sessions are frequently required to treat not only the existing lesions but new ones that may appear in the interval. For children, the use of EMLA cream before treatment can make cryotherapy much more acceptable. For the physician experienced with the use of curettage, this is the preferred method of treatment. Curettage after use of EMLA cream is less painful than cryotherapy, has an excellent cosmetic result, and can be performed rapidly.

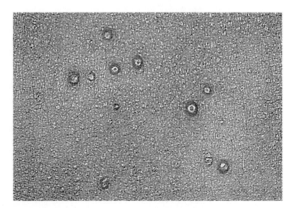

**FIG 11-12**
Molluscum contagiosum.

## Mucoceles

Mucoceles can be treated after a small amount of lidocaine with epinephrine is injected into the mucocele from inside the mouth (See Fig. 15-15). After a wait of 5 minutes for vasoconstriction, a small stab incision with a No. 11 scalpel is made into the mucocele from inside the mouth. The mucinous material is then evacuated by pressure through the incision. The mucocele is then invaginated by pressure with a cotton-tipped swab to allow application of liquid nitrogen to the base of the mucocele with a second cotton-tipped swab. The liquid nitrogen is applied heavily until there is a complete freeze of the base of the mucocele and a 2-mm halo around the perimeter of the mucocele. With this technique, healing usually occurs within 4 days, and there is a low recurrence rate. Occasionally retreatment is needed. This technique has a greater success rate than cryotherapy without incision because evacuation of the mucocele contents allows access of liquid nitrogen to the deepest portion of the of the cyst wall.

## Prurigo Nodularis

Cryotherapy can be a good tool for treating prurigo nodularis, either alone or as an adjunctive therapy with topical or intralesional corticosteroids. Prurigo nodularis is notoriously difficult to treat, and some of these lesions can be very elevated and hypertrophic (Fig. 11-13). Cryotherapy is used to freeze the core of the lesion with a light or moderate freeze. Care should be taken so that the extent of the freeze does not advance beyond the periphery of the lesion. Patients should be advised that more than one treatment may be necessary. Recurrence is very common in this condition, regardless of the treatment.

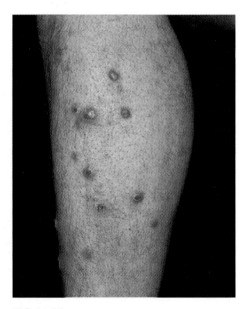

**FIG 11-13**
Prurigo nodularis. (From Habif TP: *Clinical dermatology: a color guide to diagnosis and therapy,* ed 3, St. Louis, 1996, Mosby.)

## Sebaceous Hyperplasia

Care must be taken when using cryotherapy to treat sebaceous hyperplasia to avoid overtreatment. Even with a light freeze, patients can occasionally develop hypopigmentation or depression at the site of the cryotherapy. For physicians who are experienced with cryotherapy, this modality can produce good cosmetic results. The lesions are frozen lightly to their periphery and no further. Cotton-tipped swabs may be used to apply liquid nitrogen to keep the freeze superficial. The lesions need to be frozen for only 3 to 5 seconds.

## Seborrheic Keratosis

One technique for treating seborrheic keratoses involves the use of local anesthetic followed by light electrodesiccation to the tops of the lesions to soften them and then curettage to remove the lesions in their entirety. This technique can be more time consuming than cryotherapy. Cryotherapy also has the theoretical advantage of potentially causing less hypertrophic scarring in individuals who are prone to this. Seborrheic keratoses are also treated nicely by shave excision, which carries with it the advantage of producing material for histopathology. Lesions that are morphologically questionable will need to be shaved and sent for histopathology.

For those seborrheic keratoses that are typical and characteristic in clinical appearance, cryotherapy is an acceptable treatment (Fig. 11-14). Care must be taken when treating these lesions with cryotherapy to avoid overtreatment because this will cause large blisters and considerable discomfort. The proper technique of treatment with cryotherapy involves a freeze of the entire lesion, with only a small margin of normal skin (approximately 1 mm or less) frozen around the periphery of the lesion. Blistering ensues within the first few hours generally, and healing usually requires 7 to 10 days. After healing, there can be some residual erythema for up to several weeks. The advantage of cryotherapy is that multiple lesions can be treated quite rapidly in one session without the use of local anesthesia. Patients must be warned that the procedure does cause discomfort.

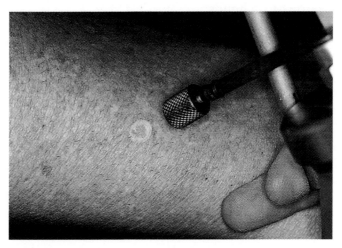

**FIG 11-14**
Seborrheic keratosis with a 1-mm halo after cryotherapy.

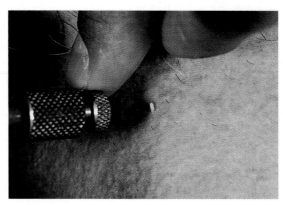

**FIG 11-15**
Cryotherapy of a small skin tag on the neck.

## Skin Tags (Acrochordons)

For most physicians, the preferred treatment method of choice for skin tags will be light electrodesiccation or snip excision. Cryotherapy is an alternative method of treatment for smaller skin tags that are hard to excise with scissors. When cryotherapy is used, the entire lesion should be frozen, with care to avoid freezing normal skin at the base of the lesion (Fig. 11-15).

## Verrucae (Warts)

Genital warts (condyloma acuminata) were discussed earlier. The following discussion of cryosurgery for warts will be divided into sections by anatomic location and morphology (hands, fingers, plantar warts, and flat warts).

### Verrucae on hands

Verrucae on hands are excellent candidates for cryosurgery. For raised verrucae, the verruca is frozen continuously to produce an iceball that encompasses the

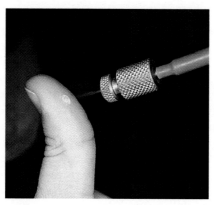

**FIG 11-16**
Cryotherapy of a single wart on a finger.

entire body of the verrucae and extends to 1 to 2 mm of normal tissue in diameter around the base of the lesion. This requires a continuous or near continuous freeze, starting with the top or the most distal portion of the lesion if the lesion is elevated. The freeze should be continued until the body of the verruca becomes an iceball. There is no need to thaw and refreeze verrucae if they are treated with this method.

### *Verrucae on fingers*

Care must be taken that the freeze does not impinge on the digital nerves that are on the lateral aspects of each finger (Fig. 11-16). In addition, care must be taken when freezing the nails or near the nail bed. Frozen areas that extend underneath nails can cause a severe amount of pain because the blister that occurs is physically limited and pressed on by the hard nail structure. In addition, freezing around fingernails can cause permanent nail destruction if the matrix is damaged. Before performing cryosurgery for periungual warts near the base of the nail, patients should be informed that they may lose the fingernail on a temporary or permanent basis.

### Plantar warts

Plantar warts present a difficult therapeutic problem. They can be resistant to multiple modalities of treatment, and they frequently recur regardless of which modality is chosen. Cryotherapy is an acceptable treatment modality for plantar verrucae but carries with it the disadvantage of considerable discomfort during and after the procedure. Patients with plantar warts that have been frozen may have difficulty walking for several days to weeks after the procedure.

The method of treatment is similar to that used for other verrucae. The lesion is frozen until there is a 1- to 2-mm halo around the perimeter of the verruca. An alternative method, which in many cases is preferable, is to use cryotherapy as an adjunct treatment for plantar verrucae. Using this method, the lesions are lightly frozen. This produces a surface slough of wart and thereby reduces the volume of the wart, enhancing the effect of topical keratolytics that are then applied by the patient at home. Several visits are required when using this technique, and on each visit the physician will use either a No. 15 or a No. 10 scalpel blade to pare the dead tissue overlaying the wart.

In Fig. 11-17, A, a single plantar wart is seen. The patient asked for treatment because he was having pain while walking. The physician chose to pare the wart first with a No. 15 scalpel (Fig. 11-17, B) and then performed cryotherapy to the base (Fig. 11-18, C). After the procedure, the patient had increased pain while walking for only 2 days. A good part of the wart sloughed off. The following week the patient was directed to use topical salicylic acid nightly until the entire wart was gone.

Patients with multiple plantar or periungual warts frequently are not good candidates for cryotherapy. These patients may require referral to a dermatologist for alternative methods of therapy, including intralesional bleomycin, topical dinitrochlorobenzene (DNCB), or pulsed dye laser. Referral for these treatments is appropriate for warts that are not responding to cryotherapy, chemical agents, or electrosurgery. Large mosaic plantar verrucae over weight-bearing areas on the feet and resistant periungual warts on the fingers will need to be treated with intralesional bleomycin or DNCB.

### Flat warts

Flat warts are usually seen in clusters on the face (Fig. 11-18), arms, or legs. These warts may actually be curable with the daily application of topical tretinoin (Retin-A) alone. If the tretinoin does not work, cryotherapy may be tried. Because flat warts are very thin and superficial, the freeze should be light with only a 1-mm halo.

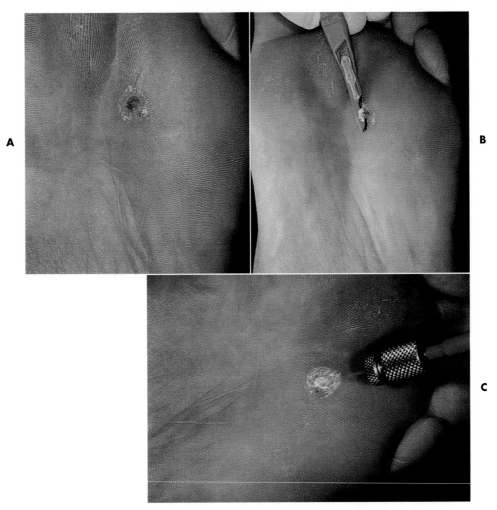

**FIG 11-17**
A, Plantar wart on the sole of the foot. B, Shaving off the most external portion of the wart with a No. 15 scalpel. C, Cryotherapy of the base of the wart.

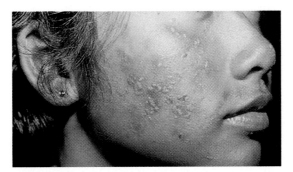

**FIG 11-18**
Flat warts of the face.

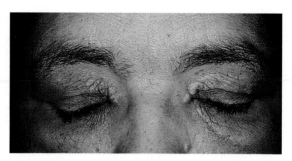

**FIG 11-19**
Xanthelasma.

### Xanthelasma

Cryotherapy of xanthelasma on the eyelids is an acceptable technique for the cosmetic removal of these benign lesions. Care should be taken when using liquid nitrogen around the eye so that cryogenic substances are not delivered to the conjunctiva and cornea. For this reason, we prefer not to use cryospray in this area. Even when using cotton-tipped swabs and liquid nitrogen, the physician must take care not to drip liquid nitrogen into the eye. Because xanthelasma are superficial lesions, cryotherapy should be light and carefully applied.

The patient in Fig. 11-19 had elevated serum lipids and extensive xanthelasma. In this case, the patient elected to not have treatment.

## TREATMENT OF PREMALIGNANT LESIONS

### Actinic Keratosis

Cryotherapy is the physical modality of choice for the great majority of actinic keratoses. It is rapid, produces an excellent cosmetic result, and has high patient acceptance. Single or multiple lesions can be treated at any given office visit. These precancerous lesions occur in areas of sun damage in individuals predisposed to this either by occupation or by skin type (Fig. 11-20). Lesions have a characteristic gritty, sandpaper-like feel. Cryotherapy is particularly suitable for patients who have either a solitary lesion (Fig. 11-21) or a few scattered lesions. For multiple lesions in one area, topical fluorouracil (5-FU) or masoprocol is usually preferred. Actinic keratoses may be frozen lightly with any of the cryosurgical modalities discussed. When using liquid nitrogen with a cotton-tipped swab, the freeze time is usually 3 to 5 seconds. Biopsies should be performed on actinic keratoses that are unusual, indurated, or hypertrophic to make sure they have not progressed to squamous cell carcinoma. If the lesion appears to extend below the surface of the skin, a biopsy is in order. The feel and the appearance of the lesion in Fig. 11-22 were suspicious. A biopsy demonstrated a Bowenoid actinic keratosis, which is not malignant, and the lesion was treated successfully with liquid nitrogen.

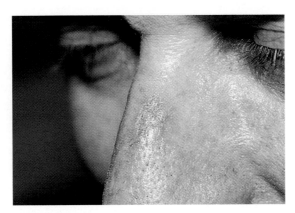

**FIG 11-20**
Actinic keratosis on the nose.

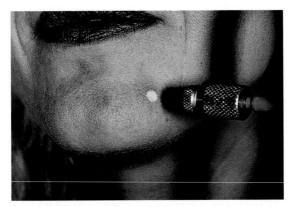

**FIG 11-21**
Cryotherapy of an actinic keratosis on the chin.

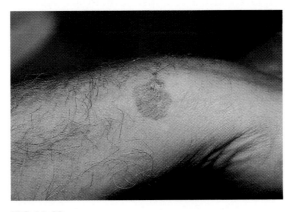

**FIG 11-22**
Bowenoid actinic keratosis. Differential diagnosis includes
actinic keratosis, SCC, or superficial BCC.

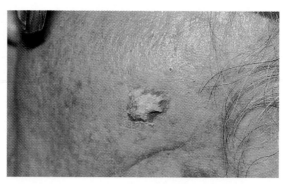

**FIG 11-23**
Cutaneous horns (may be benign, premalignant, or malignant).

### Cutaneous Horns

Cutaneous horns (Fig. 11-23) may be benign, premalignant, or malignant. Because cutaneous horns can originate from a variety of both benign and malignant neoplasms, including basal cell carcinoma, squamous cell carcinoma, seborrheic keratosis, or keratoacanthoma, it is advisable to do a biopsy before treatment. After the clinical diagnosis is known, cryotherapy can be an effective treatment. In general, cutaneous horns will require a somewhat longer freeze because they are hyperkeratotic lesions. Total freeze times of 10 to 20 seconds with liquid nitrogen may be needed. This may require multiple applications of liquid nitrogen during the same session to completely freeze the cutaneous horn. Removing the horn first by gentle shearing can decrease the freeze time needed.

## TREATMENT OF MALIGNANT LESIONS: (BCC OR SCC)

Cryosurgery is an excellent modality for superficial BCC (Fig. 11-24) and SCC and should be done only by a physician with considerable experience using cryotherapy to treat benign and malignant lesions. Some authorities recommend using a thermocouple to measure the tissue temperature when treating malignancies.

It is essential to have a definitive pathologic diagnosis before proceeding with cryotherapy. If the BCC or SCC is recurrent, or the BCC is a sclerosing (morpheaform) BCC (Fig. 11-25), cryotherapy is not an adequate curative treatment. For example, a large morpheaform BCC on the face, such as in Fig. 11-25, is especially not appropriate for cryotherapy. Specific relative contraindications by area are neoplasms of the ala nasi and nasolabial fold, anterior tragus, upper lip near the vermilion border, and over the shins. Melanoma should not be treated with cryotherapy.

Before freezing a BCC or SCC, it helps to draw a circle around the lesion, leaving a 5-mm margin. Liquid nitrogen should be applied continuously with a cryogun to the center of the lesion until the ice ball reaches the 5-mm halo drawn

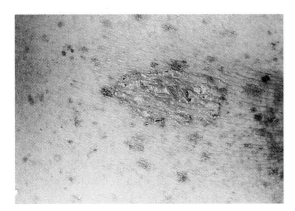

**FIG 11-24**
Superficial BCC.

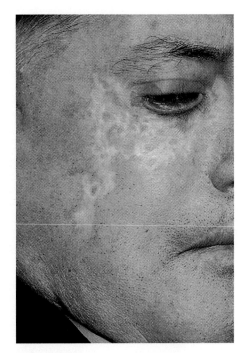

**FIG 11-25**
Morpheaform BCC. Cryotherapy is not an adequate curative treatment.

around the tumor.[1] This should produce a freeze time of 60 to 90 seconds.[1] In this way, the center of the BCC or SCC has a greater dose of cold applied to it than the periphery of normal tissue. The halo thaw time should be over 60 seconds. Some authorities recommend a second freeze of the same amount, but in our experience one freeze with a 60-second thaw time is usually adequate to achieve a cure for these superficial tumors.

## COMPLICATIONS

The two most common unpleasant side effects of cryotherapy for patients are pain and blistering. In Fig. 11-26, the patient experienced much pain during the freezing and thawing period. This was due in part to the location of the wart in the periungual and subungual areas. The area of frozen tissue shows extension below the nail. Fig. 11-26, *D*, shows the erythema and swelling present after the thawing process, during which the patient was in much pain. It may be prudent to use a long-lasting local anesthetic such as Marcaine before using cryotherapy in this location. Other modalities, such as DNCB, bleomycin, or laser may also be considered. However, this is one lesion in which the pain of the procedure may be less than the pain of the local anesthetic. Also, the risk of damage to the nail should be discussed with the patient. For a list of other complications, see Box 11-2.

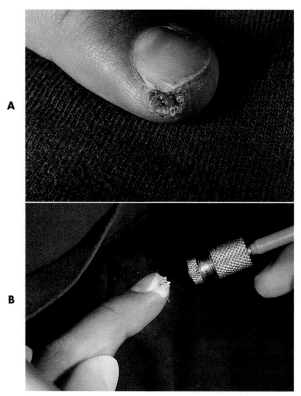

FIG 11-26
**A,** Periungual and subungual wart. **B,** Cryotherapy.

---

**BOX 11-2   Complications From Cryosurgery**

**Immediate and Routinely Expected (not true complications)**
Pain during the freezing and thawing period
Blister formation
Intradermal hemorrhage
Edema

**Immediate and Less Common**
Headache affecting forehead, temples, and scalp
Syncope

**Delayed and Rare**
Postoperative infection
Hemorrhage from the wound site
Pyogenic granuloma

**Prolonged and Rare**
Hyperpigmentation
Milia
Hypertrophic scars
Neuropathy

**Permanent**
Hypopigmentation (common)
Ectropion and notching of eyelids
Notching and atrophy of tumors overlying cartilage
Tenting or notching of the vermilion border of the upper lip
Atrophy
Alopecia

---

Modified from Zacarian S: *Cryosurgery for skin cancer and cutaneous disorders,* St. Louis, 1985, Mosby.

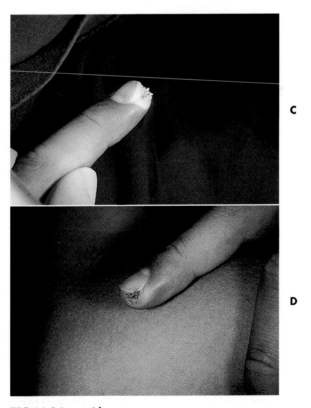

**FIG 11-26, cont'd**
C, Area of frozen tissue showing extension below the nail.
D, Erythema and swelling after the thawing process, during which the patient was in much pain.

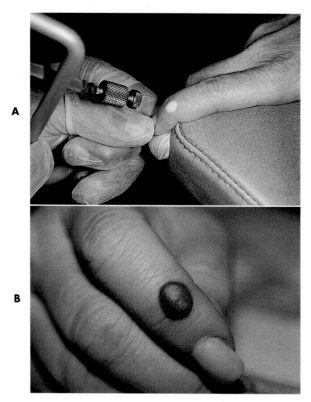

**FIG 11-27**
**A,** Cryotherapy of two small warts adjacent to each other on the finger. **B,** Blister formation accompanied by significant pain.

**FIG 11-28**
Hypopigmentation after cryotherapy.

In Fig. 11-27, cryotherapy was used to treat two small warts adjacent to each other on the finger. A few hours later the patient developed a blister accompanied by significant pain. Ultimately, the patient drained the blister with a sterile needle, relieving the pain of the tense blister. The pain decreased over time and completely resolved after 3 months. The warts disappeared and never recurred. In Fig. 11-28, there is residual hypopigmentation after cryotherapy.

**TABLE 11-5    Efficacy of Cryosurgery**

| Lesion | Cure rate |
|---|---|
| Viral warts (hands) | 75%[2] |
| Dermatofibroma | 90%[3] |
| Actinic keratosis | 99%[4] |
| Bowen's disease | 99%[5] |
| Basal cell carcinoma | 95% or greater*[5-10] |
| Squamous cell carcinoma | 95% or greater*[5,7,9,10] |

Modified from Dawber R: Cryosurgery. In Lask G, Moy R, editors: *Principles and techniques of cutaneous surgery*, New York, 1996, McGraw-Hill.
*Cure rates may be closer to 90% when inexperienced physicians perform the cryotherapy.

## EVIDENCE FOR THE EFFICACY OF CRYOSURGERY

Table 11-5 shows some representative numbers from the literature regarding the efficacy of cryosurgery. A critical review of the study methodology is beyond the scope of this book.

## WOUND CARE

After cryosurgery, the patient may continue all normal activities, including bathing and swimming. The only limitations that may occur may be secondary to pain. For example, after cryotherapy of a plantar wart on the bottom of the foot, the area may be too painful for running.

It is helpful to tell the patient how to treat blisters. Not all patients know that the roof of the blister is protective and should be left alone if possible. If the blister is tense or blocking normal activities, it can be drained with a sterile needle. If the roof of the blister is rubbed off, it is best to cover the open area with Bacitracin or Polysporin or petrolatum alone and a sterile dressing. See Chapter 18 on Wound Care for further information.

## CONCLUSION

Proper use of cryotherapy can lead to excellent cosmetic results and good cure rates with excellent patient acceptance.

## RESOURCES

Liquid nitrogen equipment: Delasco Dermatology Buying Guide (800-831-6273)
Cryogun for nitrous oxide cryotherapy: Wallach (800-243-2463)
Verruca-Freeze: Cryosurgery, Inc. (800-729-1624)

## REFERENCES

1. Torre D, Lubritz R, Kuflik E: *Practical cutaneous cryosurgery,* Norwalk, Conn, 1988, Appleton and Lange.
2. Bunney MH et al: An assessment of various methods of treating virus warts, *Br J Dermatol* 94:667, 1976.
3. Lanigan SW, Robinson TWE: Cryotherapy for dermatofibromas, *Clin Exp Dermatol* 12:121, 1987.
4. Lubritz RR, Smolewski SA: Cryosurgery cure rate of actinic keratoses, *J Am Acad Dermatol* 7:631, 1982.
5. Holt PJA: Cryotherapy for skin cancer: results over a 5-year period using liquid nitrogen spray cryosurgery, *Br J Dermatol* 119:231-240, 1988.
6. Biro L, Price E: Cryogenic anaesthesia and haemestasis, *J Dermatol Surg Oncol* 61:608, 1980.
7. Graham GF: Cryosurgery for acne. In Other AN, editor: *Cryosurgery for skin cancer and cutaneous disorders,* St. Louis, 1985, Mosby.
8. Graham GF: Statistical data on malignant tumours in cryosurgery, *J Dermatol Surg Oncol* 9:238, 1982.
9. Kuflik EG: Cryosurgery for tumors of the ear, *J Dermatol Surg Oncol* 11:1165, 1985.
10. McIntosh GS et al: Basal cell carcinoma: a review of treatment results with special reference to cryotherapy, *Postgrad Med J* 59:698, 1983.

## SUGGESTED READING

Fewkes JL, Cheney ML, Pollack SV: *Illustrated atlas of cutaneous surgery,* Philadelphia, 1992, Lippincott-Gower.
Hocutt JE: Cryosurgery. In Pfenninger JL, Fowler GC, editors: *Procedures for primary care physicians,* St. Louis, 1994, Mosby. (Especially good for nitrous oxide cryogun technique.)
Graham GF: Advances in cryosurgery during the past decade, *Cutis* 52:365-372, 1993.
Kuflik EG: Cryosurgery updated, *J Am Acad Dermatol* 31(6) 925-944, 1994.
Kuflik EG: Cryosurgical treatment of cutaneous lesions. In Roenigk RK, Roenigk HH, editors: *Dermatologic surgery: principles and practice,* ed 2, New York, 1996, Marcel Dekker.

# CHAPTER 12

# Electrosurgery

*Richard P. Usatine*

Electrosurgery is used in skin surgery to destroy benign and malignant lesions, control bleeding, and cut or excise tissue. There are many types of electrosurgical units available for use in the office setting. Modern electrosurgery units transfer current to the patient through cold electrodes. The term *electrocautery* implies that a hot electrode is being used; electrocautery is just one *type* of electrosurgery. Electrocautery is useful for some patients with pacemakers, for whom the use of modern electrosurgical current may be contraindicated.

The major techniques used in electrosurgery are electrodesiccation, fulguration, electrocoagulation, and electrosection. In fulguration, the electrode is held away from the skin so that there is a sparking to the surface (such as happens with lightning). In fact, the term *fulguration* comes from the Latin term *fulgur,* which means lightning. Fulguration produces a more shallow level of tissue destruction (Fig. 12-1, *A*). With electrodesiccation, the active electrode touches or is inserted into skin to produce tissue destruction (Fig. 12-1, *B*). Epilation is a type of desiccation in which a fine-wire electrode is inserted into a hair follicle. Electrocoagulation is used to stop bleeding in deep and superficial surgery. In electrosection, the electrode is used to cut tissue.

## ADVANTAGES OF ELECTROSURGERY

Advantages of electrosurgery include the following:

- Simple to use
- Easy to master
- Useful for a wide variety of skin lesions, especially for:
    Superficial lesions
    Tiny lesions (may not need anesthesia)
    Vascular lesions
    Basal cell carcinomas
- Rapid technique
- Controls bleeding while cutting or destroying tissue
- Equipment compact and affordable
- When used for tissue destruction, sterile conditions or sutures are not needed
- Infection rarely develops in wounds left open

## DISADVANTAGES OF ELECTROSURGERY

Disadvantages of electrosurgery include the following:

- Safety risk (electric shocks, burns, or fires)
- Hypertrophic scars, especially with poor technique

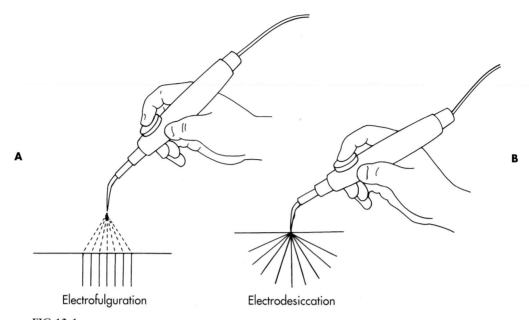

Electrofulguration          Electrodesiccation

**FIG 12-1**
**A,** Electrofulguration. The needle is held above the skin surface. **B,** Electrodesiccation. The needle touches the skin surface. (From Boughton RS, Spencer SK: *J Am Acad Dermatol* 862-867, 1987.)

- Risk of "channeling" of current down vessels and nerves
- Smoke may carry viral particles
- Delayed hemorrhage
- Unsightly wound
- Slow healing, especially if large area treated (healing can be slower than scalpel shave excision)
- Obliteration of histology because of tissue destruction
- Electrosurgical artifact at margins if used for biopsy

## ELECTROSURGERY VERSUS CRYOSURGERY

Cryosurgery is often the treatment of choice for actinic keratoses and simple warts. It is faster and easier to perform than electrosurgery for these indications because it does not require anesthesia. Cryosurgery also tends to cause less scarring than electrosurgery for both of these lesions. However, cryosurgery may be more likely to cause hypopigmentation because the cold kills the melanocytes. This is especially important in a more darkly pigmented person. Electrosurgery is more effective than cryosurgery for condyloma, especially if the condyloma are pedunculated and a cutting current can be used.

There may be a risk of developing human papilloma virus (HPV) in the respiratory tract from inhaling the plume (smoke) from an HPV lesion as it is being treated.[1-8] Intact HPV DNA has been isolated from the plume of verrucae that were treated with electrosurgery and lasers.[1-2] Therefore it is prudent for all physicians to use a smoke evacuator while performing laser and electrosurgical treatment of verrucae and other viral lesions. (See Safety Measures With Electrosurgery, p. 176.) There is even a theoretical risk of inhaling HIV particles during electrosurgery. Unfortunately, there is insufficient evidence to measure the magnitude of these risks. However, these personal risks may be one factor used to determine the physician's choice of therapy for viral lesions.

One disadvantage of cryotherapy over electrosurgery is that with cryosurgery the final result cannot be seen immediately, and there is more guesswork involved in performing the treatment. However, the degree of damage can be estimated accurately with more experience. Cryosurgery also causes more postoperative swelling, which may be uncomfortable for the patient but is only a transient phenomenon.

## ELECTROSURGERY VERSUS SCALPEL

The traditional instrument for performing excisions and shave biopsies is the scalpel. It is inexpensive, the blades are disposable, and the cuts are clean. The scalpel causes no heat-induced tissue damage that could obscure the pathology specimen. Using electrosurgery in place of the scalpel has the advantage of facilitating hemostasis while cutting. However, the lateral heat produced by the electrosurgical instrument can cause tissue damage that might cause slow healing and artifact on the edges of the biopsy specimen.

The Hyfrecator has a cutting tip, but if it is used to do a shave biopsy or cut an ellipse, the damage to the specimen is too great. Therefore if the electrosurgical unit is a Hyfrecator, we suggest doing surgical cutting with a scalpel and using the Hyfrecator for hemostasis when tissue destruction is desired (e.g., on a pyogenic granuloma). If it is important to minimize tissue destruction (e.g., after shaving a seborrheic keratosis), we suggest using a chemical hemostatic agent. Using the spark to fulgurate is less damaging than allowing the electrode to contact the tissue; therefore fulguration is the preferred mode of electrosurgery when minimal damage is desired.

Physicians who own a radiosurgery unit often use this higher-frequency instrument to perform shave or elliptical excisions on benign-appearing lesions. However, even if the unit is set on the pure cutting current at the right power setting, the cut will not match the scalpel for producing an acceptable pathologic specimen. Therefore if there is a suspicion of malignancy, we recommend doing the biopsy with the scalpel (cold steel).

For excising benign lesions, the small amount of lateral heat may not interfere with wound healing when used carefully on a low-power setting. A shave excision with electrosurgery is best performed with a loop electrode. The waveform dial can be set for either a cutting/coagulation blend or cutting only.

The Surgitron unit has a special vari-tip electrode with a small wire that is adjustable in length. This electrode is meant to be used for cutting through the entire skin thickness for elliptical and other full-thickness excisions. On the pure cutting setting, the vari-tip electrode can cut with less lateral heat and can allow the physician to do quick and bloodless excision of benign lesions. A combined cold steel and electrosurgical procedure is often optimal. Making the superficial incision (epidermis and dermis) with a scalpel and performing the deeper dissection and excision with cutting or blended cutting and coagulation settings may optimize efficiency.

In summary, no instrument can beat the scalpel for cost and minimization of tissue damage. The electrosurgery and radiosurgery units are much more expensive, especially for the initial purchase. A radiosurgery unit can be used to perform several kinds of surgery that have been traditionally performed with a scalpel. This may be beneficial if the lesion is benign and very vascular and a blend of cutting and coagulation is required. However, it cannot match the scalpel for quality of pathologic specimen, wound healing, and cosmetic results.

## ELECTROSURGERY VERSUS LASER

Electrosurgery is less expensive than laser surgery. Unfortunately, to emulate the utility of any electrosurgical device, no single laser will suffice. The standard electrosurgical units are a fraction of the cost of a laser. It is unlikely that a physician other than a specialist in skin surgery would own or rent a laser. Therefore most other physicians would be facing the choice of referring a patient for laser surgery versus doing electrosurgery in their own office. The high cost of the laser is the determining factor in the cost of the treatment. As with electrosurgery, the $CO_2$ laser may be used to cut, coagulate, and destroy tissue. It is most often used for resurfacing procedures, such as removing wrinkles. The pulsed dye laser or a similar yellow-light laser is unequivocally better than electrosurgery for treating large hemangiomas and maximizing the cosmetic result. These lasers are used very effectively to treat port-wine hemangiomas. Visible-light lasers get better cosmetic results when treating other vascular lesions, such as angiomas and telangiectasias. There is much less chance of scarring.

In some cases, it may be appropriate to allow the patient to choose between being treated with electrosurgery in the office or going to a specialist for cosmetic laser treatment. It is helpful to inform the patient of the risks and benefits of electrosurgery and laser treatment. Ultimately, the patient needs to make the final decision (especially if the goal of therapy is purely cosmetic). If a patient is seeking treatment for cosmetic reasons, it may be best to refer him or her for what they perceive is the very best therapy.

Keep in mind that any physician can buy any instrument, but electrosurgical instruments are considered standard office fixtures, and their basic use is generally learned in many residencies. Because of their cost, however, lasers are generally encountered only in subspecialty training programs, and more time may be needed to learn laser technique. The use of a laser may invoke different patient expectations.

## EQUIPMENT

### Electrosurgical Units (Fig. 12-2)

- Spark gap
  Bantam Bovie*
  Cameron-Miller Units 26-230 and 26-0345
- Solid state
  Hyfrecator (by ConMed, previously by Birtcher)
  Delasco 734 (newer version of the discontinued Hyfrecator 733)
- Surgitron radiofrequency unit (by Ellman Educational Unit)
  Bovie specialist (by Clinical Technology)
  Cameron-Miller 80-1983
- Surgistat (by Valley Lab)

Because the Hyfrecator and Surgitron are commonly used in the office setting, we will provide information somewhat specific to these two instruments. This is not meant as an endorsement of these units. However, to provide practical advice for performing electrosurgery, we have decided to highlight the specific features and accessories of the most widely used and written-about units available.

*Discontinued model.

Valley Lab produces a variety of electrosurgical devices, ranging from small office units to large powerful units generally found only in operating rooms. The Valley Lab Surgistat is a good machine for the serious surgeon, but is costly to operate because many of its accessories are disposable, including grounding pads and standard handpieces. This adds a cost of $10 to $20 per procedure.

The Surgistat allows either pure cutting current, pure coagulation, or a mix of these two. The more versatile machines have multiple blend settings that can be optimized for multiple tissue types and allow more than one device (handpiece and bipolar forceps, for example) to be used simultaneously.

## Two Types of Hyfrecator
- Hyfrecator 2000
- Delasco 734

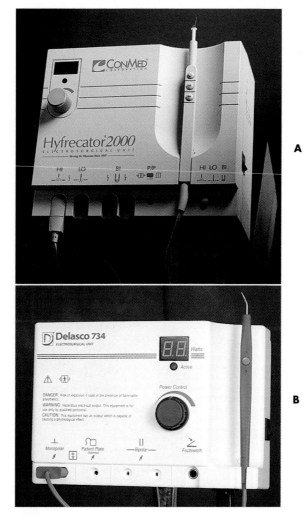

**FIG 12-2**
Hyfrecator electrosurgery units made by ConMed (**A**) and Delasco (**B**). (**A** Courtesy ConMed; **B** courtesy Delasco.)

## ACCESSORIES

### Hyfrecator

- Disposable electrodes (Fig. 12-3)
- Electrolase blunt tips
- Electrolase sharp tips (beware: these tips can cut tissue)
- Metal-hubbed needles with adapter
- Epilation needles
- Sterile sleeves for switching handle (sterile gloves or 12-inch sterile Penrose drains can be used to cover the handle in a sterile field)

### Ellman Surgitron

- Nondisposable electrodes (loops, ball, needle tips [autoclavable]) (Fig. 12-4)
- Disposable electrodes (loops, ball)

### Valley Lab Surgistat

- Sterile disposable handpieces with spatula or needle tips (these can be used interchangeably with Hyfrecator tips); handpieces have a rocker switch that allows the surgeon to easily change between cutting and coagulation in the operating field

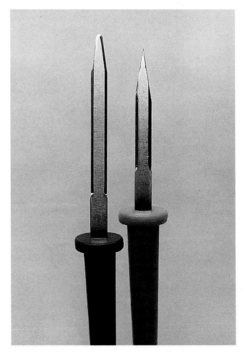

FIG 12-3
Disposable electrolase tips for the Hyfrecator. Blunt tip and sharp tip shown. (Courtesy ConMed.)

- Nondisposable bipolar forceps, with active and ground contacts located within the instrument itself so that no external grounding pad is needed; this is especially useful for point coagulation of small bleeding vessels because grasping the vessel and coagulation are done in one movement

## Smoke Evacuators

- Con-Med Hyfre-Vac
- Delasco SaftEvac (least expensive unit)
- Ellman Vapor-Vac
- Accuderm-Vac
- Buffalo Filters

## Thermal Pencil Cautery

A $7 to $10 thermal pencil cautery is a useful device to have, especially when working on the eyelids. This disposable device consists of two penlight batteries in a housing connected to a filament that heats up when activated. It can be a useful tool for treatment around the eyes and on patients with pacemakers. The devices come in high- and low-temperature varieties; low-temperature devices are preferred in skin surgery. Physicians should keep a few of these in their offices to be used as needed.

Thermal pencil cautery units are excellent for opening a subungual hematoma. When the hot electrode perforates the nail, the heated tip is cooled by the blood from the hematoma, preventing damage to the nail bed.

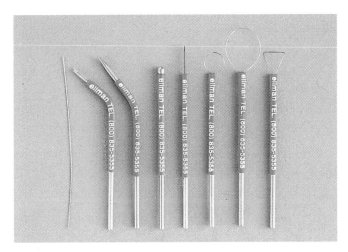

**FIG 12-4**
Reusable Surgitron electrodes. (Courtesy Ellman Educational Division.)

**TABLE 12-1    Lesions and the Modality to Use With the Hyfrecator**

| Lesions | Modality |
| --- | --- |
| **Benign** | |
| Angiomas (cherry) | Superficial D or F |
| Angiomas (spider) | D of center |
| Condyloma acuminata | F |
| Milia | D with epilation needle |
| Molluscum contagiosum | D |
| Neurofibromas | D |
| Nevi (benign) | D after shave (2-6 watts)* |
| Mucoceles | D of base after I & D |
| Pyogenic granulomas | D after shave or curettage |
| Seborrheic keratosis (including dermatosis papulosa nigra) | F |
| Sebaceous hyperplasia | Light F |
| Skin tags (acrochordon) | D or F (1-3 watts)* |
| Telangiectasias | Light quick D with needle |
| Verrucae vulgaris | F (5-15 watts)* |
| Verrucae plana | Light F |
| **Premalignant** | |
| Actinic keratoses | Light F |
| Keratoacanthomas | Shave, curette, then F/D |
| **Malignant** | |
| Shave biopsy and firm diagnosis needed before treatment | |
| Basal cell carcinomas | Curette, then F/D, repeat 2 times |
| Bowen's disease (squamous cell carcinoma in situ) | Curette, then F/D, repeat 2 times |
| Squamous cell carcinomas | Curette, then F/D, repeat 2 times |

*Power settings with Hyfrecator Plus based on the videotape *Common dermatologic procedures: utilizing the Hyfrecator Plus, with Jack E. Sebben*, New York, 1995, ConMed Video Library (800-488-6506).

*D*, Desiccation; *F*, fulguration; *F/D*, fulguration and desiccation; *I & D*, incision and drainage.

# INDICATIONS FOR USE OF ELECTROSURGERY

Indications for use of electrosurgery and radiosurgery and the recommended modalities are listed by lesion in Tables 12-1 and 12-2.

**TABLE 12-2   Settings for Radiosurgery**

| Lesions | Waveform | Power setting |
| --- | --- | --- |
| **Benign** | | |
| Angiomas (cherry) | Coagulation | * |
| Angiomas (spider) | Coagulation | * |
| Condyloma acuminata | Cut and coagulation | 2 |
| Oral mucus cysts | F of base after I & D | * |
| Seborrheic keratosis | Cut and coagulation | 2 |
| Telangiectasias | Cut and coagulation with needle | <1 |
| Verrucae vulgaris | F to produce spark | * |
| Verrucae plana | F | * |
| **Premalignant** | | |
| Actinic keratoses | Light F | * |
| Keratoacanthomas | Shave, curette, then F/D | * |
| **Malignant** | | |
| Shave biopsy and firm diagnosis needed before treatment | | |
| Basal cell carcinomas (BCC) | Curette, F/D, repeat 2 times | 5 |

*F*, fulguration; *F/D*, fulguration and desiccation; *I & D*, incision and drainage.
*Determine power setting by principles described on the next page.

## CONTRAINDICATIONS

By patient—use care if patient has:

- A pacemaker (see Pacemaker Problems, p. 178)
- Metal plates, metal pins, or metal prosthetic joints

By lesion:

- Melanoma (electrosurgery is not indicated as a treatment modality)
- BCC—if sclerosing BCC or if larger than 2 cm

By location for malignant lesions:

- Body folds—alar groove and inner canthus of eye (higher chance of deep invasion of tumor)
- SCC on non–sun-exposed skin and mucous membranes (may be more agressive biologically)

## COMPARISON OF ELECTROSURGICAL UNITS

Radiosurgery is electrosurgery using radiofrequency current. The frequencies used are in the spectrum of AM radio. Radiosurgery is performed at a much higher frequency than that used by the Hyfrecator. Radiosurgical units are more than twice the cost of the Hyfrecator, but allow for greater versatility in their use (especially for cutting). The Valley Lab Surgistat is a useful electrosurgical unit that is excellent for cutting and is not a radiofrequency unit.

Radiosurgery uses an antenna as the "indifferent" electrode. This antenna does not have to make contact with the skin. When using a Hyfrecator, it is usually unnecessary to use the indifferent electrode.

The major significant difference between radiosurgery units and a Hyfrecator is that the radiosurgery units allow for more efficient cutting with less tissue damage. To use electrosurgery only for hemostasis and tissue destruction of benign and malignant lesions, there may be no real difference between the units. Currently, all radiosurgical units are significantly more expensive than Hyfrecators. (At this time, the Surgitron and Surgistat are well over $2000 and the Hyfrecator Plus and the Delasco 734 are still less than $1000.) In fact, the authors all use Hyfrecators in our offices as the standard units for electrosurgery.

## GENERAL PRINCIPLES OF ELECTROSURGICAL TECHNIQUES

### Power Setting

Every electrosurgical unit is different from other units, and the desired setting will vary for each model, procedure, lesion, or patient. Even two supposedly identical electrosurgical models may require different settings. Therefore we will not provide exact dial or number settings for many of the procedures. The basic principle for setting the correct output power is to start low and increase the power until you are producing the desired outcome (destruction, coagulation, or cutting). When the desired outcome is destruction, the tissue should bubble or turn gray. Keep in mind that destruction of tissue below the visible area of treatment can occur. The power setting for coagulation and cutting is higher than the setting needed for tissue destruction. A general rule of thumb is to use the lowest power setting that accomplishes a given result for cosmetically sensitive procedures.

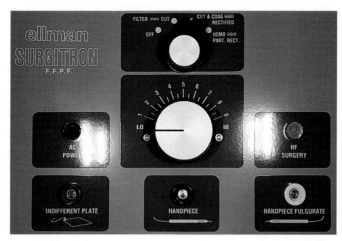

**FIG 12-5**
Surgitron dial showing different settings for the type of electrical current.

The Hyfrecator has high- and low-output terminals. The Surgitron radio-surgery unit has a dial with settings from 1 to 9 for the power setting (Fig. 12-5) and the following five different surgical modes:

1. Pure cutting current
2. Blended cutting and coagulation
3. Coagulation
4. Fulguration (similar to the Hyfrecator)
5. Bipolar coagulation (rarely used)

## Anesthesia

We recommend using local anesthesia for virtually all electrosurgery. Injecting 1% lidocaine with epinephrine before the procedure will make the electrosurgery painless. There are some physicians that advocate not using anesthesia for lesions such as telangiectasias, small angiomas, milia, and small skin tags. Topical anesthesia with ethyl chloride is contraindicated because ethyl chloride is flammable. EMLA cream can be used for anesthesia before treatment of facial telangiectasias and eliminates the effects of distortion from injectable anesthesia. Also, short bursts of low current can be less uncomfortable than anesthesia in some individuals. For other lesions, the use of a 30-gauge needle for injecting the lidocaine should be less painful than the electrosurgery.

When not using anesthesia for small lesions, it can sometimes help to stabilize the physician's hand against the patient's body (or face) so that if the patient moves, the electrode moves with the patient.

## TIPS SPECIFIC TO RADIOSURGERY

1. Activate the electrode with the foot switch before touching the patient with the electrode. This allows the current to flow fully through the electrode for faster and more efficient cutting and coagulation.
2. While cutting, use a smooth uninterrupted movement of the electrode. The intensity should be adjusted until the electrode moves through the tissue like a hot knife through butter.
3. Always use the indifferent plate (antenna). The indifferent plate should be under the patient and not far from the operative site. This indifferent plate does not have to touch the skin.
4. To avoid excessive tissue damage when cutting, minimize lateral heat.

   Lateral heat = Time that electrode contacts tissue $\times$ Intensity of power $\times$ Electrode size $\times$ Nature of the waveform/frequency

   - Electrode contact time (keep to a minimum)
   - Intensity of power
     Too high causes sparking and increases tissue destruction
     Too low causes tissue drag, which can increase lateral heat and increase risk of bleeding
   - Electrode size (smaller electrodes cause less lateral heat and require less power to operate)
   - Nature of the wave form
     Fully rectified filtered (cutting) (least lateral heat: 90% cutting, 10% coagulation)
     Fully rectified (blend of 50% cutting and 50% coagulation) (less lateral heat)
     Partially rectified (coagulation) (high lateral heat: 90% coagulation, 10% cutting)
   - Frequency: Higher frequencies cause less lateral heat. The Surgitron operates at 3.8 MHz. The fulguration port on the Surgitron and the Hyfrecator both operate at 0.5 MHz and therefore produce more lateral heat. However, because fulguration and desiccation are used to destroy tissue, the lateral heat is not a problem. It is during cutting that tissue destruction is to be avoided.

## SAFETY MEASURES WITH ELECTROSURGERY

### Potential Hazards of Electrosurgery (To Patient and Physician)

- Fire and burns
- Electric shock
- Transmission of infection through electrode, smoke plume, or spattering blood
- Pacemaker problems

### Safety Precautions to Avoid Potential Hazards

#### Fire and burns

- Do not use alcohol to prepare the skin
- Do not use ethyl chloride as local anesthetic
- Keep oxygen and other flammable material away from electrosurgical equipment
- Have fire extinguisher available
- Be careful of bowel gas in perirectal procedures

### Electric shock

- Keep electrosurgical equipment functioning properly; if there are signs of malfunction, get equipment fixed before use
- Use three-pronged plug connected to an outlet that is not overloaded
- Do not use the outlet in the treatment table
- Do not make or break contact with patient while the electrode is activated
- Make sure patient is not grasping or touching metal portions of the treatment table

It may be advantageous for the physician to touch the patient with the free hand while performing electrosurgery. However, if this contact is either made or broken during the delivery of the current, there will be a shock between the patient and the physician.

### Transmission of infection through electrode

- Always wear gloves
- Use disposable electrodes when possible
- Use disposable, metal-hubbed needles with an adapter. Ensure that the connection is tight. A loose needle that falls into an open wound or an unprotected eye can be a disaster. A Luer Lok adapter is now available from Delasco and avoids the risk of the needle falling off.
- When using reusable electrodes, clean them after each use by removing the char and sterilizing the electrodes.
- For small procedures, in which minimal electrosurgery is needed, an assistant who is not part of the sterile field can apply the electrosurgery as needed. If the physician needs control of the electrosurgical device, a sterile glove can be held open and the nonsterile Hyfrecator handle with electrode attached can be lowered into the glove, with the tip piercing a finger of the glove. The physician can then control a sterile handle. This is easier to set up than a sterile Penrose drain if control is urgently needed in the middle of a procedure.

### Transmission of infection through smoke plume or spattering blood

Transmission of infection through a smoke plume or spattering blood is a potential risk when treating lesions of viral origin. This is especially true when treating HPV infection in all types of warts. Intact HPV DNA has been recovered in the smoke plume of verrucae treated with electrosurgery and the carbon dioxide laser.[1,2,4-8] There is a case report that suggests a physician acquired an HPV infection of the larynx (laryngeal papillomatosis) from performing laser therapy on HPV-infected lesions.[3]

Although there may also be a potential risk of transmission of hepatitis, herpes, or HIV through blood splatter or smoke plume, there is even less scientific evidence showing such transmission.[7-9] Nevertheless, we recommend the following safety measures (especially if the lesion is of viral origin or the patient is known to be infected with HIV or hepatitis).

1. Use a smoke evacuator with the intake nozzle held within 2 cm of the operative area. It is essential to use the evacuator when treating any viral lesion.
2. The physician and treatment team should wear surgical masks and eye protection (most important when treating HPV). Special surgical masks that filter down to 0.5 microns are available and should be used for extensive cases.
3. Consider using a different treatment modality based on evaluation of the risks and benefits of treatment.

### Pacemaker problems

Electrosurgery should be avoided in patients with pacemakers (or cardiac monitoring equipment). Thermal pencil cautery is not contraindicated in patients with pacemakers; these devices are not as versatile as other electrosurgical units but distribute no current to the pacemaker. If there is no alternative to electrosurgery, consult a cardiologist to discuss the risks and benefits for the patient based on the type of pacemaker and the stability of the patient. (There is a good, detailed discussion of this risk in *Cutaneous Electrosurgery* by Jack Sebben.[10])

## TREATING SPECIFIC LESIONS

### Benign Lesions

The benign lesions we are treating can be divided into three basic groups: viral lesions, cosmetic lesions, and precancers. It is especially important to do no harm when treating cosmetic lesions. The treatment methodology for benign lesions must minimize scarring and complications.

### Angiomas (cherry)

Cherry (often called *capillary* or *senile*) angiomas (Fig. 12-6, *A*) are cosmetic lesions that are asymptomatic and have no malignant potential. If the patient insists on having some treatment, electrosurgery is probably the most effective inexpensive treatment. Various lasers can treat cherry angiomas at a higher cost to the patient but with a lower chance of scarring.

We use local anesthesia with epinephrine before treating most cherry angiomas. The largest cherry angiomas may be easier to treat by shaving them first and then electrodesiccating the base. Smaller cherry angiomas can be lightly electrodesiccated. The char can be wiped off with gauze or a curette.

### Angiomas (spider)

Spider angiomas (Fig. 12-6, *B*) are also cosmetic lesions that can be left alone or effectively treated with laser therapy. For patients who request treatment but are unable to afford laser therapy, electrosurgery is an effective alternative. Because injecting lidocaine and epinephrine may obscure the lesion, it is acceptable to treat spider angiomas without anesthesia. Alternatively, the use of EMLA topical anesthesia is ideal in this situation.

Electrodesiccation of the central feeding vessel should eradicate the entire angioma. This can be done with an epilation needle, a metal-hubbed needle with an adapter, or a blunt electrode. If a blunt electrode is used, we recommend press-

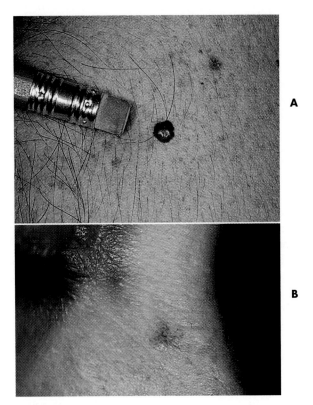

**FIG 12-6**
**A,** Cherry angiomas. **B,** Spider angiomas.

ing it against the central feeding vessel to maximize efficacy. No curettage is needed after this electrosurgery. The very lowest setting that causes blanching of the vessel should be used. Using excessive energy that can cause permanent indentations should be avoided. It is normal to see skin flushing around the treatment site in the office.[4] No special aftercare is needed. However, the patient should not scrub the treatment site vigorously while in the healing stage.

Unfortunately, the recurrence rate is high. There is also a tendency to leave a small residual scar.[5]

### Condyloma acuminata

If there are multiple, small condylomata in a moist area, it may be better to use topical chemicals for treatment. In the office, this may include trichloroacetic acid or podophyllin. The patient may also be sent home with a prescription for Condylox (a purified podophyllin preparation). However, lesions that occur in drier areas (such as the shaft of the penis or buttocks) often do not respond to topical chemical treatments. These lesions may respond better to a combination of cryotherapy and topical chemicals. Condyloma acuminata can also be successfully treated with electrosurgery.

A local anesthetic should always be used before electrosurgery in the genital area. Also, because patients may fear electrosurgery to these areas, it is important to explain that electrosurgery can treat the condyloma with a single treatment that should heal in 7 days and usually causes little scarring. This may be particularly appealing to the patient that has failed multiple treatments with various chemicals and/or cryosurgery.

There are two major methods that can be used for electrosurgery of condyloma. One is to use light electrofulguration or electrodesiccation. The other is to perform radiosurgery with a loop electrode using a blend of a cutting and coagulating current. If the condyloma is large, an alternative is to do a shave excision with a cold scalpel and electrodesiccate the base. The goal is to destroy the pedunculated lesion with minimal effect to the surrounding normal skin. Note that with cryotherapy we suggest a 1- to 2-mm halo, and with electrosurgery we do not suggest a halo.

When performing radiosurgery, an appropriate-sized loop electrode should be used to treat the condyloma. The unit should be set for cut and coagulation with the power at setting 2. The condyloma should be debulked on the first pass and then the edges should be lightly "feathered" to ensure there is no remaining tissue and to blend the treated skin into the surrounding normal tissue.

It is especially important to wear a mask and use a smoke evacuator when treating lesions that contain HPV. Extensive and recurrent condylomata may be referred for laser therapy or surgical excision.

### Milia

Milia are only cosmetic lesions. The preferred method of treating milia is needle or scalpel incision and expression of the keratin with a comedone extractor. This may not require anesthesia and is easy to accomplish with a medium-gauge needle or a No. 11 blade. (See Chapter 13 for further information on this procedure.) An alternative therapy is to use the epilation needle with an electrosurgical unit to open the milia, allowing for self-extrusion of the keratin. This procedure may be done without anesthesia.

### Molluscum contagiosum

The lesions of molluscum contagiosum (See Fig. 11-12) are caused by a virus and can regress spontaneously after months. Accepted treatments include curettage, cryotherapy, topical agents, and electrodesiccation. In our experience, curettage is the most effective treatment. Very light electrodesiccation with or without anesthesia is an alternative treatment. If curettage is used without anesthesia, it is easy to stop the minor bleeding with aluminum chloride or Monsel's solution. If desiccation is used, there is no need for additional hemostasis.

Of all the accepted treatments, the risk of scarring is probably greatest with electrodesiccation. Therefore it is probably best to avoid using electrodesiccation to treat molluscum in the genital area. Curettage alone gives the most controlled and effective treatment. Cryotherapy and the application of topical agents are easiest to perform.

For small children who will not sit still for any of these "painful" procedures, you may elect not to treat or to have the parents apply topical agents such as Duofilm or Retin-A daily at home. "Tincture of time" is a reasonable option for children. Another alternative is to use EMLA cream under occlusion for 1 hour and then proceed with curettage or cryotherapy. Another alternative is to apply cantharone with a pointed stick. This is painless at application and if applied only to the lesion and no surrounding skin may be minimally uncomfortable when it blisters 24 hours later.

### Mucocele (oral mucus cyst)

Oral mucus cysts (See Fig. 15-15) are mucin-containing cysts that occur on the lip. These cysts are usually on the lower lip, and often follow trauma to the lip, such as biting the lip. After injecting 1% lidocaine with epinephrine from inside the mouth, it is helpful to wait 5 minutes to get maximum vasoconstriction. The lip is a very vascular area so it is worth waiting for the epinephrine to work. With a No. 15 or No. 11 blade, the cyst should first be opened before using electrosurgery.

In Chapter 11, we recommend opening the cyst from inside the mouth with a No. 11 scalpel before treating with liquid nitrogen. Before electrosurgery, the physician should make a stab incision with a No. 11 blade or excise the roof of the cyst with a shave approach using a No. 15 blade from inside the mouth. The mucin should then be expressed, and the base of the cyst treated by light electrodesiccation. Extensive electrodesiccation of the lip can lead to scarring.

If the mucocele recurs, the cryotherapy or electrosurgery can be repeated if needed or the mucocele can be excised and the defect sutured.

### Neurofibroma

Neurofibromas are soft, benign tumors that are elevated above the skin surface. Patients may request their removal for cosmetic purposes or because of fear that the lesion is not benign. Two electrosurgical methods for removal are shave with scalpel and then hemostasis with chemical or electrocoagulation or shave with a wire loop electrode or a sharp electrode using cutting and coagulation current.

Before treating neurofibromas, physicians should tell patients that these lesions can regrow or that the area of the excision can become indented.

### Nevi (benign)

If there is any suspicion that a presumed nevus is malignant, a full-thickness biopsy of the lesion must be performed to rule out melanoma. It is not acceptable to do this biopsy with electrosurgery because the heat-induced tissue destruction can interfere with the pathologic diagnosis. We recommend sending all pigmented lesions excised by any method to the pathologist. Therefore you should be certain of the benign nature of the lesion before treating nevi with electrosurgery.

For treatment of a nevus, we always recommend doing a cold scalpel shave excision before applying the Hyfrecator. The Hyfrecator can then be used to destroy the residual nevus cells. Hyfrecation can also be used to remove any remaining rim of tissue. See Chapter 6 for further information on this procedure.

Although radiosurgery is used to shave off nevi, we do not recommend this procedure. There is a greater risk of hypopigmentation when the lesion is removed with electrosurgery than with a cold scalpel.

### Pyogenic granuloma

Pyogenic granulomas are very vascular benign tumors (Fig. 12-7, *A*). They occur most commonly on the fingers, face, lips, and gingiva. Pyogenic granulomas often occur at the site of minor trauma and are more common in pregnancy. These vascular lesions are ideal for electrosurgical treatment.

Before treatment, the physician should inject 1% lidocaine with epinephrine to cause blanching of the skin at the base of the lesion. Epinephrine is needed because of the extreme vascularity of these lesions. If the pyogenic granuloma is on a finger, it is possible to use epinephrine as long as the injection is not directly into the digital artery. Some physicians place a temporary tourniquet around the base of the finger to control bleeding during the procedure. If choosing this approach, the tourniquet should not be kept on for more than 10 minutes.

Fig. 12-7 shows treatment of a pyogenic granuloma on the lip of a woman after pregnancy. We waited 5 minutes after the injection of local anesthesia to have the benefit of the epinephrine for vasoconstriction. Fig. 12-7, *B* shows the vasoconstriction and swelling during the administration of anesthesia. In Fig. 12-7, *C*, the elevated portion of the lesion was shaved off with a cold scalpel. (Alternatively, a loop electrode using a cutting/coagulation current could have been used.) We recommend sending the specimen for pathology to rule out the remote possibility that the lesion is an amelanotic melanoma. We curetted the base of the lesion with a 2-0 to 3-0 sharp dermal curette to remove the remaining tissue. Before attempting to stop the bleeding with electrosurgery, it helps to dry the base by applying pressure with cotton-tipped swabs. Pooled blood will diminish the efficacy of electrosurgery. In Fig. 12-7, *D*, the base was then treated with electrodesiccation. (It may be necessary to use the higher power of electrocoagulation for these vascular lesions.) It may be necessary to repeat the curettage and desiccation a number of times to destroy the whole pyogenic granuloma and to stop the bleeding. If some tissue remains, the pyogenic granuloma will regrow. Silver nitrate applied to the base of these lesions after thorough curettage may minimize regrowth.

The pyogenic granuloma in Fig. 12-7 recurred twice after electrosurgery. We then proceeded to excise the lesion and to suture the lip. The final result can be seen in Fig. 12-7, *F*.

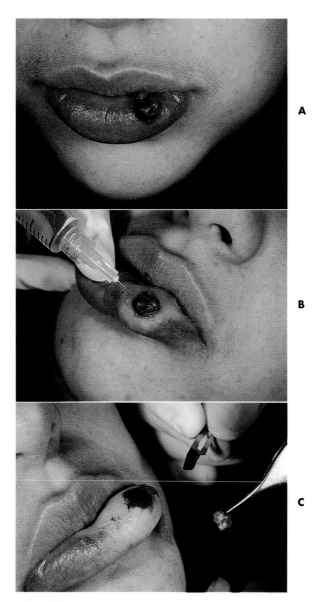

**FIG 12-7**
Pyogenic granuloma. **A,** Pyogenic granuloma on the lip after pregnancy. **B,** Vasoconstriction and swelling during administration of local anesthesia. **C,** Shave excision with No. 11 blade.

*Continued*

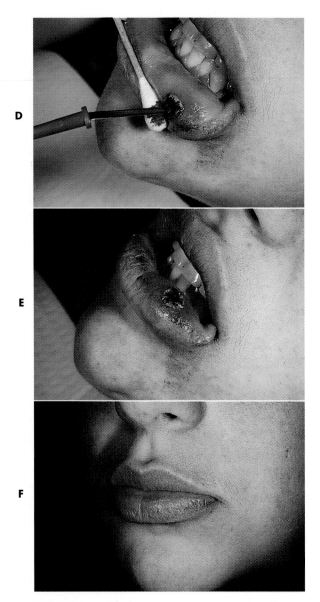

**FIG 12-7, cont'd**
Pyogenic granuloma. **D,** Electrocoagulation with Hyfrecator and disposable electrode. Note that the cotton-tipped swab is rolled ahead of the electrode to dry the field immediately before the electrocoagulation. **E,** Full electrodesiccation of the base of the lesion and complete hemostasis. **F,** Lip healed after recurrent lesion was excised with a scalpel and sutured. No scar is visible.

### Sebaceous hyperplasia

Sebaceous hyperplasia of the face is a common condition as people age. It is asymptomatic and not dangerous, but patients often ask for treatment for cosmetic reasons. Occasionally it may be unclear whether what appears to be sebaceous hyperplasia may actually be a BCC. If the diagnosis is uncertain, a biopsy is indicated. It is easiest to do a shave biopsy with a scalpel or loop electrode and send the specimen for pathologic diagnosis.

If the diagnosis is certain because the sebaceous hyperplasia is typical, the condition should be treated with tissue destruction using cryosurgery or electrodesiccation. Either of these approaches will not yield a specimen for pathology. When using electrodesiccation, a low power setting should be used to avoid scarring. The physician should remember that the overall principle here is "do no harm" because this is a purely cosmetic lesion. The physician should also explain to the patient that there is a risk of scarring, and the alternative is to do nothing. Another approach is to apply 50% trichloroacetic acid with a pointed stick to the lesions, making sure not to apply it to the normal skin. Remember that patients with cosmetic-type lesions can be much more concerned about leaving any residual mark.

### Seborrheic keratosis

If there is any question about whether a presumed seborrheic keratosis is malignant, we recommend performing a biopsy with a scalpel or punch to get a good specimen for pathology. If the lesion is shaved or excised with electrosurgery, the heat-induced tissue destruction may interfere with the pathologic diagnosis. When removing a seborrheic keratosis with shave biopsy using a scalpel, hemostasis can be easily achieved with aluminum chloride or Monsel's solution, and electrosurgery is not needed.

When dealing with a classic seborrheic keratosis, another technique is to lightly fulgurate the lesion with the Hyfrecator and then wipe it off with a gauze or curette. Because this does not provide tissue for pathology, this approach should not be used if the lesion has suspicious features (i.e., may be a melanoma). The advantage to this technique is that the desiccated seborrheic keratosis is easily removed from the skin below, without going deeper than necessary. This allows for good control of the depth of removal and can minimize scarring.

When using radiosurgery to shave these lesions, it may help to outline the lesion with a surgical pen. A loop electrode can be used to shave off the lesion with a single initial pass at a cut and coagulate setting of 2. The skin can be scraped, like an artist painting with a brush, while keeping the electrode at a 90-degree angle to the skin surface. Gentle strokes are used to feather the edges of the lesion into the normal skin. A moist 4 × 4 gauze can be used between passes of the electrode to remove tissue and moisten the skin. Moistening the skin reduces tissue drag for more efficient lesion removal. The easiest way to moisten the gauze is to run it under tap water and then wring it out. Because the electrical current kills potential infectious organisms, there is no need to use sterile water or saline to moisten the gauze. Remember that radiosurgery will still cause more tissue destruction than just a surgical blade, so that the chance of hypopigmentation or scarring may be greater.

### Skin tags (acrochordons)

There is no absolute cut-off to differentiate between large, medium, and small skin tags. We define the smallest skin tags as those lesions that are too small to be grasped easily with a forceps and therefore are difficult to shave or snip off. The largest wide-based lesions are those that would be difficult to remove with a single snip of a sharp iris scissor. These are best shaved off with a scalpel.

To treat a small or medium skin tag with electrosurgery, light electrodesiccation or fulguration should be used. After the lesion is charred, the char can be
removed with a gauze or curette, or it can be allowed to fall off on its own.

Figs. 12-8 and 12-9 show electrosurgical treatment of skin tags near the eye and
on the lower lid. The eyelid is a location where it is important to be very careful
when using chemicals for hemostasis. When used carefully, light electrodesiccation
allows for hemostasis without endangering the eye. For radiosurgery of a skin tag,
a loop electrode on cut and coagulation at a setting of <2 should be used. The skin
tag should be shaved off with the loop alone or grasped with the forceps in the
loop first. Modes of treatment by skin tag size are listed in Table 12-3.

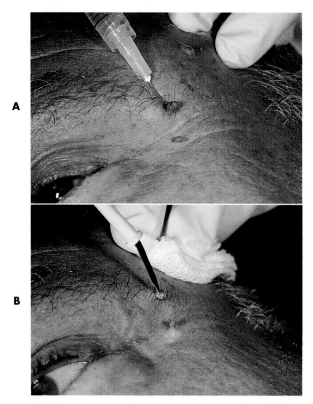

**FIG 12 -8**
Skin tags near the eye. **A,** Injecting the base of this pedunculated skin tag with lidocaine and epinephrine. **B,** Electrodesiccation with Hyfrecator.

**TABLE 12-3    Treatment of Skin Tags by Size**

| Size | Anesthesia | Treatment |
| --- | --- | --- |
| Large, wide base | Yes | Shave |
| Medium base and size | Yes | Shave, snip, cryotherapy, or electrocurgery |
| Smallest | Yes or no | Electrosurgery or snip with fine scissors |

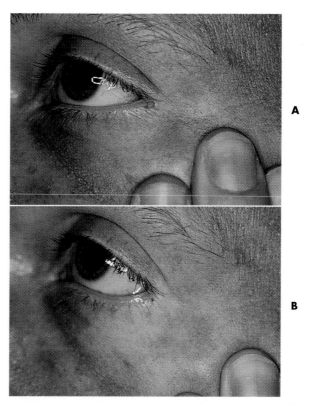

**A**

**B**

**FIG 12 -9**
Skin tag on lower lid. **A,** Skin tag before injection of local anesthesia. **B,** Lower lid after snip excision and electrodesic-cation of the remaining tissue (chemical hemostatic agents are avoided so close to the eye).

### Telangiectasias

Telangiectasias (Fig. 12-10) are purely cosmetic lesions that occur commonly on the face and legs as people age. Laser treatment may produce the best cosmetic result, but it is expensive. If the patient requests treatment by another method to save money, the physician should discuss the risks and benefits of electrosurgical treatment and obtain informed consent before proceeding. If the patient chooses to undergo electrosurgery, the following guidelines should be considered:

1. A fine-needle electrode or sharp tip of the Electrolase electrode should be used on a low-energy setting.
2. The fine needle should be inserted into one to two sites per telangiectasia. Longer telangiectasias may need treatment at three to four sites.
3. Facial telangiectasias respond better to electrosurgery than ones on the leg. We do not recommend using electrosurgery for telangiectasias on the leg.
4. Local anesthesia may obscure the lesion so treatment may need to be done without anesthesia, though EMLA cream can be useful.
5. The physician may choose to use a foot switch to avoid accidentally moving the hand switch on activation.
6. The physician should rest the hand holding the needle electrode against the patient, so if the patient moves the physician's hand will move with the patient.

When not using anesthesia for telangiectasias, we recommend placing the electrode against the skin to alert the patient of the sensation before activating it. This will avoid the element of surprise. It also may help to warn the patient that tearing of the eyes may occur as a reaction to treatment near the eyes.[4]

The Surgitron has special fine-needle electrodes for treating telangiectasias. The intermediate-needle electrode should be adequate for almost all telangiectasias. The Surgitron should be set for cut and coagulate and a power setting of <1. This is one of the few situations when it is recommended to activate the electrode after it has made contact with the patient. The needles are Teflon-coated, except for the tip, to allow for insertion into the blood vessel and to avoid burning the overlying skin. The tip should be inserted into the center of the telangiectasia and then the electrode should be activated for less than half a second (Fig. 12-11). The telangiectasia will blanch if the treatment is successful. Treatment should be repeated every 1 to 2 mm along the telangiectasia. When setting the power dial, the dial should be turned up from zero toward one, and stopped when there is some resistance from the dial. This is the minimum power setting and the appropriate setting for this procedure.

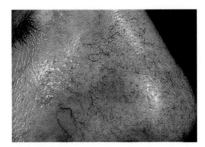

**FIG 12-10**
Telangiectasias on nose.

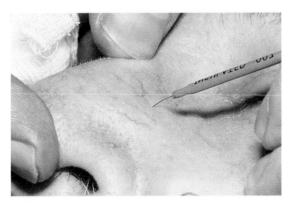

**FIG 12-11**
Teflon-coated electrode inserted into telangiectasia for treatment with Surgitron. (Courtesy Ellman Educational Division.)

### Warts

Patients seek treatment for warts (lesions caused by HPV) because the warts can cause pain, can be unsightly, and can spread to other parts of the body or to other individuals. HPV can infect many parts of the body. In this section, we will only address those HPV infections of the skin: verruca vulgaris, plantar warts, and flat warts. See p. 180 for information on condyloma acuminata.

In general, most warts can be treated effectively and easily with cryotherapy as described in Chapter 11. Patients may even use topical agents effectively at home. However, some warts are refractory to chemical treatments and cryotherapy. Electrosurgery has the advantage of allowing the physician to get good cure rates with a single in-office treatment. With electrosurgery, the complete removal of the visible wart can be seen at the time of treatment. With cryotherapy, one can only predict the clinical response based on the size of the halo and the freezing time used. Cryotherapy is more likely to require multiple visits for treatment and may actually be more painful in the days that follow the treatment.

Electrosurgery of warts always requires local anesthesia. If treating a finger (Fig. 12-12), local infiltration with epinephrine-free anesthetic or a digital block should be used. In some cases, local infiltration with lidocaine and epinephrine can be used if the digital artery is avoided. Fulguration or electrodesiccation are used to destroy the wart (Fig. 12-12, B). The desiccated tissue is then wiped away with a moist gauze or a curette (Fig. 12-12, C). If any wart tissue remains, the remaining tissue should receive additional electrosurgery and be wiped away until the final deep layer shows a uniform clear dermis (Fig. 12-12, D and E).

If the wart is large and protuberant, the initial wart can be shaved off with a cold scalpel or a loop electrode. The base can then be burned and wiped away. Care should be used not to burn the surrounding tissue and cause painful permanent scarring.

To treat verruca with radiosurgery, the handpiece should be plugged into the fulguration port and the mode set on cut and coagulation. The power dial should be turned up slowly until there is enough current to produce a spark. Otherwise, treatment is no different from what was described for the Hyfrecator.

### Verrucae (hands)

Special care should be taken if the wart is over a digital nerve. It is important to avoid channeling of the current down the digital nerve or causing local nerve damage. Periungual warts may be better treated by DNCB or intralesional bleomycin as discussed in Chapter 11.

### Plantar warts

We do not recommend electrosurgical treatment of large plantar warts because of the potential risk of permanent, painful scarring. Small plantar warts can be treated with electrosurgery or cryotherapy. See Chapter 11 for additional information on plantar wart treatment. Laser treatment is a reasonable alternative for plantar warts.

### Flat warts

Flat warts are usually seen in clusters on the face, arms, or legs. These warts may actually be curable with the daily application of topical tretinoin solution (Retin-A) 0.05% applied precisely to the warts. Retin-A can be used in combination with topical fluorouracil (Efudex) in cases refractory to Retin-A alone. If the tretinoin does not work, cryotherapy is probably the next best treatment option. If the patient only has a few flat warts in a noncosmetically sensitive area, it may be reasonable to use light fulguration or desiccation to treat these warts (especially if tretinoin and cryotherapy did not work). Resistant and recurrent warts may respond to laser treatment.

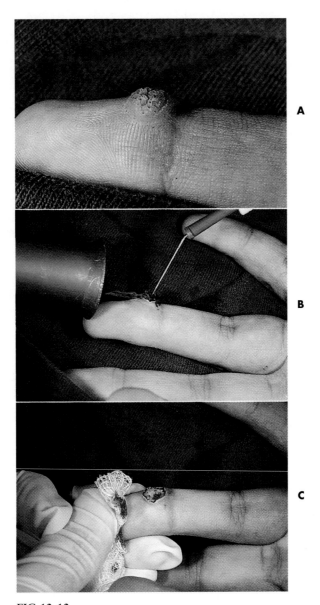

**FIG 12-12**
Verruca. **A,** Large wart on finger that had not responded to
cryotherapy. **B,** Electrodesiccation of the wart. **C,** Wiping
off the desiccated wart with a (moist) gauze pad.

*Continued*

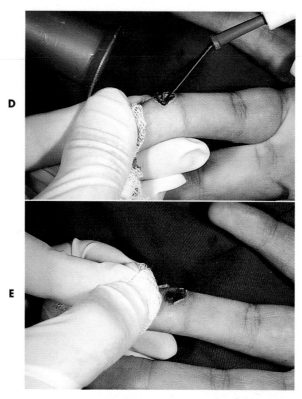

**FIG 12-12, cont'd**
Verruca. **D,** Burning the remaining wart tissue. Note the smoke going into the blue smoke evacuator. **E,** Final result of electrosurgical treatment.

# PREMALIGNANT LESIONS

## Actinic Keratosis

Cryosurgery is our preferred method to treat obvious actinic keratoses. It does not require anesthesia and is less likely to cause scarring than electrosurgery. If the lesion is thick or indurated, a biopsy should be done by the shave technique rather than treating the lesion blindly. Although radiosurgery could be used for such a shave biopsy, we prefer to use a cold-scalpel approach. If it is certain that the lesion is an actinic keratosis and no cryosurgical equipment is available, light fulguration can be used as an alternative treatment. Plain curettage is another alternative. Care should be exercised to avoid unnecessary scarring.

## Keratoacanthoma

A keratoacanthoma can extend deeply into the dermis. Keratoacanthoma on the face has a higher risk of metastasizing, and once diagnosed should be fully excised with clear margins. A keratoacanthoma can be excised initially and diagnosed with a deep shave using a scalpel or a radiosurgical cutting electrode. After shave excision, the base of the lesion can be curetted and then treated with electrosurgery or cryotherapy (See Chapter 11). Curettage and desiccation can successfully treat the fringe of tissue remaining at the perimeter and base. A complete description of curettage and desiccation treatment can be found on p. 194.

# MALIGNANCIES

In general, most suspected malignancies should undergo biopsy for pathologic diagnosis before definitive treatment. However, if the lesion is small and an elliptical biopsy is used for diagnosis, there maybe no need for a second procedure if the surgical margins are clear. Before performing electrosurgery on a suspected BCC or SCC, we suggest a shave biopsy for definitive diagnosis. If the lesion may be a melanoma, a full-thickness biopsy should be performed with an ellipse or punch and no further treatment with electrosurgery.

Although electrosurgical treatment can be good, definitive treatment for some BCC and SCC, it is not the treatment of choice for all BCC and SCC. The pathology result will help decide the appropriate treatment. If a suspected BCC comes back as sebaceous hyperplasia, it would not have been good to have done extensive and destructive electrosurgery with its risk of scarring and other complications. Electrosurgery is most effective for superficial BCC, Bowen's disease, and SCC in situ on the trunk and extremities.

There are contraindications for using electrosurgery to treat BCC or SCC based on the histology and location. Sclerosing or morpheaform BCC and SCC in non–sun-exposed areas are more aggressive and should be fully excised. BCC or SCC that occur in body folds, such as the alar groove and the corner of the eye, are more likely to be invasive and should not undergo electrosurgery.

## BCC or SCC: Curettage and Dessication

The skin surrounding the BCC should be injected with 1% lidocaine and epinephrine. A sharp dermal curette, such as a 2-0 or 3-0, should be used to scrape out the BCC. This procedure works because the BCC is softer than the surrounding normal skin. The abnormal tissue can be removed by scraping with the curette in all directions (Fig. 12-13). This will be more likely to get small pockets of tumor. It is helpful to use the curette on the border of the BCC to get the rim of outlying tissue. Then fulguration or desiccation of the base of the lesion and 2 mm of the surrounding normal tissue can be performed for an extra margin of cure.

There is a debate in the literature whether one cycle of curettage and desiccation is enough or whether two to three cycles are needed. Some experienced dermatologists have reported good cure rates with one cycle, but most of the cure rate studies have been done with three cycles. Studies have also shown that inexperienced physicians have greater recurrence rates. Therefore we recommend doing all three cycles to diminish the recurrence rate. In Fig. 12-14, it was helpful to use the curettage and desiccation technique because it avoided having to cut near the temporal branch of the facial nerve (See Fig. 19-6).

We recommend using the curette to scrape out the abnormal, softer tissue of a BCC before using electrosurgery. When using a radiosurgery unit, the fulguration port should be used with the power dial set to 5 or greater. The ball electrode works best for radiosurgery.

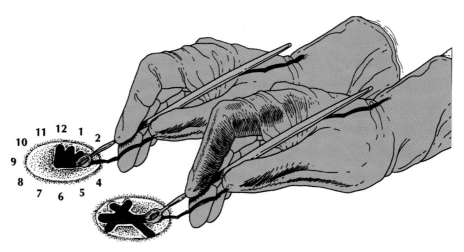

**FIG 12-13**
Two methods of scraping in all directions with a curette. (From Fewkes JL, Cheney ML, Pollack SV: *Illustrated atlas of cutaneous surgery,* Philadelphia, 1992, Lippincott-Gower.)

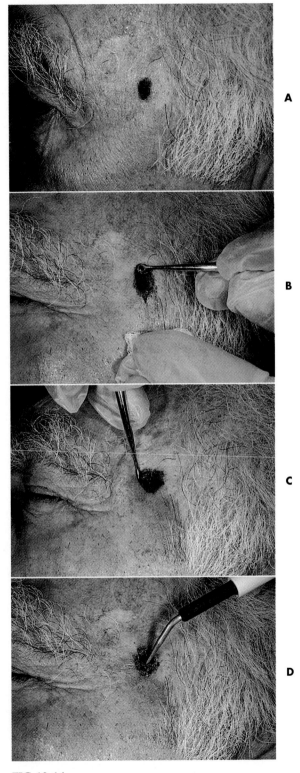

**FIG 12-14**
Curettage and desiccation of BCC on the face. **A,** BCC after shave biopsy; dark color is from Monsel's solution used for hemostasis. **B,** Curettage up and down. **C,** Curettage side to side. **D,** Electrodesiccation with Hyfrecator.

*Continued*

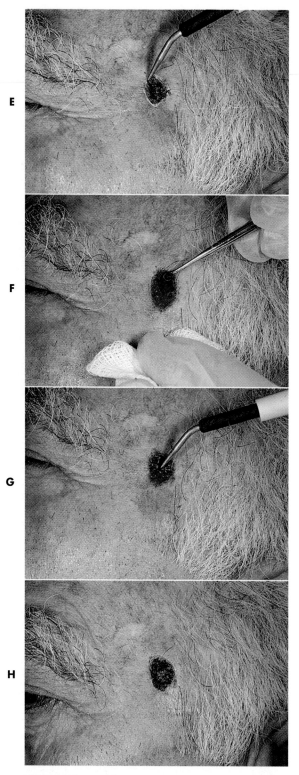

**FIG 12-14, cont'd**

Curettage and desiccation of BCC on the face. **E,** Electrodesiccation including margin. **F,** Second curettage. **G,** Second electrodesiccation. **H,** Final result after three cycles of curettage and desiccation. Note that the curettage and desiccation is a not a deep procedure and therefore in this location will not damage the facial nerve. An elliptical excision would carry an increased risk of nerve damage to the temporal branch of the facial nerve.

## ELECTROSURGERY NEAR THE EYE

Electrosurgery near the eye is a special circumstance. The physician should remember that when performing fulguration the spark will jump the shortest distance to tissue. To cauterize on the lid or in the canthi, the physician should ensure that the tip is very close to the site being treated. If the tip is far from the intended treatment site and a portion of the globe is closer to the active tip of the electrosurgical device, the current can arc to the globe and cause damage to the eye. Also, for contact electrosurgery in the area, the power should not be set too high because cautery of vessels on the bulbar conjunctivae or deeper in the eye is not desirable. If a globe protector is to be used, it should be made of nonconductive plastic.

## PRACTICING ELECTROSURGERY

Regardless of the electrosurgery unit to be used, it is possible to practice the techniques with a piece of uncooked beef steak (Fig. 12-15). The steak should be a fresh, inexpensive cut of steak that is not too fatty. Fatty meat should not be used for practice because it will smoke more. Pig's feet can even be used (e.g., after a suturing workshop). It is not necessary to use a smoke evacuator while practicing on meat, but there will be the smell of a barbecue.

### Practicing With the Hyfrecator

To practice with the Hyfrecator, the meat should be set on the indifferent electrode or touched with the nonoperating hand while practicing. Begin with the handpiece plugged into the low setting. Practice activating the handpiece and coming close to the steak until the sparks of fulguration appear. Turn up the current to see how the sparking and tissue destruction (cooking of the steak) increase. Try the same exercise with the electrode touching the beef to produce electrodesiccation. Then plug the handpiece into the high setting. Observe the increased destruction of tissue. If planning to treat fine vascular lesions, consider practicing with a fine metal needle and tip adapter.

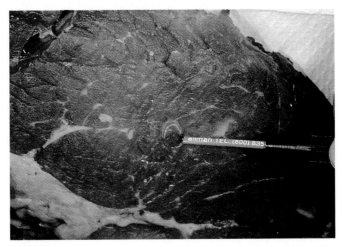

**FIG 12-15**
Practicing electrosurgery on steak.

## Practicing Radiosurgery (Surgitron)

To practice with the Surgitron, the meat should be placed on a paper towel sitting on top of the "antenna." Begin with a loop electrode in the handpiece, and set the unit to cut with a power setting of 2. Cut off a piece of meat, keeping the loop at a right angle to the tissue (Fig. 12-15). Activate the electrode before touching the meat to get a more smooth cut with minimal tissue damage. Compare how this looks and feels, waiting until the electrode is touching the skin before activation. Try this with a forceps holding the meat before activating the loop. Be sure to grasp the tissue with the forceps through the loop before starting the cutting.

The cut and coagulation setting should also be tried to feel how the electrode moves slightly more slowly through tissue with this setting. The vari-tip electrode can also be used to practice making incisions on the "cut" setting. Turn the power dial up to 8 and make a cut. See how the electrode produces a lot of sparking. This sparking causes unnecessary tissue damage. Now turn the power dial down to 1 and see how the electrode gets stuck while moving through the tissue. This tissue drag causes unnecessary tissue damage by increasing the amount of time the electrode is in contact with the tissue. Now try making cuts at power output settings of 6, 5, 4, and 3. Determine which setting will allow the electrode to move through the meat without sparking or drag. This type of intermediate setting is what is needed when using electrosurgery for cutting.

Coagulation can be accomplished with any electrode. Practice this with the ball electrode and the coagulation setting. Use a light touch, barely touching the tissue while moving the electrode gently over the area to be coagulated. Any electrode can be held to a forceps or hemostat grasping the bleeding area to accomplish coagulation.

## CONCLUSION

Electrosurgery is a powerful and versatile tool for skin surgery. It is important for the physician to become familiar with his or her electrosurgical unit. We have attempted to provide principles and guidelines for the treatment of skin lesions with electrosurgery. Electrosurgery should only be used on areas that are cosmetically sensitive (e.g., face, hands, and breasts) by physicians experienced in the techniques described in this chapter. Through the application of these principles and guidelines and the acquisition of experience, a physician should be able to safely tap the power of electrosurgery in the office.

## REFERENCES

1. Sawchuk WS et al: Infectious papillomavirus in the vapor of warts treated with carbon dioxide laser or electrocoagulation: detection and protection, *J Am Acad Dermatol* 21(1):41-49, 1989.
2. Garden JM et al: Papillomavirus in the vapor of carbon dioxide laser-treated verrucae, *JAMA* 259(8):1199-1202, 1988.
3. Hallmo P, Naess O: Laryngeal papillomatosis with human papillomavirus DNA contracted by a laser surgeon, *Eur Arch Otorhinolaryngol* 248(7):425-427, 1991.
4. Ferenczy A, Bergeron C, Richart RM: Carbon dioxide laser energy disperses human papillomavirus deoxyribonucleic acid onto treatment fields, *Am J Obstet Gynecol* 163(4):1271-1274, 1990.
5. Andre P et al: Risk of papillomavirus infection in carbon dioxide laser treatment of genital lesions, *J Am Acad Dermatol* 22(1):131-132, 1990.

6. Ferenczy A, Bergeron C, Richart RM: Human papillomavirus DNA in $CO_2$ laser-generated plume of smoke and its consequences to the surgeon, *Obstet Gynecol* 75(1):114-118, 1990.

7. Berberian BJ, Burnett JW: The potential role of common dermatologic techniques in transmitting disease, *J Am Acad Dermatol* 15:1057-1058, 1986.

8. O'Grady KF, Easty AC: Electrosurgery smoke: hazards and protection, *J Clin Engineering* 21(2):149-155, 1996.

9. Colver GB, Peutherer JR: Herpes simplex virus dispersal by Hyfrecator electrodes, *Br J Dermatol* 117:672-679, 1987.

10. Sebben J: *Cutaneous electrosurgery,* St. Louis, 1989, Mosby.

## SUGGESTED READING

DeWitt DE, Pfenninger JL: Radiofrequency surgery. In Pfenninger JL, Fowler GC, editors: *Procedures for primary care physicians,* St. Louis, 1994, Mosby.

Fewkes JL, Cheney ML, Pollack SV: *Illustrated atlas of cutaneous surgery,* Philadelphia, 1992, Lippincott-Gower.

Hainer BL: Electrosurgery for cutaneous lesions, *Am Fam Phys* 44:5, 81S-90S, 1991.

Pollack SV: *Electrosurgery of the skin,* New York, 1991, Churchill Livingstone.

Roenigk RK, Roenigk HH: *Dermatologic surgery: principles and practice,* ed 2, New York, 1996, Marcel Dekker.

Siegel D, Kriegel D: Electrosurgery. In Lask G, Moy R, editors: *Principles and techniques of cutaneous surgery,* New York, 1996, McGraw-Hill.

# CHAPTER 13

# Incision and Drainage

*Richard P. Usatine*

When incision and drainage (I&D) is used appropriately, it is a medical and surgical necessity and not an elective procedure. It is the treatment of choice for all types of abscesses, and when a definitive diagnosis of abscess is made there are no reasonable alternatives to opening and draining the purulent material. An abscess is defined as a localized collection of pus in a cavity that can occur in many areas of the body. In this chapter we will deal only with abscesses that occur in or directly below the skin. These abscesses include furuncles, carbuncles, and the abscesses around fingernails (acute paronychias). A furuncle or boil is an abscess that starts in a hair follicle or sweat gland. A carbuncle occurs when the furuncle extends into the subcutaneous tissue. We will not address peritonsillar and perinephric abscesses and other such internal infections.

Most skin abscesses are caused by *Staphylococcus aureus*. Other organisms that can cause abscesses of the skin include streptococcal species, gram-negative bacteria, and anaerobes.[1-3] External abscesses most often occur on the hands, feet, extremities, buttocks, and breast. An abscess in the breast of a nonlactating woman should prompt evaluation to rule out cancer.

## ADVANTAGES

The advantage of I&D is that it drains the pus that must be removed from an abscess to allow for healing of that lesion. Systemic antibiotics, whether parenteral or oral, do not adequately penetrate an abscess to cure the infection. If there is significant surrounding cellulitis, systemic antibiotics may be needed as an adjunct to I&D. Diagnosis may be easy when the skin overlying the abscess is red, warm, tender, swollen, and fluctuant.

When there is uncertainty whether a red, warm, swollen area of the skin is cellulitis or an abscess, it is reasonable to do a diagnostic needle aspiration. If pus is aspirated, this is not a definitive treatment for the abscess. The purulence can reaccumulate unless the abscess is fully opened. The bottom line is that I&D is the only reliable treatment for an abscess.

## DISADVANTAGES

Patients often experience pain and discomfort from I&D. It is difficult to get complete anesthesia around the abscess, even with good local anesthesia, because of the acidic environment of the abscess. Anesthesia that is injected peripheral to the area of inflammation may give good anesthesia of moderate duration because it is not enzymatically hydrolyzed as rapidly as anesthesia injected directly over the abscess. Also, pressure is needed to drain the purulence, and this can often be painful for patients. However, there is no effective, less painful alternative to I&D for a true abscess.

## INDICATIONS

Indications for I&D include the following:

- All skin abscesses
- Furuncle/carbuncle
- Inflamed epithelial cyst
- Paronychia with abscess (Fig. 13-1)
- Milia

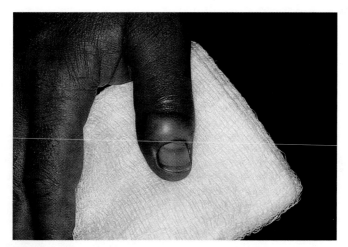

**FIG 13-1**
Abscess on finger (paronychia).

## CONTRAINDICATIONS

I&D should not be performed on facial furuncles located in the danger triangle of the face.[1] Otherwise, there are no contraindications for I&D. Caution should be exercised when performing I&D around vital structures such as the eye and neck and in areas overlying important nerves and blood vessels.

## EQUIPMENT

Equipment used to perform I&D (Fig. 13-2) includes the following:

- 1% lidocaine with epinephrine or ethyl chloride spray
- 27- to 30-gauge needle and 3-ml syringe for anesthesia
- Scalpel with No. 11 blade (essential for the incision)
- Cotton-tipped swabs
- Hemostat, preferably curved
- Forceps (for packing the dead space)
- Scissors (to cut the gauze [Nu-Gauze])
- 4 × 4 gauze pads to remove pus from field
- Nu-Gauze (width based on size of abscess; comes in ¼-inch and ½-inch iodinated or noniodinated form)
- Culture materials may be needed if the patient has diabetes, is HIV positive, or is immunocompromised

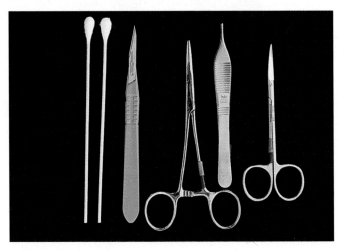

**FIG 13-2**
Instruments for I&D from left: Cotton-tipped swabs, No. 11 scalpel, hemostat, forceps, scissors.

## CONSENT

It is important to explain to patients that this procedure is required for the adequate treatment of an abscess. Once the patient understands that the abscess must be drained, you should explain that there are no alternatives to this procedure. Verbal consent should be adequate unless you are concerned with other circumstances that might increase the risk of litigation.

Occasionally patients will not consent to I&D and request a trial of oral antibiotics. If the abscess is small and not endangering vital structures and the patient is not systemically ill, the physician may contract with the patient for a trial of antibiotics along with warm compresses that may encourage spontaneous drainage of the abscess, with the provision that the patient understands the importance of close follow-up. This may actually be an appropriate treatment plan for a small paronychia or inflamed cyst when it appears to have little to no pus. If the abscess is large, a needle aspiration may prove to the patient the need for full drainage.

## TECHNIQUE

1. Determine how the skin lines run over the abscess. Plan the incision to run parallel to these skin lines to minimize scarring.
2. (Optional) Prep skin with antiseptic agent. Mark the incision site with a surgical marker if desired. This is not a sterile procedure, so a drape is optional.
3. Inject 1% lidocaine with epinephrine into the skin at the site to be opened, using a 27- to 30-gauge needle. (Try to avoid injecting into the abscess cavity because this will increase the pressure and pain to the patient. Use the minimum necessary volume of anesthesia.) Insert the needle peripheral to the central abscess and anesthetize the skin above the abscess until the skin blanches. If the abscess is deep, as with an infected, deep epithelial cyst, you can redirect the needle to anesthetize the deeper surrounding soft tissue. Another approach to anesthetizing the area is to use a field block.[4] A field block is depicted in Fig. 3-5. If the abscess is under a lot of pressure and feels tense, drain off some of the pus with a No. 18 needle on a 10-ml syringe to prevent the abscess from squirting. Proper eye protection should be worn before opening any abscess under pressure. For a small superficial abscess, such as a paronychia, ethyl chloride spray may be used for local anesthesia, spraying until a white frost is visible at the site for puncture.

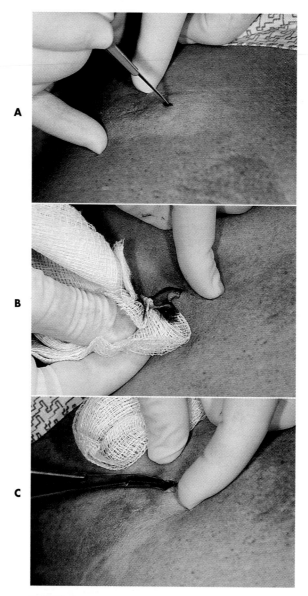

**FIG 13-3**
I&D of an inflamed epidermal cyst. **A,** Opening inflamed cyst with No. 11 scalpel. **B,** Expressing pus from cyst. **C,** Using a hemostat to probe the cyst.

4. Make a stab incision with the No. 11 scalpel (Fig. 13-3, *A*) Direct the point of the scalpel straight into the abscess, with the handle held at a 90-degree angle to the skin. Use the long blade of the scalpel to extend the incision until it is wide enough to easily express the pus.

5. Apply pressure around the abscess to expel the purulence (Fig. 13-3, *B*) This takes time. Have patience. If a culture needs to be obtained from the abscess, the pus that is expelled at this time is the optimal source for sampling.

6. If there is no pus, reassess the situation and determine if the incision was deep enough and in the area of maximum fluctuance (Fig. 13-3, *C*).

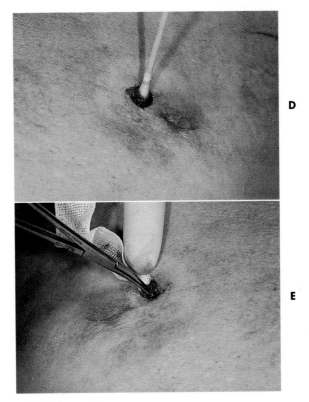

**FIG 13-3, cont'd**
I&D of an inflamed epidermal cyst. **D,** Using cotton-tipped swab with peroxide to clean pus and keratin from cyst. **E,** Packing empty cyst with Nu-Gauze. *Note: A larger incision would have facilitated easier drainage and packing of this lesion.*

7. Use cotton-tipped swabs dipped in hydrogen peroxide to break up loculations and clean out the remaining pus (Fig. 13-3, *D*). Alternatively, a hemostat or a small curette may be used to break up loculations. Because an abscess is rarely symmetric, probe with the swab or another instrument for fingers of extension. It is important to clean out these areas of extension.
8. Repeat steps 5 and 7 if needed.
9. (Optional) Lavage abscess with hydrogen peroxide, local anesthetic, or saline.
10. If the abscess was large, pack the dead space with Nu-Gauze for hemostasis and to keep incision open (Fig. 13-3, *E*). *Note: A larger incision would have facilitated easier drainage and packing of this lesion.*
11. Apply external dressing with 4 × 4 gauze to absorb drainage.

## AFTERCARE

Patients may shower daily and reapply outer gauze. They should not take a bath or swim and immerse the wound in water until the incision is closed. Follow-up visits and removal of packing can be handled in many different ways. There is no evidence to support one practice over another. Choices include the following:

1. Patient returns to the office in 1 to 2 days (1 day if abscess was on face).
   a. Remove packing and repack loosely (especially if purulence remains)
   b. Remove packing and don't repack (especially if erythema is resolving and there is no drainage)
   c. Partially remove packing and leave some gauze in place to remove further at next visit.
2. If the original abscess was small and not in a dangerous location, the patient may be directed to pull out the gauze wick at home and come into the office only if there is significant pus or blood.

### Additional Follow-up

The patient should be directed to not reinsert packing if it falls out. If the physician chooses to repack the wound, the patient should seek follow-up care every few days. Timing and number of follow-up visits should be determined by the severity of the abscess and the speed of resolution. Some physicians recommend warm soaks twice daily after the packing is out. Healing may take 7 to 21 days.

## COMPLICATIONS

Possible complications of I&D include the following:

- Spread of infection locally or systemically (cellulitis, lymphangitis, bacteremia, sepsis)
- Bleeding
- Recurrence of abscess
- Scarring

Patients should be warned to call or come for evaluation if they note new fever or chills or increased redness, swelling, or streaking. Patients who are diabetic, HIV positive, or immunocompromised should receive close follow-up care the day after the procedure if they are not hospitalized.

There is a risk of bleeding if you do not pack the dead space with gauze. If packing is done, there is very little risk of bleeding. The risk of bleeding can be greater in highly vascular areas. If the packing is not working to control the bleeding, electrocoagulation can be used to provide hemostasis. Make sure there is no alcohol or ethyl chloride in the area before using electrocoagulation.

If the physician does not open a large enough hole, the incision can seal up again before the abscess fully drains. This is most likely to happen in an unpacked wound or if the packing is removed too soon in an abscess that was not opened adequately. This may also occur if there was inadequate probing for loculations or inadequate aftercare. Scarring may occur but it can be minimized by following skin lines when making the initial incision. Although larger incisions may have a greater chance of leaving a scar, this must be balanced with the need to get adequate initial drainage and avoiding premature closure of the opening.

## SPECIAL CIRCUMSTANCES

### Paronychia of the Toe

Paronychia is an infection of the nail fold. On the finger, it is often a staphylococcal infection with a small abscess. On the toe, it is often an inflammatory process caused by an ingrown toenail. Although ingrown toenails are common on the big toe, a small abscess may occur as seen in Fig. 13-4. More commonly, the toe paronychia often requires partial toenail removal, which is not strictly an I&D.

In Fig. 13-4, it was decided to use ethyl chloride for topical anesthesia before draining the small paronychia. When the point of maximal fluctuance turned white from the ethyl chloride, a No. 11 blade was inserted into the abscess. The pus drained freely and the area did not need to be packed. Systemic antibiotics were not needed, and the patient was directed to soak his foot in warm water 2 times per day. If a toenail paronychia is recurrent and associated with an ingrown nail, ablation of the lateral horn of the nail and its associated matrix can be performed at the same time as the toenail removal.

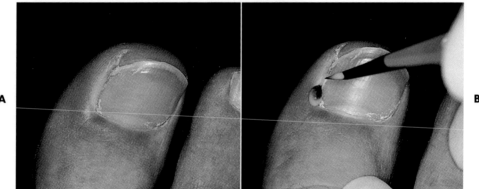

**FIG 13-4**
Paronychia of the toe. **A,** Small abscess at nail fold. **B,** Drainage of pus using No. 11 scalpel.

## Paronychia of the Finger

Chronic paronychia of the finger is often associated with a *Candida* infection and does not need to be cut open. If the acute paronychia is fluctuant (Fig. 13-5, *A*), I&D is indicated. If the nail fold is red and there appears to be no pocket of pus in an acute paronychia, treatment can proceed with warm soaks and oral antibiotics.

In a paronychia of the finger, ethyl chloride can be used for used for local anesthesia. It is quick and easy and spares the patient from a needle stick. In Fig. 13-5, *B*, the blade is pointed directly into the large pocket of pus. If the area of fluctuance is small and only superficial, it may help to hold the blade flat with the nail fold and skin. These incisions are usually too small to pack. Patients can be directed to soak finger the twice daily for a few days to ensure adequate drainage of purulence.

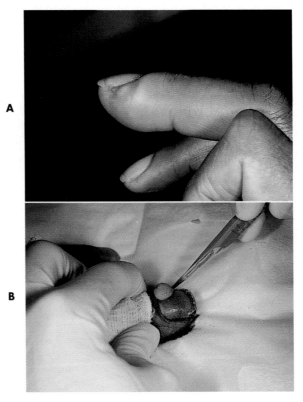

**FIG 13-5**
Paronychia of the finger. **A,** Swelling of distal finger.
**B,** Drainage of purulence with No. 11 scalpel.

## Inflamed Epithelial Cyst

The fact that a physician is dealing with an inflamed epithelial cyst may be evident by the presence of a central punctum. This is confirmed when white keratinaceous material is expressed along with pus from the incision site. If the cyst wall can be removed, recurrence of the cyst may be prevented. Most often when an epithelial cyst is inflamed, the cyst wall is obscured. When this occurs, the physician should discuss the pros and cons of having the patient return to remove the remaining cyst after the infection heals. If the cyst is inflamed and does not appear to be full of pus, oral antibiotics may be prescribed and the cyst excised when the inflammation/infection cools down.

## Milia

To perform I&D on milia, make a small opening in the milia with a needle or a No. 11 scalpel (Fig. 13-6, A). Because the opening is small and superficial, use of local anesthesia is not necessary. Express the contents (keratin) of the milia with a comedone extractor (Fig. 13-6, B).

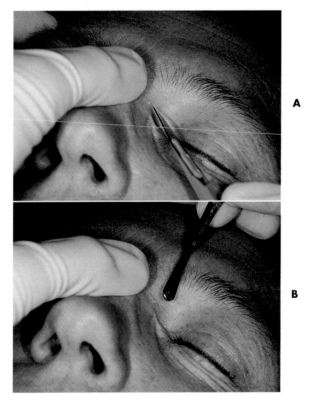

**FIG 13-6**
I&D of small milia. **A,** Approaching the milia carefully with No. 11 scalpel. **B,** Comedone extractor removes keratin from opened milia.

## USE OF ANTIBIOTICS

The use of antibiotics to treat a skin abscess is controversial. Most authors agree that full drainage of a simple abscess should be adequate treatment. Because the surrounding erythema may be caused by inflammation only, it should resolve with I&D. However, if there appears to be a true bacterial cellulitis, an oral antibiotic is indicated. Because most skin abscesses are caused by *S. aureus*, the antibiotic should provide good staphylococcus coverage (i.e., dicloxacillin and cephalexin). If the patient is diabetic, HIV positive, or immunocompromised, consider doing a culture and gram stain and starting empiric antibiotics in addition to I&D.

## CONCLUSION

I&D is an essential procedure that should be mastered by any physician taking care of basic skin problems. It is easy to learn, and it is the treatment of choice for skin abscess.

## REFERENCES

1. Derksen DJ: Incision and drainage of an abscess. In Pfenninger JL, Fowler GC, editors: *Procedures for primary care physicians,* St. Louis, 1994, Mosby.
2. Moy JG, Pfenninger JL: Peripheral nerve blocks and field blocks. In Pfenninger JL, Fowler GC, editors: *Procedures for primary care physicians*, St. Louis, 1994, Mosby.
3. Sanford JP, Gilbert DN, Sande MA: *The Sanford guide to antimicrobial therapy,* Vienna, Va, 1996, Antimicrobial Therapy Inc.
4. Graber R: Procedures for your practice: incision and drainage of cutaneous abscesses, *Patient Care* Dec 15, pp 163-168, 1986

# CHAPTER 14

# Intralesional Injections

*Richard P. Usatine*

Intralesional injections of steroids are used to decrease inflammation in lesions such as cystic acne and granuloma annulare, to flatten keloids and hypertrophic scars, and to increase hair regrowth in alopecia areata. In dermatology, bleomycin is used for intralesional injections of verrucae. However, this chapter will focus on the use of steroids for injections of various skin lesions. Although, triamcinolone (Kenalog) suspensions are most often used for these injections, other injectable steroids may be used. Choosing or mixing the appropriate-strength steroid and injecting the steroid into the correct location are the most crucial aspects of this process.

## INDICATIONS

Indications for the use of intralesional injections include the following:

- Keloids
- Hypertrophic scars
- Acne cysts
- Granuloma annulare
- Hidradenitis suppurativa

Other lesions that are commonly injected with steroids include alopecia areata, psoriasis, and lichen planus. Although we do not cover these lesions in this chapter, further information is available on the injection of these conditions in Habif's *Clinical Dermatology: A Color Guide to Diagnosis and Therapy.*[1]

## CONTRAINDICATIONS

Intralesional injection of steroids should be avoided if lesions are too extensive.

## EQUIPMENT (FIG. 14-1)

- Injectable steroids (triamcinolone acetonide 3 mg/ml, 10 mg/ml, 40 mg/ml)
- Needles (25 g to 30 g)
- Syringes (1 ml or 3 ml [Luer Lok preferable])
- Vials of sterile saline for injection (for dilutions)

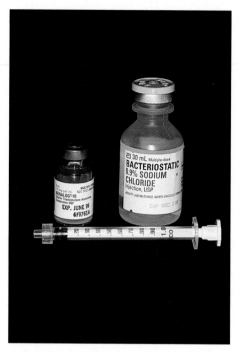

**FIG 14-1**
Equipment for intralesional injections: triamcinolone 10 mg/ml, bacteriostatic sodium chloride, and a 1-ml Luer Lok syringe for injection.

Special 1-ml Luer Lok syringes and triamcinolone acetonide 3 mg/ml (Tac-3) are manufactured specifically for intralesional injection. Special labels are available that can be applied to vials of normal saline when used for dilution of triamcinolone. These labels have instructions on how to dilute triamcinolone and are available through Delasco.

## INFORMED CONSENT

Patients should be informed of the risks of skin atrophy, incomplete resolution of the lesion, and changes in skin pigmentation. If the appropriate steroid strength and dose is used, the risk of atrophy should be minimal. Consider having the patient sign a consent form, especially if the lesion is on the face.

## STEROID STRENGTH

Once the appropriate-strength steroid for the injection has been chosen, the standard-strength preparations may need to be diluted to produce the desired

**TABLE 14-1   Recommended Strength of Steroid for Intralesional Injections**

| Lesion | Triamcinolone mg/ml |
| --- | --- |
| Keloids and hypertrophic scars | 10-40 mg/ml (start with weaker strength for first injection [10 mg/ml if on the face]) |
| Cystic acne of face | 1-2 mg/ml |
| Cystic acne (not on face) | 2-3 mg/ml |
| Granuloma annulare | 3-10 mg/ml |
| Hidradenitis suppurativa | 2-5 mg/ml |

**TABLE 14-2   Needle Size for Injection**

| Lesion | Needle size (gauge) |
| --- | --- |
| Keloid (hypertrophic scars) | 25-27 |
| Acne | 30 |
| Granuloma annulare | 25-30 |
| Hidradenitis suppurativa | 27-30 |

strength. Recommendations for steroid strength are listed in Table 14-1. Triamcinolone acetonide suspension is available in three strengths: 3, 10, and 40 mg/ml. It is essential to dilute the steroid for a number of injections, especially for injections of cystic acne of the face. Dilution may be done for each patient just before giving the injection or may be done in a sterile vial of saline and saved for the injection of multiple patients over time. Unless you are giving intralesional injections frequently, it is probably better to perform the dilution for each patient. Vials that you create by dilution can lose their potency and have a higher theoretical risk of contamination.

Triamcinolone is most often diluted with sterile normal saline for injection. Alternatives include sterile water or 1% lidocaine (without epinephrine). The isotonicity of sterile saline makes it the preferred solution for dilution.

A 1-ml Luer Lok or tuberculin syringe is useful for making a single dilution before injection. To create a 2 mg/ml concentration, draw 0.4 ml of sterile saline into a l-ml syringe and add 0.1 ml of 10 mg/ml triamcinolone. You will need to turn the syringe upside down a number of times to mix the new suspension. It is recommended that the saline be drawn up first because it is more acceptable to get a little saline into the triamcinolone than vice versa. Recommended needle sizes by lesion are listed in Table 14-2.

## TECHNIQUE BY LESION

### Keloids and Hypertrophic Scars

A hypertrophic scar is one in which the scar tissue is raised and prominent over the area that was cut, burned, or frozen. It may show prominent suture marks and can be redder or differently pigmented compared with the surrounding tissue. Hypertrophic scars frequently regress over a few years. A keloid looks like a bad hypertrophic scar that grew beyond the limits of the original surgery. This growth allows keloids to become quite raised and enlarged. There are even histologic differences between hypertrophic scars and keloids. For the purpose of intralesional injection, however, they are treated identically. Keloids are more

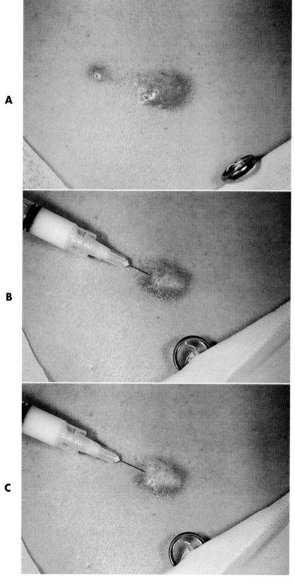

FIG 14-2

Injection of a keloid on the chest. **A,** Two keloids from acne scars on the chest of a 35-year-old woman. **B,** Needle inserted into the body of the larger keloid. **C,** White steroid is filling the keloid.

often symptomatic, and patients may note pain, tenderness, and hyperesthesia, especially in the early stages of keloid development.[1]

Persons with darker skin are at higher risk (15 to 20 times normal) of developing keloids than light-skinned persons. Keloids most commonly occur on the chest and shoulders, but can occur anywhere on the skin. Keloids can occur after acne and ear piercing. Hypertrophic scars may itch but rarely are as symptomatic as keloids. Keloids and hypertrophic scars can be treated with steroid injections, cryotherapy, and surgery. However, because hypertrophic scars often regress, surgical excision is often unnecessary.

We recommend starting with 10 mg/ml of triamcinolone for the first treatment of a keloid or hypertrophic scar. The needle should be introduced into the body of the keloid at a 20- to 30-degree angle with the skin. It is important that the tip of the needle is within the keloid and not below it. Proper needle position should result in a whitening of the keloid as the white suspension is injected into the keloid (Fig. 14-2). If the needle is too deep, reposition it and restart the injection. Inject firmly while advancing the needle and observing the keloid blanch.[1]

In Figs. 14-2 and 14-3, a 35-year-old woman developed keloids from acne scars on her chest and arm. The patient requested injection. In both sites, 40 mg/ml triamcinolone was injected into the keloids with a 30-gauge needle inserted into the body of the keloid. The white steroid is seen filling the keloid after the injection is complete. In Fig. 14-2, *E*, the smaller keloid is gone and the larger keloid is flatter 5 months after the single injection. The patient received a second injection at this time.

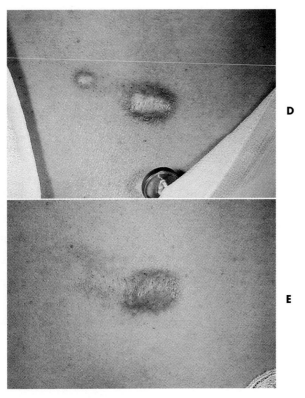

**FIG 14-2, cont'd**
Injection of a keloid on the chest. **D**, Steroid injection completed. **E**, 5 months after single injection, the smaller keloid is gone and the larger keloid is flatter. The patient received a second injection at this time.

In Fig. 14-3, *B*, the keloid on the arm resolved completely with significant skin atrophy. The skin was indented and thinned from the steroid. In retrospect, the injection of the arm keloid distended the keloid too much and the 40 mg/ml triamcinolone was too potent for this site. This suggests that it is better to start with 10 mg/ml for the first injection of a keloid to determine how the patient will respond. You can always use a more potent concentration in subsequent injections if the lower concentration fails.

Large keloids may need multiple injections at one time to adequately infiltrate the lesion. Sometimes the needle can be pulled back and reoriented for the next injection from the same puncture site. The quantity injected should be just enough to blanch the entire keloid white. Hypertrophic scars are injected using the same technique. A 3-ml LuerLok syringe facilitates the injection into these firm structures.

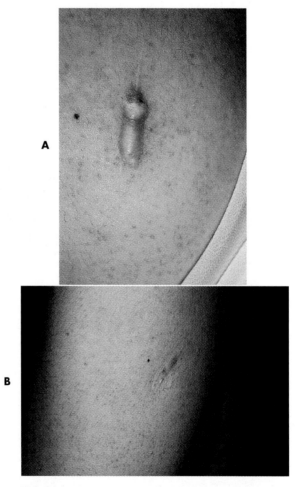

**FIG 14-3**
Keloid on arm before and after injection that resulted in skin atrophy. **A,** Keloid from acne scar on upper arm of the same 35-year-old woman in Fig. 14-2. This injection distended the keloid too much and the 40 mg/ml triamcinolone was too potent for this site. **B,** Skin atrophy 5 months after the single injection.

If the keloid is older and/or firmer, it may not respond to injection therapy as well as softer and newer lesions (Fig. 14-4). It may help to pretreat the keloid with cryotherapy.[1,2] Various recommendations are found in the literature for the amount of freezing to use before injection. Habif recommends applying liquid nitrogen for 2 to 4 seconds and waiting 10 to 15 minutes before injecting the steroid.[1] Zuber and Pfenninger recommend a 10- to 15-second freeze and a waiting period of 20 to 60 minutes.[2] We freeze a keloid or hypertropic scar to obtain a 3- to 5-second freeze time and then wait 2 minutes before doing the injection. We do not freeze a margin of normal tissue. We attempt to confine the iceball to the very center of the lesion with a 3- to 5-second freeze. This minimizes pain and also prevents the destruction of normal tissue around the lesions. After liquid nitrogen or another freezing modality is applied to the scars, they are allowed to thaw and develop edema. This generally takes 1 to 2 minutes, which allows the easier introduction of intralesional corticosteroids into the pulp of these lesions. Multiple treatment sessions usually are required, but we attempt to space the time between treatments to at least 2 to 3 weeks. Spacing treatments too closely will increased the risk of atrophy caused by the intralesional steroids.

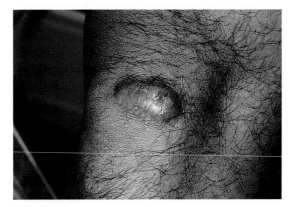

**FIG 14-4**
Old keloid on leg, refractory to injection alone. Cryotherapy and injection should be used.

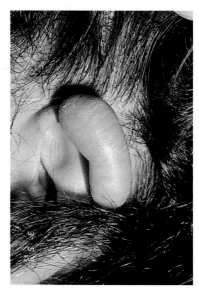

**FIG 14-5**
This keloid on an ear is too large for
injection alone.

Fig. 14-5 shows a keloid on the ear that is too large for injection alone. Successful treatment of this keloid will require a surgical excision and injection of the base with steroid. Because of its size and location, this is a good lesion to refer to a specialist.

## Acne Cysts

Acne cysts can be injected with 1 to 3 mg/ml of triamcinolone using a 30-gauge needle on a 1-ml syringe at a 90-degree angle with the skin (Fig. 14-6). If the acne cyst is on the face, 1 to 2 mg/ml should be used. Enough liquid should be injected to see and feel the cyst become distended but no more than 0.1 ml for any one cyst. One injection site per acne cyst should be adequate. If the cyst is large and tense, you may incise the cyst with a small stab incision from a No. 11 scalpel after the injection to drain the cyst contents. However, in most cases it is unnecessary to drain the cyst after the steroid injection.

## Hidradenitis Suppurativa

Injecting hidradenitis suppurativa is similar to injecting an acne cyst but one lesion may be injected with up to 5 mg/ml of triamcinolone. Because the cysts are often larger than acne, a 3-ml syringe may be needed to provide more volume for injection. Large, purulent cysts can be drained with a No. 11 scalpel if needed.

## Granuloma Annulare

Granuloma annulare (See Fig. 5-11) should be injected in a process similar to injecting a keloid or hypertropic scar, using a less diluted triamcinolone suspension of 5 mg/ml. A few injection sites may be needed to cover the entire annular lesion.

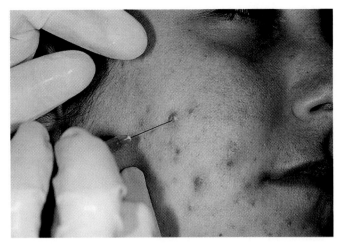

**FIG 14-6**
Steroid injection (1.5 mg/ml of triamcinolone) in an acne cyst on the face.

## COMPLICATIONS

Complications include skin atrophy (Fig. 14-3, *B*) and pigmentary changes, especially hypopigmentation. If skin atrophy occurs, it is worth waiting a number of months to see if the atrophy will resolve. After 4 months the patient could receive injections of their own fat to restore the depressed area. This can be performed with a liposuction and injection technique. One author suggests that an injection of normal saline into the depressed area has been successful in reducing atrophy. Although this has not been rigorously tested, the author claims that it may dilute any remaining steroid crystals and he has had empiric success with this technique.

## AFTERCARE

No special aftercare is needed other than follow-up for inspection of the results and consideration of additional treatments.

## CONCLUSION

A number of dermatologic conditions respond well to the intralesional injection of steroid suspensions. The basic technique is very useful in the treatment of conditions such as keloids, hypertrophic scars, acne cysts, granuloma annulare, and hidradenitis suppurativa.

## REFERENCES

1. Habif TP: *Clinical dermatology: a color guide to diagnosis and therapy,* ed 3, St. Louis, 1996, Mosby, p 167 (acne), p 637 (keloids and scars).
2. Zuber TJ, Pfenninger JL: Treatment of hypertrophic scars and keloids. In Pfenninger JL, Fowler GC, editors: *Procedures for primary care physicians,* St. Louis, 1994, Mosby.

# CHAPTER 15

# Diagnosis and Treatment of Benign and Premalignant Lesions

*Edward L. Tobinick**

Familiarity with the treatment modalities of the most common benign cutaneous lesions is essential for all physicians who have primary care responsibilities. Benign cutaneous lesions are conveniently grouped into three categories: those with predominantly epidermal involvement, those with predominantly dermal involvement, and those that are subcutaneous (Table 15-1). There are a variety of modalities available to treat each of these benign lesions, including electrosurgery, cryosurgery, punch biopsy, shave biopsy, excision, topical agents, incision and drainage, and intralesional injection of steroids. This chapter discusses in detail the treatment of individual lesions.

## EPIDERMAL LESIONS

This section encompasses benign growths that either wholly or predominantly involve the epidermis. Several of these lesions, such as actinic keratoses and lentigines, are flat. Others, such as verrucae and seborrheic keratoses, can be quite raised (despite the fact that they involve only the epidermis) because of epidermal hyperplasia. In general, epidermal lesions can be removed with a minimum of scarring if they are properly treated. In addition, because of their superficial location, they are amenable to removal with the use of topical agents, such as trichloroacetic acid, as well as the more destructive physical modalities, such as electrosurgery.

### Acrochordons (Skin Tags)

Acrochordons (Fig. 15-1) are most commonly found on the neck, axilla, and groin. Multiple lesions frequently develop with pregnancy, and some of these will resolve spontaneously after delivery. Many typical acrochordons (those that have a thin neck and are small [1 to 3 mm]) are most easily removed by snip excision using a small pair of sharp scissors. Spraying each lesion with ethyl chloride before snipping provides adequate anesthesia. Aluminum chloride can then be used for hemostasis. Tiny acrochordons and broad-based lesions are amenable to light electrosurgery. Cryosurgery is an alternative treatment. Broad-based acrochordons, particularly those in the groin and the axilla, can be very vascular and are best shaved or snipped off after injection with lidocaine and epinephrine. An electrosurgical unit should be available for hemostasis if the topical hemostatic agent does not work.

*Illustrations by Richard P. Usatine.

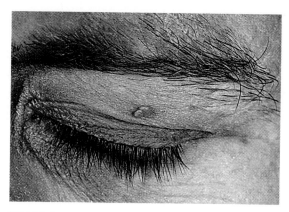

**FIG 15-1**
Acrochordon on upper eyelid.

**TABLE 15-1    Overview of Treatment of Benign Cutaneous Tumors**

| Type of lesion | Preferred modalities* | Optional modalities* |
|---|---|---|
| **Epidermal Lesions** | | |
| Acrochordons | Scissors snip excision, electrosurgery | Cryosurgery |
| Actinic keratoses | Cryosurgery, topical chemicals, curretage +/− cautery (allows tactile feel) | Electrosurgery, shave biopsy |
| Condyloma acuminata | Topical chemicals | Electrosurgery, shave biopsy |
| Cutaneous horn | Shave biopsy | |
| Freckles | Cryosurgery | |
| Lentigines | Cryosurgery | Punch biopsy, if atypical |
| Molluscum contagiosum | Curettage | Cryosurgery, shave biopsy, topical chemicals |
| Plantar verruca | Topical chemicals, intralesional bleomycin | Cryosurgery, laser surgery, immunotherapy |
| Porokeratosis | Paring, cryosurgery | |
| Seborrheic keratoses | Curettage, cryosurgery, shave biopsy, electrosurgery | |
| Verruca plana | Topical chemicals, cryosurgery | Light electrosurgery, immunotherapy |
| Verruca vulgaris | Topical agents, cryosurgery | Electrosurgery, shave excision, intralesional bleomycin, laser therapy, immunotherapy |
| Xanthelasma | Cryosurgery | |

*The distinction between preferred and optional treatment modalities is based on the authors' experiences and is meant to serve as a guideline only. The optimal method of treatment varies and depends on many individual factors, including anatomic location, size of the lesion, cosmetic and cost considerations, and other individual factors. This table is designed as a general guide because in most cases there is not one single correct way to biopsy or remove a lesion. Within a given category, individual skill and preference will often determine the actual treatment modality. If you are not sure of the best approach for a given patient or anatomic site, consider consultation.

*Continued*

## TABLE 15-1   Overview of Treatment of Benign Cutaneous Tumors—cont'd

| Type of lesion | Preferred modalities* | Optional modalities* |
| --- | --- | --- |
| **Dermal Lesions** | | |
| Angioma, telangiectasia | Electrosurgery, laser therapy | Shave (angioma) |
| Dermatofibroma | Punch (if small), shave plus cryosurgery | Excision, intralesional corticosteroids |
| Hypertrophic scars and keloids | Cryosurgery, intralesional steroids | Excision or shave (with caution) plus intralesional steroids, silicon gel, sheeting |
| Keratoacanthoma | Shave biopsy, then curretage and dessication, excision | Cryosurgery |
| Milia | Incision and drainage | Shave, electrosurgery, punch |
| Mucocele | Cryosurgery or electrosurgery after incision and drainage | Shave, punch, or elliptical excision |
| Nevi | Shave biopsy, punch biopsy, elliptical excision | |
| Neurofibroma | Shave excision, punch, or elliptical excision | Cryosurgery, electrosurgery |
| Prurigo nodularis | Cryosurgery, topical medications | Electrosurgery, shave excision, intralesional steroids |
| Pyogenic granuloma | Shave, curettage, then electrosurgery or excisional biopsy | |
| Sebaceous hyperplasia | Cryosurgery, light electrosurgery, shave biopsy | Punch biopsy |
| **Subcutaneous Tumors and Cysts** | | |
| Epidermal cyst | Small elliptical excision, incision and drainage if ruptured | Incision and drainage plus intralesional steroids |
| Pilar cyst | Linear or small elliptical excision | |
| Lipoma | Linear excision, small incision and extrusion, elliptical excision | Liposuction |

*The distinction between preferred and optional treatment modalities is based on the authors' experiences and is meant to serve as a guideline only. The optimal method of treatment varies and depends on many individual factors, including anatomic location, size of the lesion, cosmetic and cost considerations, and other individual factors. This table is designed as a general guide because in most cases there is not one single correct way to biopsy or remove a lesion. Within a given category, individual skill and preference will often determine the actual treatment modality. If you are not sure of the best approach for a given patient or anatomic site, consider consultation.

## Actinic Keratoses

Actinic keratoses (Fig. 15-2) are most commonly seen in light-skinned individuals in areas that have been chronically overexposed to sunlight, particularly the face, scalp, and dorsum of the hands. Many of these patients have a great number of lesions scattered diffusely in the areas of actinic damage. These patients are best treated with topical fluorouracil cream or solution, 5% applied twice daily for a period of 4 weeks on the face and 6 weeks on the arms, scalp, and back of the hands. Shorter courses may result in only transient improvement. This topical chemotherapy has the advantage of treating incipient lesions and allowing

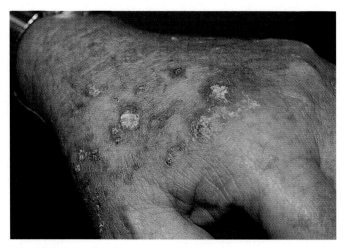

**FIG 15-2**
Multiple actinic keratoses on the dorsum of the hand. Some lesions are
hypertrophic and require biopsy to rule out SCC.

patients to treat themselves. The disadvantage of fluorouracil treatment is that
severe redness and inflammation can result. The skin may look terrible, and the
patient may become very self-conscious.

An alternative plan for treating patients with topical fluorouracil is to have the
patient use it every third night instead of every day. Using the 1% cream instead
of the 5% cream may cause less irritation. This plan will require that the patient
be treated for many months before the lesions may resolve. Masoprocol (Actinex)
is a newer topical medicine used to treat actinic keratosis. It works like fluorouracil cream but may result in less irritation. However, masoprocol may cause
a higher incidence of allergic contact dermatitis.

Patients with solitary or a small number of lesions can be treated with
cryosurgery, which is rapid, produces an excellent cosmetic result, and has high
patient acceptance. Either one or multiple lesions can be treated at any given
patient session. Actinic keratoses may be lightly frozen to produce a 1- to 2-mm
halo. When using liquid nitrogen, the freeze time is usually 3 to 5 seconds.

Lesions that are hypertrophic or have palpable induration or infiltration should
usually undergo biopsy to rule out progression to squamous cell carcinoma (SCC).
The thicker, red scaling lesions that have not responded to two or three liquid
nitrogen treatments should undergo shave biopsy to both remove the lesion and
to obtain a pathologic diagnosis. Borderline lesions can sometimes be treated with
more aggressive cryosurgery or curettage and dessication. These patients should
be seen regularly for follow-up examinations to check for response to previous
treatments and to look for new actinic keratoses or skin cancers.

## Condyloma Acuminata

Condyloma acuminata (See Fig. 11-9) are sexually transmitted warts. They are
contagious, and some serotypes (e.g., 16, 18, 31, 33) are associated with an
increased incidence of cervical carcinoma in women. Warts are removed to prevent their growth and their spread to others. Because of their transmissible
nature, the therapeutic goal should be complete eradication. Condyloma can be
challenging to treat because they have a tendency to recur regardless of the treatment modality, and they are frequently multiple. Patients who have not had

access to care or who have been hesitant to seek professional consultation can have hundreds of large lesions that can occasionally be disfiguring. For isolated lesions on the penile shaft or on the vulva, cryosurgery is the ideal treatment (See Chapter 11). Care must be taken when treating multiple lesions in sensitive areas because cryosurgery can produce a considerable amount of discomfort and local swelling. Additionally, therapy that is unnecessarily aggressive can result in damage to vital structures (penile vessels and nerves) or painful webbing (labia).

Topical chemicals are appropriate for certain patients with condyloma acuminata. Used topically, podophyllin is particularly effective for lesions in moist areas. Physicians should beware of using podophyllin for lesions that are very extensive, and keep in mind that podophyllin by itself is generally not effective for lesions on dry areas such as the shaft of the penis. Podophyllin is useful to shrink extensive lesions before surgical removal. Condylox, a newer preparation of podophyllotoxin, appears to be more effective than podophyllin and also can be used postoperatively after the use of cryosurgery or electrosurgery to prevent recurrence. However, Condylox produces a considerable amount of local irritation, so it must be used with extreme care. Condylox and podophyllin are contraindicated in pregnant women. Trichloroacetic acid can also be used and is favored by many for use with vulvar and intravaginal condyloma. Extensive intravaginal condyloma are generally best handled by a gynecologist and occasionally will require laser treatment. Biopsy is important in large lesions to rule out the possibility of malignant degeneration.

Electrosurgery can be used to treat lesions that have failed to respond to cryosurgery or treatment with topical agents. Care must be taken when using electrosurgery to avoid damage to deeper elements of the dermis that may result in scarring. Healing with electrosurgery may be prolonged, especially for extensive lesions.

## Cutaneous Horns

Cutaneous horns (Fig. 15-3) are keratotic papules most frequently found in areas of actinic damage, such as the face, ears, scalp, and the backs of hands. *Cutaneous horn* is a descriptive term based on clinical appearance, but the underlying pathology can be varied, including seborrheic keratosis, SCC, basal cell carcino-

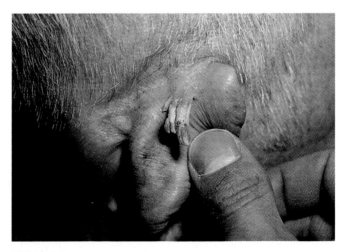

**FIG 15-3**
Cutaneous horn on the back of the ear. Histologic examination is necessary to identify the underlying lesion.

ma (BCC), or keratoacanthoma. For this reason, the proper treatment is to perform a deep shave biopsy, making sure to include the entire base of the lesion.

## Freckles (Ephelides)

Freckles are confined to the uppermost epidermis, necessitating very judicious use of destructive treatments to avoid scarring. Freckles are best left untreated and will often fade during the winter months or when sun exposure is limited. If a patient is insisting on treatment, cryosurgery is the only treatment we recommend. When using liquid nitrogen, care should be taken that freckles are frozen without freezing normal skin. Generally, freckles require only a 2- to 5-second freeze with liquid nitrogen. When treating these hyperpigmented macules for cosmetic reasons, we always warn our patients that there is a risk of hypopigmentation. We also will generally start with one or two lesions as a test before treating multiple lesions. When using liquid nitrogen, the applicator of choice is a cotton-tipped swab, but a cryogun can be used with a small aperture if available.

## Lentigo Simplex

Lentigo simplex (Fig. 15-4) is a benign pigmented macule that can vary in size from 0.2 to 2 cm. Many of these lesions are sun induced and are called *solar lentigines* (pleural for *lentigo*). Many lentigines are seen on the hands, face, and arms of older persons and are often called *sun spots* or *liver spots* by the general population. Atypical lentigines, such as those with variegation of color or large size, will usually require biopsy before treatment to differentiate them from lentigo maligna or early melanoma (See Figs. 9-1, 9-2, and 9-9). Lentigines in children are generally not sun induced. In Fig. 15-4, a 12-year-old girl noted that a dark spot on her shoulder was itching and growing. A 3-mm punch biopsy was performed to excise the lesion fully and rule out melanoma.

If a lentigo is small and regular in shape and color, it may be treated with liquid nitrogen using the same procedure as for freckles. Alternatively, the pigment of solar lentigines may be lightened with topical tretinoin, hydroquinones, or azelaic acid.

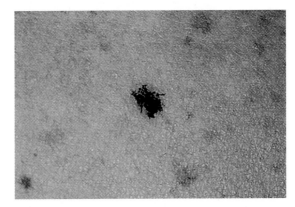

**FIG 15-4**
Lentigo simplex on the shoulder. The dark, irregular lentigo
is surrounded by lightly pigmented freckles.

## Molluscum Contagiosum

Molluscum contagiosum lesions (Fig. 15-5) are caused by a pox virus that is transmissible. These lesions are common in children and also are seen in adults. Molluscum contagiosum are epidermal lesions and, if treated carefully, will generally resolve with little or no scarring. Care must be taken to avoid aggressive electrosurgery or the use of other modalities that can cause scarring because these lesions frequently are in cosmetically sensitive places, such as the face or the genital area. In our experience, curettage is the preferred treatment. Before curettage, the lesions can be individually anesthetized with a small amount of injectable lidocaine; in children we use EMLA cream to achieve cutaneous anesthesia without injection. Curettage is less painful than cryosurgery, gives an excellent cosmetic result, and is extremely rapid to perform. Multiple sessions are usually required to treat molluscum contagiosum because of the subsequent appearance of new lesions after the first treatment episode. After curettage, the use of a hemostatic agent such as aluminum chloride or Monsel's solution will usually be adequate to stop the minor bleeding. If not, very light electrodesiccation may be used to obtain complete hemostasis.

For small children that will not sit still for any of these procedures, topical agents such as Retin-A, cantharidin, or salicylic acid preparations may be used. Many of these patients will spontaneously resolve their molluscum contagiosum after a number of months. For adults with sexually transmitted molluscum, however, we prefer complete eradication of all existing lesions, with careful follow-up to detect and treat any new lesions that occur. The physician should remember that molluscum contagiosum and condyloma acuminata are not necessarily solitary diseases, and evaluation for other sexually transmitted diseases should be made.

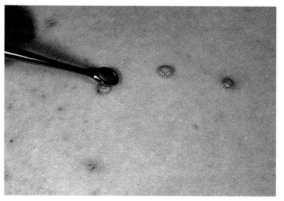

**FIG 15-5**
Curettage of molluscum contagiosum.

## Plantar Verrucae

Plantar verrucae (Fig. 15-6) are a challenging therapeutic problem. Frequently multiple, these lesions can even be confluent ("mosaic") and extensive. There probably is truth to the belief that plantar verrucae can be transmitted from the shower floor, so our first advice to patients with verrucae is to wear rubber sandals in the shower to prevent transmission or reinfection. Relief can be achieved by a simple paring of the warts with a No. 15 scalpel blade. Another method of treatment is the intralesional injection of bleomycin,[1] which usually must be repeated a second or third time 2 weeks after the initial treatment. Because bleomycin is a potentially toxic chemotherapeutic agent, this therapy requires experience on the part of the physician and should not be used during pregnancy.

Topical salicylic acid preparations, particularly "the old standby" 40% salicylic acid plasters, are safe and effective for treating plantar warts but are also time consuming. Cryosurgery (See Chapter 11) and electrosurgery (See Chapter 12) are alternatives, as is laser therapy, but each of these treatments has particular disadvantages (pain, scarring, and cost, respectively).

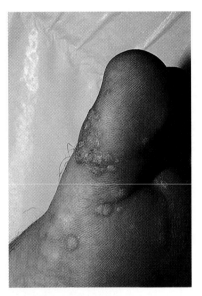

**FIG 15-6**
Multiple plantar verrucae.

## Porokeratosis

Porokeratosis (Fig. 15-7) is generally a solitary lesion that occurs on the sole of the foot, where it presents as a slow-growing, hyperkeratotic papule that can be mistaken for a plantar wart. Porokeratosis is a benign lesion that is caused by hypertrophy of the stratum corneum around the duct of a sweat gland. Porokeratosis can be differentiated from a plantar wart by its lack of pinpoint bleeding areas when pared. The preferred treatment is shave removal, generally with a No. 15 blade. Slow paring is recommended, to avoid bleeding or discomfort. These lesions are usually thick, and their removal will eliminate the discomfort that they cause when walking.

## Seborrheic Keratoses

Seborrheic keratoses (Figs. 15-8 and 15-9) are benign epidermal lesions that occur in many shapes and sizes. Most commonly, they have a stuck-on, warty appearance and do not require a biopsy for diagnosis. However, they can also be indistinguishable from malignant melanoma, requiring biopsy and histopathologic examination for final diagnosis. We have seen several malignant melanomas that were present within a field of multiple seborrheic keratoses; careful examination was required before they were discovered. Many patients have multiple keratoses, sometimes so many that treatment is impractical. More often, however, there are several scattered lesions.

Some patients will be satisfied to learn that the lesions are benign and do not require treatment. Lesions that are very suggestive of malignant melanoma should be excised in their entirety as discussed in Chapter 16. More often, the physician is confronted with lesions that are suggestive but not diagnostic of seborrheic keratosis. These lesions can undergo shave biopsy.

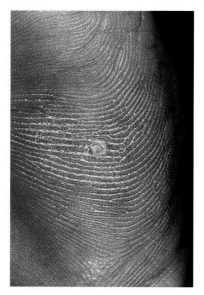

**FIG 15-7**
Porokeratosis. These lesions are frequently misdiagnosed as plantar verrucae. They lack the characteristic thrombosed capillaries of plantar verrucae.

Treatment of seborrheic keratoses of which the identity is certain can be done with either cryosurgery, electrosurgery, curettage, shave removal, or a combination of these treatment modalities. For seborrheic keratoses on individuals who have a tendency to form keloids or in areas that are cosmetically sensitive, such as the face or center of the chest in women, we generally prefer cryosurgery (See Chapter 11).

Cryosurgery may be the quickest way to treat multiple lesions. The disadvantage of this technique is that it may be difficult to judge the freeze needed to obtain complete removal in one session. The melanocytes in the skin are very sensitive to cold injury, and hypopigmentation can occur. Cryosurgery wounds also create more edema, redness, and inflammation than the other techniques.

A preferred technique for treating seborrheic keratoses on the back and trunk involves the use of lidocaine and epinephrine followed by light electrodesiccation or fulguration to the tops of the keratotic lesions, thereby softening them. This is followed by light curettage with a small (3 or 4 mm) curette. A hemostatic agent

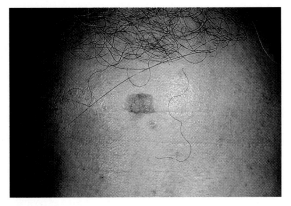

**FIG 15-8**
Seborrheic keratosis on the forehead. There is a smaller sebaceous hyperplasia inferior to the keratosis. The patient elected to not treat these benign lesions.

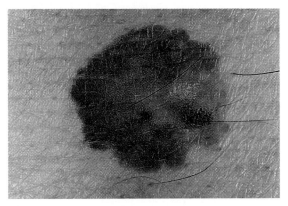

**FIG 15-9**
Seborrheic keratosis (proved by punch biopsy). Because the large size, irregular borders, and variegated color can mimic melanoma, a 2-mm punch biopsy was performed within the darkest portion of the lesion.

such as aluminum chloride is then applied to the area. If care is used to avoid excessive electrosurgery, this technique can yield excellent cosmetic results.

Because a seborrheic keratosis is superficial and "stuck on," the difference between the keratosis and the normal skin below it is detectable when using the curette. If the lesion is lightly cauterized first, it may be wiped off with gauze, and the curette may not be needed.

Shave removal with a No. 15 blade, or for larger lesions a No. 10 blade, is also effective and can leave an excellent cosmetic result if care is taken to avoid a large divot.

## Verruca Plana

Verruca plana, or flat warts (See Fig. 11-18), are typically a difficult therapeutic problem. They tend to respond poorly to treatment, and it is easy for the cosmetic effect of treatment to look worse than the warts themselves. Nevertheless, flat warts do slowly respond to several agents.

Multiple flat warts on the face are a common problem. Multiple flat warts are also common on the legs in women, and are probably spread by shaving. In both of these situations, we recommend patients use separate shaving devices: one for the area over the warts and one for areas that are wart free. Multiple warts can respond to topical tretinoin or topical fluorouracil, either singly or in combination. Patients with isolated lesions can be treated with cryosurgery or light electrodesiccation.

## Verruca Vulgaris (Common Warts)

Warts caused by human papilloma virus (Fig. 15-10) are a common condition and can present the physician with a difficult therapeutic problem. On the one hand, these warts are benign, generally asymptomatic, and can spontaneously disappear. On the other hand, they can be cosmetically disfiguring, can interfere with ambulation, and are potentially contagious. The physician should remember that these are epidermal lesions that can potentially be removed with little scarring. These lesions have a high propensity for recurring, regardless of which technique is used for their removal; not uncommonly, they will recur time and time again, even when treatment is in the best of hands. The challenge for the physician is to simultaneously do the most good and the least harm. These lesions can be among the most challenging of any cutaneous condition encountered by a physician.

General guidelines regarding warts are helpful. Particular attention should be paid to warts on the fingers and hands of young women. These are cosmetic areas and need to be treated with respect for the cosmetic outcome. Likewise, warts that occur in areas where function is important, such as on the soles of competitive runners and the palmar surfaces and fingers of workmen and musicians, also require careful treatment. In all of these circumstances, treatments should be avoided that will cause functional disability or adverse cosmetic consequences, such as scarring from electrosurgery.

An effort should always be made to avoid unnecessary discomfort, particularly with children. Cryosurgery can be very painful. Many patients find that slow injection of lidocaine with a 30-gauge needle is preferable to the pain felt after cryosurgery. When treating children, a nonpainful approach should be considered, such as using salicylic acid preparations, before beginning any procedure that causes pain.

Keep in mind that warts can disappear after treatment with nonphysical modalities. Placebos have a success rate with warts, as do other oral therapies,

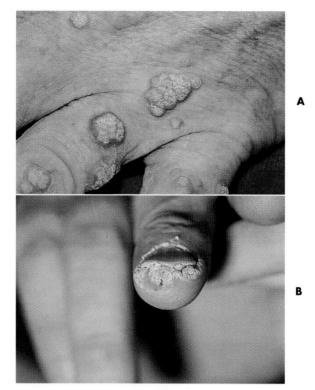

**FIG 15-10**
**A,** Verruca vulgaris on the hand. Treatment of multiple verruca is often challenging. **B,** Periungual verruca. Cure is difficult. Multiple treatment sessions are always necessary.

such as the use of $H_2$ blockers and other immunostimulants. Topical therapies with fluorouracil cream and formaldehyde solution definitely have a place, particularly with resistant warts. Intralesional injection of bleomycin (contraindicated during pregnancy) is extremely effective[1] and is used extensively to treat plantar warts and periungual warts. Pulsed dye and other lasers seem to be effective and also have a place in treating resistant warts.

When a physical modality is indicated, we prefer cryosurgery (See Chapter 11). Electrosurgery (See Chapter 12) is generally reserved for resistant lesions, and in those cases it is used gingerly to avoid scarring.

## Xanthelasma

Cryotherapy of xanthelasma (See Fig. 11-19) on the eyelids is one acceptable technique for the cosmetic removal of these benign lesions. Care should be taken when using liquid nitrogen around the eye to avoid delivering cryogenic substances to the conjunctiva and cornea. For this reason, we prefer not to use cryospray in this area. Even when using cotton-tipped swabs and liquid nitrogen, care must be taken not to drip liquid nitrogen into the eye. Because xanthelasma are superficial, cryotherapy should be light and carefully applied. Excision is the most definitive therapy, and superficial laser treatment is another alternative.

## DERMAL LESIONS

Benign lesions that primarily involve the dermis require more destructive modalities for their removal than do epidermal lesions. Often, there is a degree of epidermal change, such as thinning, that is visible when the surface of the lesion is carefully inspected, particularly under magnification. In addition to the techniques involving the scalpel, cryosurgery and electrosurgery are also effective treatments for these deeper lesions.

### Angiomas (Cherry and Spider) and Telangiectasias

Cherry angiomas (See Fig. 11-8), spider angiomas (See Fig. 12-6, *B*), and telangiectasias (See Fig. 12-10) on the face and chest respond well to light electrosurgery (Chapter 12). For spider angiomas, electrodesiccation of the central feeding vessel should eradicate the whole angioma. This can be done with an epilation needle, a metal-hubbed needle with an adapter, or a blunt electrode. If a blunt electrode is used, we recommend pressing it against the central feeding vessel to maximize efficacy. The very lowest setting that causes blanching of the vessel should be used. Telangiectasias on the leg are usually treated with the injection of sclerosing agents, such as hypertonic saline. Lasers are the treatment of choice for extensive facial telangiectasias and large hemangiomas. Lasers used to treat these conditions include pulsed dye lasers, yellow light lasers, or 532-nm diode lasers. All of these treatments can potentially cause scarring, and the vessels can recur. Cherry angiomas can easily be treated with shave excision and chemical and/or electrosurgical hemostasis.

### Dermatofibromas

The ideal treatment for small dermatofibromas (4 mm or less) (Fig. 15-11) is punch excision (Fig. 15-12). Larger lesions require a small elliptical excision. Large dermatofibromas (more than 1 cm) are more difficult to treat by excision because in their usual location on the lower extremities, the surgical defect can be difficult to close. The preferred treatment for these larger lesions is shave removal of the bulk of the lesion, followed by cryosurgery to the remaining fibroma. Patients must be advised that the cosmetic outcome is never certain, and that lesions can recur.

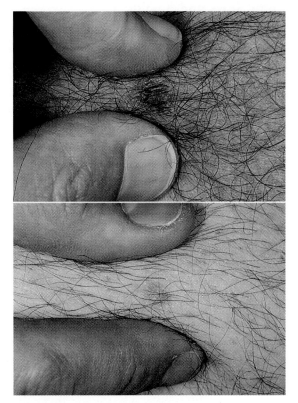

**FIG 15-11**
Dermatofibromas. These characteristically dimple when squeezed because of their hard, fibrosing nature.

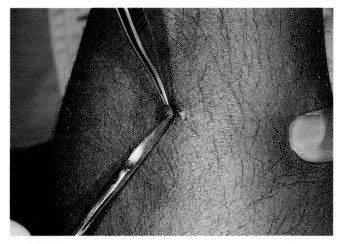

**FIG 15-12**
Small dermatofibroma on the forearm being removed after a punch excision. Care must be taken during the punch to not cut into the underlying ulnar bone.

## Hypertrophic Scars and Keloids

Although hypertrophic scars and keloids are predominantly dermal, the epidermis is obviously affected, usually by atrophy and pigmentary change. These scars can be challenging to treat, particularly if they involve facial structures such as the ears. Difficult or refractory cases should be referred to specialists. Keloids often will respond to intralesional steroids (Fig. 15-13), which must be carefully injected to ensure that steroids are contained within the scar (See Chapter 14). Cryosurgery can also be helpful. Lasers and excision are also occasionally used but are beyond the purview of most physicians. Topical steroids (especially Cordran tape) is useful in treating some individuals.

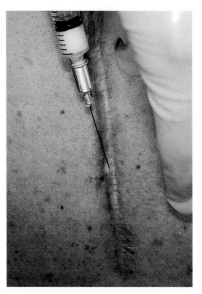

**FIG 15-13**
Injection of intralesional steroid into a keloid formed above the sternum after coronary bypass surgery.

## Keratoacanthomas

Keratoacanthomas (Fig. 15-14) are clinically identified by their characteristic keratotic, papular appearance and their rapid growth, frequently doubling in size over the course of 2 weeks. The preferred method of treatment is complete removal during the initial visit. Excisional biopsy of the entire lesion is the preferred treatment for small lesions. The specimen is sent for histopathologic confirmation to rule out the possibility of an SCC. Large lesions are more difficult to treat. We will usually choose to perform curettage and dessication, with care to thoroughly remove all the tumor. Alternative nonsurgical treatments are also effective, including intralesional and/or topical fluorouracil and intralesional bleomycin.[2] Although keratoacanthoma can resolve spontaneously, large aggressive lesions can destroy normal tissue during their growth phase and are particularly problematic when located near vital structures on the face.

## Milia

A common cosmetic problem, milia are superficial white cysts that are most often seen singly or in multiples on the face. These tiny cysts can be removed through a 1-mm incision made with a No. 11 blade (See Fig. 13-6). The soft white material in the cyst can then be expressed with a comedone extractor. Local anesthesia is often not necessary, but is helpful if the cyst is adherent to the surrounding tissue (See Chapter 13).

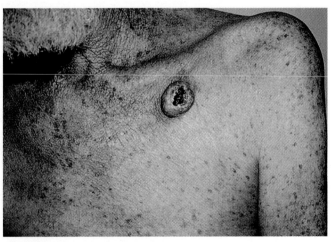

**FIG 15-14**
A large keratoacanthoma, inferior to the clavicle. These lesions can grow large and destroy adjacent tissue structures if untreated.

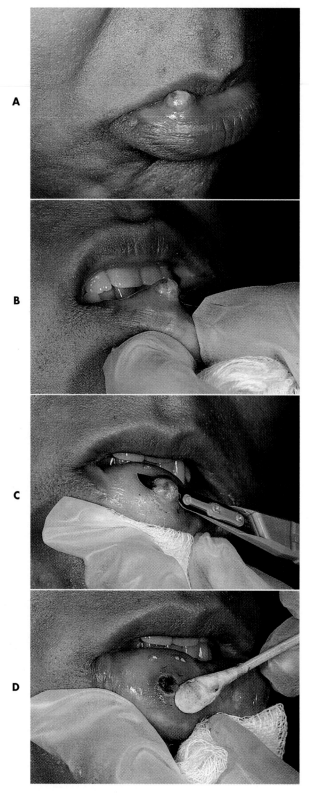

**FIG 15-15**

**A,** Large mucocele on the lip that recurred after previous incision, drainage, and cryosurgery. **B,** The lip is stabilized for administration of local anesthesia with lidocaine and epinephrine. **C,** The protruding tip of the mucocele is shaved off with a No. 15 blade. **D,** Preliminary hemostasis is achieved with Monsel's solution.

## Mucocele

Mucoceles are not uncommon on the inner surface of the lower lip (Fig. 15-15). They are mucin-filled cysts and have a marked tendency to recur. The simplest treatment is cryosurgery, which is more effective if the cyst is first drained by making a small incision with a No. 11 blade. In Fig. 15-15, the mucocele was large and protuberant, so a No. 15 blade was used to shave off the protuberant portion of the mucocele before cryosurgery and electrosurgery were used. In this case, the mucocele recurred and the treatment was repeated successfully. Mucoceles commonly recur and treatment may be repeated. Occasionally, recurrent lesions will need to be excised fully and the lip sutured.

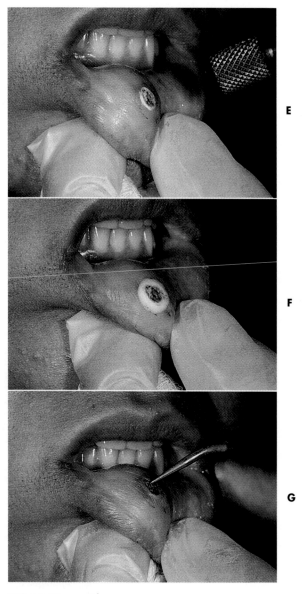

**FIG 15-15, cont'd**
**E,** Liquid nitrogen is sprayed to destroy the underlying lesion. **F,** Cryospray is continued until there is a 2-mm halo of normal tissue frozen around the affected area. **G,** Electrosurgery is used to achieve final hemostasis after cryosurgery.

## Nevi

Common moles (benign nevi) (Figs. 15-16, 15-17, and 15-18) have three typical variants: junctional, compound, and intradermal (Table 15-2). Junctional nevi are flat and hyperpigmented. Intradermal nevi are raised and often flesh colored. Compound nevi are often raised and hyperpigmented. However, it is not possible to determine whether a raised nevus is an intradermal or compound nevus just by looking. All three nevus types are benign and rarely turn into a melanoma. Some patients have atypical-appearing nevi that have suspicious features. These have been called *dysplastic nevi* (See Fig. 5-4) and are currently best referred to as *atypical moles*. In 1992 the NIH Consensus Conference report [3] described the clinical appearance of atypical nevi as follows:

> Atypical moles vary in size and are often larger than common moles. Atypical moles have macular and/or papular components and have borders that usually are irregular and frequently are ill-defined. Their color is variegated, ranging from tan to dark brown often on a pink background.

**TABLE 15-2    Characteristics of Common Moles (Benign Nevi)**

| Type | Clinical characteristics |
| --- | --- |
| Intradermal | Raised, flesh colored (sometimes pigmented) |
| Junctional | Flat and uniformly pigmented |
| Compound | Flat to raised, flesh colored or brown |
| Atypical nevi | Larger than 5 mm, macular and/or papular components, borders that usually are irregular and frequently are ill-defined, variegated color that ranges from tan to dark brown often on a pink background |

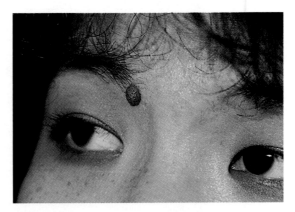

**FIG 15-16**
Benign nevus. This lesion is amenable to either elliptical excision or shave excision. Each technique can potentially produce an excellent cosmetic result. However, an ellipse may leave suture marks and a visible linear scar, and a shave may leave residual pigmentation or may result in recurrence of the nevus.

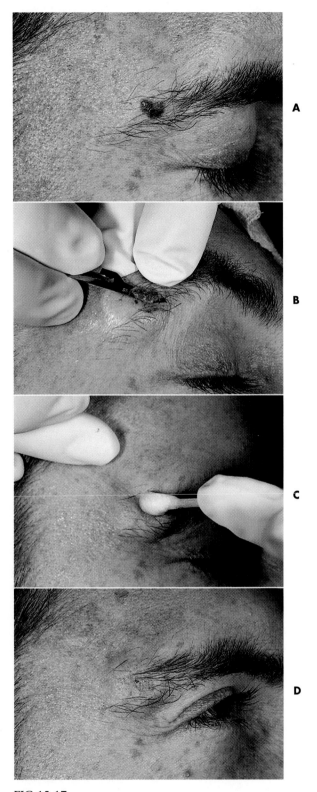

**FIG 15-17**
Shave excisional biopsy of a pigmented lesion. **A,** Pigmented papule with variegated pigmentation in the lateral eyebrow. **B,** After the lesion is elevated by superficial injection of lidocaine, it is removed with the shave technique using a No. 15 blade. **C,** Hemostasis is achieved by applying aluminum chloride with a cotton-tipped swab. **D,** Immediately postoperative, showing the resultant shallow defect, which should heal with an excellent cosmetic result. Pathology showed a benign nevus.

Removal of a suspicious, atypical mole is usually best accomplished by using an elliptical excision to obtain a full-thickness biopsy. This allows for appropriate measurement of thickness if the lesion turns out to be a melanoma.

Many benign nevi can be excised by using the shave excision technique. The most common type of nevi on which this technique can be used is raised, flesh-colored nevi. These nevi are clearly benign, and because a majority of the lesion is above the surface of the skin, these lesions can be removed by shave excision. It is important to tell the patient that the lesion can recur after using this technique, but the cosmetic result created by shave excision can be better than a linear scar created by excisional biopsy. Removal of benign nevi by shave excision requires that the shave is not deep into the dermis. If the wound is indented below the surface of the skin, an indented scar may be created.

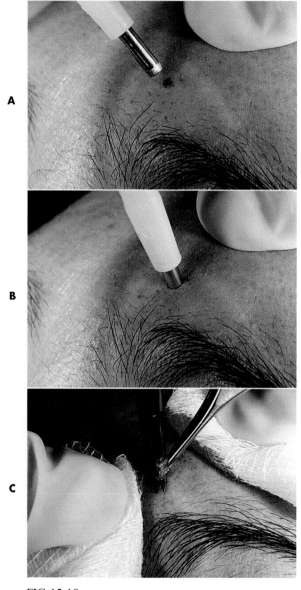

**FIG 15-18**
**A,** Punch excision of recurrent nevus superior to the eyebrow. **B,** Skin is retracted perpendicular to the skin tension lines and 3-mm punch is advanced. **C,** Biopsy specimen is removed with forceps.

Some nevi are flat but appear to be benign. Their borders are regular, their shape is symmetric, and their color is uniform. Some of these flat nevi can be removed by the shave excision technique. However, the wound may create an indented scar because it is necessary to do a deep shave to remove the nevus. The advantages of using a shave excision technique on truncal or extremity nevi are that the cosmetic results are usually equivalent to excisions, and the procedure is easier for physician and patient because sutures are not needed. The risk of overusing the shave biopsy happens when the lesion unsuspectingly turns out to be a melanoma. It then becomes difficult to obtain an adequate assessment of the level of tumor invasion. Small flat nevi may be excised with the punch technique.

Moles can become irritated, can interfere with shaving, or can be removed purely for cosmetic reasons. Benign-appearing raised nevi are best removed by the shave

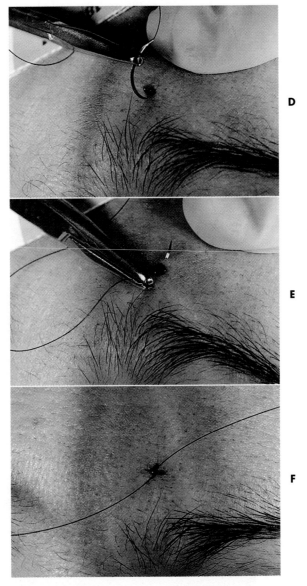

**FIG 15-18, cont'd**
D, Defect becomes circular and 6-0 nylon suture is placed.
E, The needle is advanced through both edges of the wound.
F, One suture pass closes the wound, which is converted into a line. Suture will be removed in 4 to 5 days.

technique. If the nevus has suspicious features, a full-thickness excision or biopsy should be done. The tissue removed should be submitted for pathologic examination, preferably to a dermatopathologist, to rule out melanoma. Failure to diagnose melanoma is a common medicolegal problem. Patients should be advised that the moles may regrow and pigment may return (especially after a shave excision). This occurs less often if the nevi are excised, either by punch or by ellipse. Excision, done meticulously, can provide a superior cosmetic result in some circumstances; in other circumstances, shave removal is superior. Light electrodesiccation to the base of a compound or intradermal nevus may help prevent regrowth.

In Fig. 15-18, the patient had a raised nevus over her eyebrow. It was excised using the shave technique, and the pathology was benign. However, in 2 months the nevus recurred. This time the nevus was small and flat. In Fig. 15-18, *A*, the physician is about to excise the recurrent nevus with a 2-mm punch. The defect was sutured (Fig. 15-18, *D* to *F*), and the pathology was benign. This time the nevus did not recur.

## Neurofibromas

Neurofibromas (Fig. 15-19) are common benign tumors that occur as isolated lesions or at multiple sites. A single lesion may look like an intradermal nevus. Most commonly, neurofibromas are 3 to 6 mm in diameter, but large lesions (greater than 1 cm) are not unusual. Small lesions are most easily removed with the shave technique. After shaving a neurofibroma, it is common for the tissue below the shaved area to "pouch out."

Shave biopsy is adequate for diagnosis, but neurofibromas often recur after shave removal, with a less than satisfactory cosmetic result. Therefore excision or punch biopsy with very small (1mm) margins is usually preferable. Generally, excision is best for larger lesions because they involve the deep dermis and tend not to heal well when shaved.

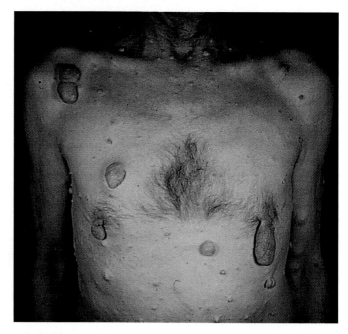

**FIG 15-19**
Neurofibromatosis. Many large neurofibromas are present

## Prurigo Nodularis

Prurigo nodularis (See Fig. 11-13) is a type of chronic eczema that manifests with pruritic nodules (itchy bumps). Cryosurgery, with or without the addition of intralesional or topical steroids, is the treatment of choice for these lesions. Cordran tape, which is unique in being the only tape with cortisone impregnated within it, is also useful for treatment of this condition, which tends to be recurrent and resistant to treatment.

## Pyogenic Granuloma

Pyogenic granulomas (See Fig. 12-7) are vascular benign tumors that grow rapidly and bleed easily. They occur most commonly on the fingers, face, lips, and gingiva. Pyogenic granulomas often occur at the site of minor trauma and are more common in pregnancy. Electrosurgery, with or without preceding curettage, is the initial treatment of choice for pyogenic granuloma. Care must be taken to reach the base of the lesion and destroy it because of the great tendency of these tumors to recur. Recurrent tumors can be retreated with curettage followed by electrosurgery, or they may be excised. Histology should be confirmed to rule out amelanotic melanoma.

## Sebaceous Hyperplasia

Sebaceous hyperplasia (Fig. 15-8) are common benign tumors, most often seen on the face in middle-aged and older adults. If diagnosis is uncertain, it is best to perform a shave biopsy because these lesions can closely resemble BCC. Usually, however, their yellow hue, slight central depression, and occurrence on the face in multiple locations is characteristic enough to make their identification certain, and biopsy is not necessary. Reassurance of their benign nature is adequate for many patients. Others request removal for cosmetic reasons. Options include light electrodesiccation, either before or after shave removal of the bulk of the tumor, or cryosurgery.

Care must be taken when using any of these modalities to remove sebaceous hyperplasia to avoid overtreatment. Even with a light freeze or light electrodesiccation, patients can occasionally develop hypopigmentation or depression at the site of the former lesion. The safest modality for removing sebaceous hyperplasia is cryosurgery. The lesions are frozen lightly to their periphery and no further. Cotton-tipped swabs may be used to apply liquid nitrogen to the lesion to keep the freeze superficial. The lesions need to be frozen for only 3 to 5 seconds.

# SUBCUTANEOUS LESIONS

Two benign subcutaneous tumors are commonly seen in practice: lipomas and epidermal cysts. They both may be excised by a similar surgical approach. Pilar cysts are a type of epidermal cyst found on the scalp. They are usually easier to remove than other epidermal cysts because the cyst wall is well demarcated from the surrounding tissue. All benign subcutaneous tumors can be either solitary or multiple; many patients with multiple tumors have a family history of such lesions. These tumors can be large and require surgical expertise for proper removal.

Surgical removal of these tumors begins with either a linear incision for small tumors (generally those less than 1.5 cm in diameter) or a small ellipse for large tumors. The length of the ellipse should generally be about equal to the diameter of the tumor. The incision or ellipse is made above the center of the tumor. The tumor is then freed by blunt dissection with blunt-tipped tenotomy scissors and then removed en masse through the opening in the skin. The surgical defect is examined for any bleeding vessels, which are then electrocoagulated. The skin defect is then closed with sutures or surgical staples. Surgical staples are quick and easy to use to close the scalp after removing a pilar cyst. The major disadvantage to the use of surgical staples is the cost.

Because surgery is being done in the subcutaneous space, certain precautions need to be taken. Care is necessary to avoid deeper structures, such as vessels and, in particular, nerves. (See Chapter 19 for drawings of superficial nerves that should be avoided during surgery.) Also, sterile technique is particularly important. Adequate anesthesia before surgery is required, with care to inject into and around the dermis surrounding the lesion. Anesthesia injected into the lesion itself will be ineffective. After removing cysts and lipomas, a pressure dressing should be applied (See Chapter 18).

## Epidermal Cysts

Epidermal cysts (Fig. 15-20) are common skin cysts that are often called *sebaceous cysts,* although the cyst lining is more epithelial than sebaceous gland in origin. The contents of the cyst are usually foul-smelling keratin, a skin protein. The cause of most cysts is unknown.

Patients usually complain about epidermal cysts when the cysts are enlarging or when they are inflamed or infected. If the cyst manifests signs of infection, incision and drainage are necessary. Local anesthesia with 1% lidocaine with epinephrine should be injected into the overlying skin. Incision and drainage are accomplished by carrying a small incision made with a No. 11 blade through the skin surface and into the cyst cavity and then expressing the cyst contents with pressure (See Fig. 13-3).

Surgical packing is not necessary for infected skin cysts that are opened widely, especially if the patient takes oral antibiotics after the incision and drainage.

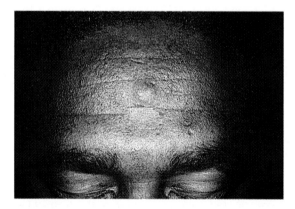

**FIG 15-20**
Epidermal cyst in the center of the forehead. Close examination will reveal the central dilated pore. Lipomas in this location can closely resemble epidermal cysts but lack the central pore. The central pore should be included in the small ellipse that is made to remove the cyst to help prevent recurrence.

Antibiotics such as cephalexin or dicloxacillin may help clear the infection. If the incision is small and the physician believes it may close before adequate drainage has taken place, the wound may be packed with gauze. This usually requires more follow-up visits by the patient to have the gauze changed or removed. Some physicians do not prescribe systemic antibiotics after drainage, believing instead that drainage alone is adequate treatment. Once all of the inflammation has resolved, surgery to excise the cyst wall may prevent further infections.

Excision of a cyst can be one of the more difficult skin surgery procedures. The physician will often try to excise the cyst through a small incision, making hemostasis difficult. It can also be difficult to excise all of the cyst wall if the cyst has already ruptured. Easy removal of these cysts is usually best accomplished by first numbing the area by placing the needle between the skin and the cyst wall so that hydrodissection is accomplished. It also important not to inject directly into the cyst to ensure that rupture will not occur before excision. Anesthesia also needs to be placed deep to the cyst. A smaller ellipse over the cyst makes it easier to get good visibility. The ellipse will remove the extra skin caused by the cyst stretching the skin. The ellipse is then carefully excised down to the cyst wall using a No. 15 blade. Once the cyst wall is seen, blunt tenotomy scissors are used to dissect the cyst wall from the surrounding tissue. If scar tissue is present, a No. 15 blade may be used to separate the cyst from the tissue.

If the cyst ruptures during removal, the entire contents of the cyst should be squeezed out with pressure. All of the cyst wall is then excised using either scissors or the blade. Hemostasis can always be achieved by getting good visualization using skin hooks. Cotton-tipped swabs are important tools for applying pressure for hemostasis. Electrocoagulation can be used to stop any bleeding that is not controlled with pressure alone. In the final repair, it helps to use deep absorbable sutures to close the dead space left by the cyst removal. This decreases the risk of hematoma formation and infection. The skin can then be closed with nylon suture using a running stitch or in an interrupted fashion.

Intact epidermal cysts can be treated with the surgical method outlined above, with the important proviso that an attempt should be made to include the central pore opening of the cyst in the ellipse of skin that is removed. Some physicians prefer to remove an epidermal cyst intact through an incision large enough to allow for this. However, even when attempting this approach, the cyst can rupture. Removing cysts in this manner is especially difficult for large lesions that tend to produce atrophy of the skin overlying the tumor.

Other physicians make a smaller incision and drain the cyst through this opening before dissecting the cyst wall from the surrounding tissue. One easy way to do this for small superficial cysts is to use a 3- to 5-mm punch to open up the cyst to allow for drainage and removal of the cyst wall. The small defect can then be closed with a single suture.

Because the cyst contents can be irritating to the tissues, it is important to fully remove these contents before suturing the wound closed. If the cyst is large, the dead space should be closed with absorbable deep sutures to prevent hematomas and infection (See Chapter 8). A pressure dressing should be applied.

Epidermal cysts that have ruptured are more difficult to manage because the surrounding inflammation and fibrosis make it difficult to see and dissect the cyst wall. In this situation, the physician is limited to performing incision and drainage, with expression of as much keratin and purulent material as possible. See Chapter 13 and Fig. 13-3 for description of this procedure.

## Pilar Cysts

Pilar cysts (Fig. 15-21) are common tumors of the scalp that are easily removed if the surgical approach outlined above is followed, with the additional step of shaving the scalp before the procedure. We begin by shaving a small area of the scalp overlying the cyst, trying to limit the shaved area to smaller than a quarter.

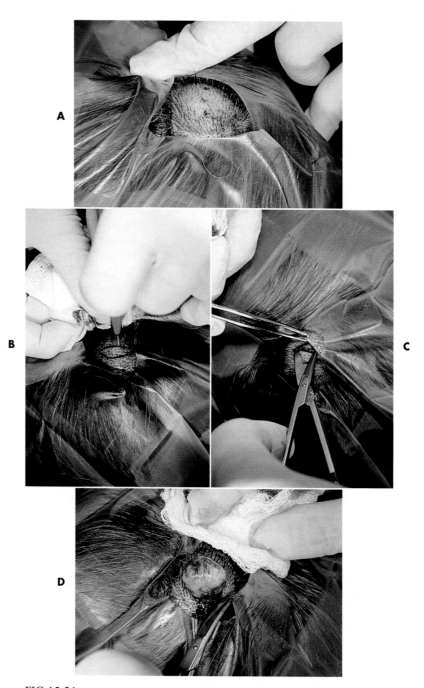

**FIG 15-21**
Excision of a pilar cyst on the scalp. **A,** Preoperative view. A 1.5-cm cyst produces a protuberance on the scalp surface. The area is shaved preoperatively, and the approximate dimensions of the cyst are delineated with a surgical marker. **B,** A small ellipse approximately equal in length to the diameter of the cyst is excised over the center of the cyst with a No. 15 scalpel, with care not to enter the underlying cyst. **C,** An iris scissors is used to bluntly dissect the cyst from surrounding tissue. **D,** The cyst is delivered through the excisional opening using pressure on the surrounding scalp.

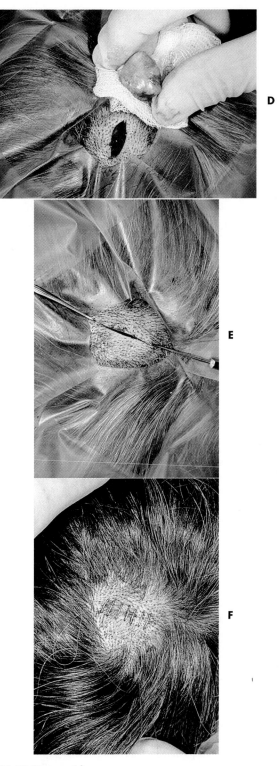

**FIG 15-21, cont'd**
E, The cyst is shown intact. Any small bleeding vessels are
electrocoagulated. F, One skin hook is placed in each end of
the ellipse to facilitate closure of the wound and placement of
the surgical staples. G, Final appearance of the wound closed
with surgical staples. The staples are removed in 2 weeks. The
wound site is dressed with a gauze pressure dressing.

Pilar cysts can be removed without shaving the hair, which is a matter of physician and patient preference.

After shaving, Betadine is applied to the surface of the scalp, and local anesthesia of lidocaine with epinephrine is injected. After a wait of 10 minutes for vasoconstriction, the linear incision or small ellipse is performed. If sterile technique is broken, we will give the patient a short course of oral antibiotics. The patient is sent home with a pressure dressing applied around the scalp, to be left on overnight. Postoperative discomfort is usually mild. Staples are removed after 2 weeks.

## Lipomas

Lipomas can occur anywhere on the cutaneous surface, but are most common on the trunk and extremities. Patients may require nothing more than reassurance about their benign nature. If removal is elected, lipomas can be excised as outlined earlier, usually through a linear incision. Removal of lipomas on the trunk and extremities is usually straightforward, but on the forehead they are more challenging. Lipomas in this location are generally submuscular, so the incision must be carried through the muscle to reveal the lipoma. In this location, it is imperative to place the incision in the crease lines of the forehead, thereby helping to achieve a better cosmetic result. Unless a physician has considerable experience excising lipomas and doing surgery on the face, we recommend referring patients with lipomas on the forehead to a dermatologist.

## CONCLUSION

A potent armamentarium of techniques is available for treating benign tumors of the skin. Shave and punch biopsy, elliptical excision, incision and drainage, intralesional injection of steroids, cryosurgery, laser surgery, topical medications, and electrosurgery all have their place in dealing with the wide variety of cutaneous and subcutaneous lesions that are commonly encountered in practice. Familiarity with the common lesions and the preferred techniques will help the physician choose the proper modality for any given lesion.

## REFERENCES

1. Munn SE et al: A new method of intralesional bleomycin therapy in the treatment of recalcitrant warts, *Br J Dermatol* 135:969-971, 1996.
2. Schwartz RA: Keratoacanthoma, *J Am Acad Dermatol* 30:1-19, 1994.
3. NIH Consensus Conference: Diagnosis and treatment of early melanoma, *JAMA* 268:1314-1319, 1992.

## SUGGESTED READING

Epstein E, Epstein E Jr, editors: *Skin surgery*, ed 6, Philadelphia, 1987, WB Saunders.
Fewkes JL, Cheney ML, Pollack SV: *Illustrated atlas of cutaneous surgery*, Philadelphia, 1992, Lippincott-Gower.
Kuflik EG: Cryosurgery updated, *J Am Acad Dermatol* 31(6):925-944, 1994.
Lask G, Moy R, editors: *Principles and techniques of cutaneous surgery*, New York, 1996, McGraw-Hill.
Pollack SV: *Electrosurgery of the skin*, New York, 1991, Churchill Livingstone.
Robinson JK: *Fundamentals of skin biopsy*, St Louis, 1986, Mosby.
Roenigk RK, Roenigk HH: *Dermatologic surgery: principles and practice*, ed 2, New York, 1996, Marcel Dekker.

# CHAPTER 16

# Diagnosis and Treatment of Malignant Lesions

*Edward L. Tobinick*

An essential part of the practice of medicine is the accurate diagnosis of skin cancer. Early detection, diagnosis, and treatment of skin cancer can not only be lifesaving but can prevent local damage to essential superficial organs, such as the eyes, ears, nose, and mouth. More than 500,000 new cases of skin cancer are reported in the United States every year. The most common, in descending order of frequency of occurrence, are basal cell carcinoma (BCC), squamous cell carcinoma (SCC), and malignant melanoma.

Malignant melanoma has one of the highest rates of incidence of all malignancies of young adults. Non-melanoma skin cancers are much more common, and their incidence continues to increase, with approximately 1 million new cases per year in the United States. This rate exceeds the combined incidence of cancers of the lung, breast, colon, rectum, prostate, and bladder and all lymphomas.[1] This chapter discusses the clinical features, diagnosis, differential diagnosis, and treatment of melanoma, BCC, and SCC.

## NON-MELANOMA SKIN CANCER

### Diagnosis of BCC and SCC

BCC can be among the most difficult cutaneous lesions to diagnose. Contributing to this problem are the multiple forms that it can take.[2] The three most important are the nodular, sclerosing, and superficial variants.

Nodular BCCs (Fig. 16-1) begin as small, firm, dome-shaped papules, with a smooth surface reflecting loss of the normal pore pattern. The surface has a pearly white, translucent appearance. Telangiectasias are often visible. As these lesions enlarge, they may ulcerate centrally (Fig. 16-2) or peripherally, leaving a small bloody crust or a scar at the site of ulceration. In brown-eyed individuals, nodular BCCs can be deeply pigmented (Fig. 16-3) with shades of brown or black and can closely resemble melanoma.

Sclerosing BCCs (Fig. 16-4) (also called *morpheaform* because of their resemblance to localized scleroderma) are ivory or colorless, flat, macular tumors, with an atrophic surface and a hard, indurated consistency.[3] They may resemble scars, and are easily overlooked.

Superficial BCCs (Fig. 16-5) and SCC in situ appear as red or pink scaling plaques, occasionally with shallow erosions or crusts. Differentiation between these two similar lesions usually requires biopsy.

SCCs of the skin (Fig. 16-6) present as slowly growing papules or nodules on the cutaneous surface, particularly the face and scalp. They are frequently hyper-

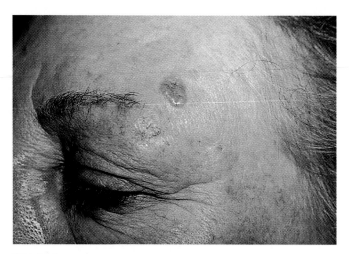

**FIG 16-1**
Nodular BCC on the temple.

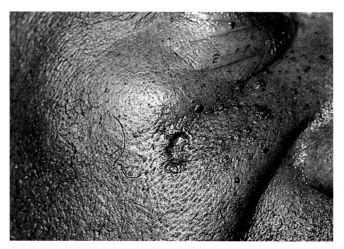

**FIG 16-2**
Nodular BCC, ulcerated, on the cheek.

keratotic and can be friable and bleed easily. About 2300 deaths caused by non-melanoma skin cancer occur each year in the United States.

## Clinical Behavior of Non-Melanoma Skin Cancer

BCCs grow by direct extension and invasion of contiguous structures. Although their growth can be rapid, it is usually rather slow, with a doubling time of at least 6 months. The sclerosing variety is the most dangerous because these tumors tend to be deeply invasive and are often neglected until they have caused extensive damage. Sclerosing tumors frequently invade muscle, nerve, and bone. Nodular BCCs are less aggressive but will grow to involve deeper structures, such as bone, if they are not treated. The sclerosing variety often ulcerate and can bleed.

Nodular and sclerosing tumors most commonly occur on the face, head, and neck. Superficial BCCs most often develop on the trunk and the extremities, enlarge peripherally, and rarely penetrate the dermis.

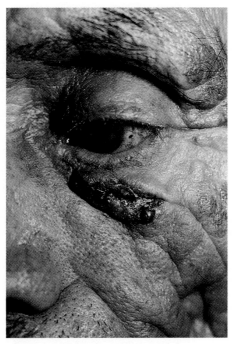

**FIG 16-3**
Nodular BCC, pigmented, on the lower eyelid.

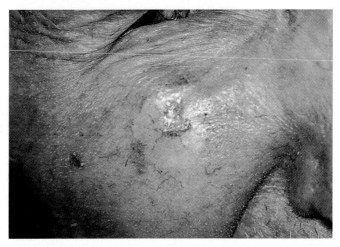

**FIG 16-4**
Sclerosing (morpheaform) BCC on the cheek.

SCCs occur in the same distribution as BCCs. They can occur anywhere on the body surface, but are most common on the head and neck. Cutaneous carcinomas on the lips, around the ears, and on the scalp have a higher chance of being SCC than in other sites. As with BCCs, SCCs initially grow by direct extension. Of particular importance is the significant tendency for SCCs to metastasize to local lymph nodes and then to distant sites. SCC on mucous membranes, including those in the oral cavity, on the lips, and on the ears, have an increased risk of metastasis. The risk of metastasis is increased for larger, advanced lesions. BCCs rarely metastasize; most mortality from BCCs is caused by lesions that have been

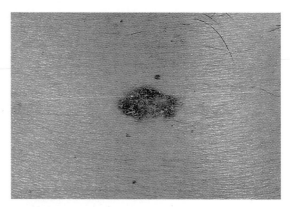

**FIG 16-5**
Superficial BCC on the neck.

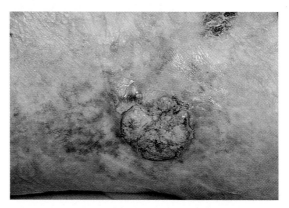

**FIG 16-6**
SCC on the thigh.

neglected and, because of their large size, invade vital contiguous structures, particularly the brain.

Early diagnosis is particularly important in facial cancers. The nose is the most frequent site of BCC, accounting for one third of reported cases in women and one fifth of those in men. Reconstruction is difficult at this site because of limited skin mobility and the esthetic importance of nasal contours, such as the alar rim. Because little fat is present, extension of the carcinoma into underlying bone and cartilage is not uncommon. Tumors on the alar groove and the nasolabial fold have a tendency to burrow deeper before lateral spread is evident.

It is crucial to diagnose tumors on the eyelids early to avoid ectropion or other functional impairment. When the medial canthus is involved, prompt diagnosis facilitates cure before the cancer spreads to the lacrimal duct, the eyelids, or deeper into the orbit.

## Differential Diagnosis of BCC and SCC

### Nodular BCC

- Intradermal nevus
  Stable size
  Soft
  No crusting or ulceration

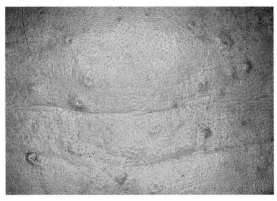

**FIG 16-7**
Sebaceous hyperplasia on the forehead.

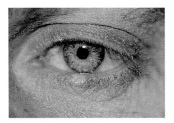

**FIG 16-8**
Molluscum contagiosum. A single
lesion on the lid margin.

- Sebaceous hyperplasia
    Yellow coloration
    Stable size
    Umbilication without ulceration
- Molluscum contagiosum
    No telangiectasia
    Usually multiple lesions
    Expressible core

Nodular BCCs can be difficult to differentiate from several benign cutaneous lesions (See the list above). For example, intradermal nevi appear as skin-colored, protuberant papules on the face in adults. They begin as flat, pigmented moles that gradually lose their color and elevate as the individual ages. These lesions are distinguished from BCCs predominantly by their growth pattern. They also tend to be somewhat softer, and there is no crusting or ulceration.

Sebaceous hyperplasia (Fig. 16-7) closely mimics small BCCs, but this lesion has a distinctive yellow tinge, often has a small central depression, and neither enlarges nor ulcerates. Both intradermal nevi and sebaceous hyperplasia may have overlying telangiectasias.

Molluscum contagiosum can occasionally occur as a solitary lesion, mimicking BCC. Fig. 16-8 shows a molluscum lesion on the eyelid margin that does not have typical features and requires biopsy. A biopsy in this location is technically difficult and is beyond the purview of most primary care physicians. The usual presentation of molluscum is of multiple, firm, discrete, flesh-colored papules, with a tiny central pore or umbilication (See Figs. 15-5 and 11-2). Telangiectasias are lacking. Facial lesions are most commonly seen in children but can occur in adults.

After consideration of the natural history of any given individual lesion and careful evaluation of its appearance, preferably under magnification, definitive identification is frequently possible without biopsy. Examination of cutaneous lesions with magnification can be accomplished in one of several ways. Many dermatologists wear visors that allow them to perform procedures with both hands free. The recommended magnification for these visors is in the range of 1.5 to 2.5, but is subject to individual preference. Keep in mind that higher magnification requires a closer position to the patient, which may not be convenient. Alternatives to visors include magnifying glasses, hand-held loupes, or even ophthalmoscopes. For some difficult lesions, biopsy will still be necessary. A shave biopsy is the procedure of choice to distinguish between nodular BCC and all of the benign lesions described above (intradermal nevus, sebaceous hyperplasia, and molluscum contagiosum). The shave biopsy is fast and easy to perform and is ideal for biopsy of these raised lesions. (See Chapter 6 for further information on shave biopsy.)

Superficial BCC and SCC in situ (Bowen's disease) can resemble nummular eczema or psoriasis. Nummular eczema can usually be distinguished by its coin-like shape, transient nature, and itchiness. Psoriasis seldom appears on the face; when it does, it is usually accompanied by lesions on the trunk, scalp, or nails that form a distinctive clinical picture (See Fig. 9-11). Differentiating superficial BCC from Bowen's disease requires biopsy. An actinic keratosis that is crusting can also mimic ulcerative BCC.

## Biopsy Technique for the Diagnosis of BCC and SCC

Shave biopsy is preferred for the diagnosis of most lesions suspected to be a BCC or an SCC. Subsequent treatment with curettage and desiccation is not hindered because the shave does not produce a full-thickness wound such as when a punch biopsy is performed. A punch specimen is usually preferred for a suspected sclerosing BCC, which is flat and may be deeply invasive. Although a deeper shave may be adequate for making the diagnosis of sclerosing BCC, a punch biopsy is still preferred in most cases.

Superficial BCC or SCC may be biopsied with a shave or punch technique. Although these lesions are generally flat and scaling, they are often slightly raised and have enough substance to make a shave biopsy feasible. Either a somewhat deeper shave or a 3-mm punch biopsy should provide adequate tissue for diagnosis of a superficial BCC or SCC.

## Treatment of Non-Melanoma Skin Cancer

The primary goals in the treatment of cutaneous carcinoma are cure, preservation of function, optimal cosmetic results, and minimal operative risk and patient inconvenience. These goals can be achieved only after careful, individual evaluation, with consideration of the location, size, growth pattern, and clinical variety of the cancer; the patient's general health; the surgeon's skill; the operative facility available; and the wishes of the patient.[4] The treatments that we will discuss are dependent on a definitive pathologic diagnosis being established first with an initial shave or punch biopsy.

As seen in Box 16-1, elliptical excision with immediate repair offers the advantages of excellent cosmesis and rapid healing, and the pathology specimen will show if the margins are free of tumor. Sutures for facial lesions are removed in 3 to 7 days. There is no crusting or oozing as with electrosurgery. Although operative risks such as hematoma are minimal with careful technique, patients receiving anticoagulants should not undergo excisional surgery unless it is absolutely necessary. Most excisions are now performed in the office with local anesthesia. Thus the risks and expense of general anesthesia and hospitalization are avoided.

---

### BOX 16-1    Treatment Modalities for Non-Melanoma Skin Cancer

**Elliptical Excision**
Treatment of choice for nodular BCCs and medium SCCs

*Advantages*
Optimal cosmetic result when repair is immediate
Rapid healing
Margin control

*Disadvantages*
Time consuming
Technically difficult
Potential surgical complications: bleeding, hematoma, infection

**Electrosurgery**
Treatment of choice for small nodular and superficial BCCs and small SCCs

*Advantages*
Quick
Easily achieved hemostasis

*Disadvantages*
Prolonged healing
No margin control
Cosmetic result variable

**Cryosurgery**
Treatment of choice for superficial BCCs

*Advantages*
Quick
Good cosmetic result

*Disadvantages*
Prolonged healing
No margin control

**Mohs' Micrographic Surgery**
Treatment of choice for sclerosing and recurrent BCCs and large SCCs

*Advantages*
Meticulous margin control
Highest cure rates
Best possible cosmetic results

*Disadvantages*
Time consuming
Technically difficult
Unnecessarily destructive for smaller lesions
Potential excisional surgical complications
Higher cost

**Radiation**
Treatment of choice for patients who are not operative candidates

*Advantages*
Good cosmetic results

*Disadvantages*
Multiple treatment sessions
High cost
Radiation damage, including telangiectasias, scarring, possible carcinogenesis

Electrosurgery involves destruction of the lesion by electrodesiccation after removal of most of the lesion mass through curettage. An experienced physician can use the curette to seek the lesion edges by feel because BCCs are softer and more friable than normal tissue. The technique of curettage and dessication is most suitable for small nodular and superficial cancers. It is not suitable for those that have extended beyond the dermis because the curette cannot follow the lesion into fat. This limitation is particularly important on the face, where fat may lie within 3 mm of the skin surface. The advantages of electrosurgery are easily achieved hemostasis, speed, and minimal operative complications. The disadvantages are variable cosmetic results for larger lesions and prolonged healing time (2 to 6 weeks).

Cryosurgery involving the application of liquid nitrogen through either a spray or a probe, is most suitable for superficial BCCs and for some small tumors of the nodular type. This technique has several advantages: it is rapid, poses minimal operative risk, and yields excellent cosmetic results. The disadvantages are lack of margin control and prolonged healing time (usually 2 to 6 weeks). Neither cryosurgery nor electrosurgery is favored for carcinomas that have indistinct clinical margins or for those that are likely to be deeply invasive, such as sclerosing tumors, lesions that have recurred after previous surgery, and tumors in danger areas such as the medial canthus and the alar groove.

Mohs' micrographic surgery involves the removal of tumor by scalpel in sequential horizontal layers. Each tissue sample is frozen, stained, and microscopically examined. This technique is the treatment of choice for BCCs with poorly defined margins, especially those on the nose or eyelids. It is unnecessary for small lesions with well-defined margins. Repair of defects left after Mohs' micrographic surgery can be either immediate or delayed, and is accomplished by adjacent tissue transfer, skin grafting, linear closure, or healing by secondary intention.

Radiation is currently used for only a small percentage of BCCs. It can produce excellent cosmetic results, although late hypopigmentation is common. Radiation is especially useful when operative intervention is difficult. Multiple treatment sessions are required, and the costs are higher than Mohs' micrographic surgery or excisional surgery.

## MALIGNANT MELANOMA

### Diagnosis and Differential Diagnosis of Melanoma

The proper diagnosis of pigmented lesions is essential for their management. Of particular concern is the need for early diagnosis of melanoma because it is now well established that early diagnosis and surgical removal will frequently be curative. Melanoma has been increasing inexorably in the United States during the last half of this century. The estimated number of cases of invasive melanoma in the United States in 1996 was 38,300.[5] In addition, there were an estimated 30,000 to 50,000 new cases of melanoma in situ for 1996.[6] In 1997 there will be an estimated 40,300 new cases of melanoma in the United States and 7300 deaths from melanoma.[7]

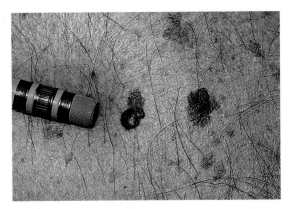

**FIG 16-9**
Seborrheic keratoses on the trunk.

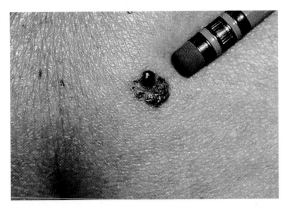

**FIG 16-10**
Benign hemangioma resembling melanoma (pseudomel-anoma).

The key to diagnosing melanoma is the skin biopsy. Early recognition of melanoma can be difficult. Early melanomas can closely resemble several benign skin lesions, most commonly benign nevocellular nevi, seborrheic keratoses (Fig. 16-9), hemangiomas (Fig. 16-10), and dermatofibromas (See Fig. 15-11). Histopathology can distinguish between these entities when they are clinically difficult to differentiate. The pathologic diagnosis of melanoma and lentigo maligna can be exceedingly difficult. Biopsies of lesions suspected of being melanoma or lentigo maligna should be sent to the best dermatopathologist available. Benign pigmented lesions are much more common than melanoma. Unusual pigmented lesions are most often uncommon variants of these benign lesions, rather than melanomas.

The ABCDE guidelines (Box 16-2) were developed to help physicians diagnose melanoma[8,9] (Fig. 16-11). Of the ABCDE guidelines, the most important is **D**, for diameter (Fig. 16-12). Most benign pigmented lesions (with the important exceptions of seborrheic keratoses, congenital nevi, and atypical moles) are less than 6 mm in diameter. Most melanomas diagnosed in the United States have a diameter greater than 6 mm. In general, melanomas larger than 1 cm in diameter have a poorer prognosis because they tend to be thicker. There is a window of opportunity, then, to diagnose early melanoma in this diameter range (6 to 10 mm), when removal will result in cure in a high percentage (80% to 100%) of cases.

The other four criteria, **ABCE**, can be used to evaluate lesions larger than 6 mm. If a lesion of this size is asymmetric, if the border is irregular, if it is composed of more than one shade of brown or more than one color, and if part of it is palpable, then a biopsy should be done (seborrheic keratoses and congenital nevi excepted) and sent for pathologic examination. Note that the recommendation for biopsy does not require that all five (ABCDE) criteria are met. Melanomas can fail to satisfy all five criteria.

A caveat to remember involves patient-related symptoms or signs. Pigmented lesions that change in size or color or ones that itch, are tender, or bleed need careful evaluation. When the patient presents with these complaints or has taken notice of a particular lesion, a detailed examination of the lesion in question, preferably under magnification, is required. If the lesion is removed, it should be sent for pathologic examination, even if it fails to meet the ABCDE criteria.

Three other special situations are worthy of discussion. First is the problem of seborrheic keratoses. These common lesions can meet all five ABCDE criteria and yet not require biopsy. Most seborrheic keratoses have a characteristic warty, "stuck-on" appearance, that allows them to be identified (See Fig. 5-7). Second is the issue of congenital nevi. These are frequently large and can meet all five ABCDE criteria (See Fig. 5-6). Their distinguishing feature, however, is the fact that they have been present since birth. Biopsy is indicated if a change in color, a new growth within the mole, or bleeding without trauma occurs within a preexisting mole. Third is the issue of atypical moles (dysplastic nevi), which is discussed in detail in Chapter 5.

---

> **BOX 16-2    The American Cancer Society ABCDE Guidelines for Diagnosis of Malignant Melanoma**
>
> **Asymmetry:** Benign nevi are symmetric; melanomas tend to have pronounced asymmetry.
> **Border:** Benign lesions usually have smooth borders; melanomas tend to have notched, irregular outlines.
> **Color:** Benign lesions usually contain only one color; melanomas frequently have a variety of colors.
> **Diameter:** Melanoma is usually larger than 6 mm in diameter.
> **Elevation:** Malignant melanoma is almost always elevated, at least in part, so that it is palpable.
> OR
> **Enlarging:** A pigmented lesion that is enlarging is more suspicious for melanoma.

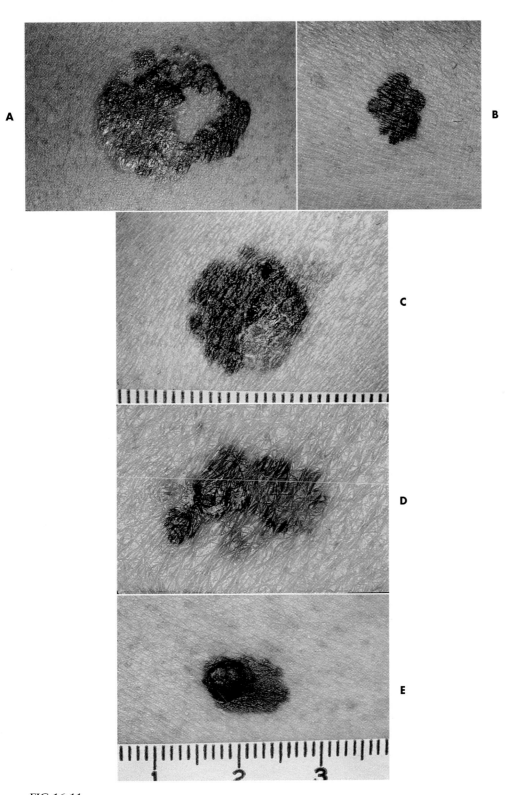

**FIG 16-11**
ABCDE guidelines for diagnosing malignant melanoma. **A,** Asymmetry. **B,** Border. **C,** Color. **D,** Diameter. **E,** Elevation. (Courtesy The Skin Cancer Foundation, New York.)

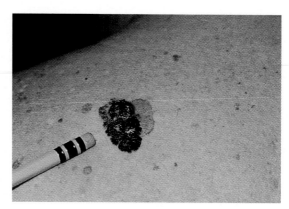

**FIG 16-12**
Large malignant melanoma on the back.

Family members of patients with melanoma have an increased risk of developing melanoma, especially if they have multiple atypical moles (dysplastic nevi). Current recommendations are that patients with multiple atypical moles be photographed and followed. Atypical moles that change require biopsy, but removal otherwise is not routinely recommended.

Incisional biopsies of skin cancers probably do not cause metastasis of the lesion or affect the prognosis, but they may interfere with accurate histopathologic staging, particularly in malignant melanoma.[10]

## Guidelines for Biopsy of Pigmented Lesions

### Biopsy indicated

- Change in preexisting nevus: itching, bleeding, change in size or color
- Pigmented lesion satisfying all of the ABCDE criteria (congenital nevi, seborrheic keratoses, and atypical moles excluded)

### Biopsy possibly indicated

- De novo pigmented lesion satisfying any combination of the ABCDE criteria need careful evaluation. *(Note: 50% of malignant melanomas arise de novo. These melanomas usually start as lesions smaller than 6 mm in diameter. We have diagnosed malignant melanomas as small as 2 mm in diameter.)*

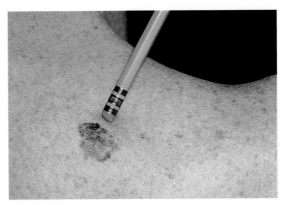

**FIG 16-13**
Superficial spreading malignant melanoma on the back.

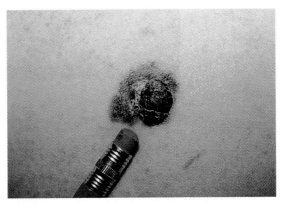

**FIG 16-14**
Nodular malignant melanoma arising in a congenital nevus.

## Clinical Variants of Melanoma

The five commonly recognized variants of melanoma include the following:

1. Superficial spreading malignant melanoma: This is the typical form of melanoma, presenting as an elevated papule satisfying most, if not all, of the ABCDE criteria (Fig. 16-13).
2. Nodular malignant melanoma: These lesions present as nodules or papules, with their most prominent clinical feature being their elevation above the surface of the skin (Fig. 16-14).
3. Acral lentiginous melanoma: These pigmented lesions occur on the palms or soles, frequently in dark-skinned patients, and carry a poor prognosis.

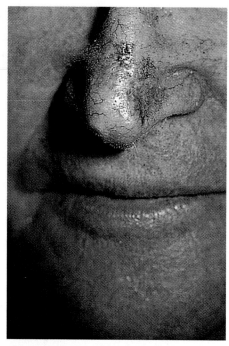

**FIG 16-15**
Lentigo maligna on the nose.

4. Melanoma in situ (lentigo maligna): These slow-growing, macular lesions have variegated pigmentation (usually two shades of brown), are typically larger than 1 cm in diameter, and are present for many years. They are curable if confined to the epidermis (Fig. 16-15).
5. Amelanotic melanoma: A nonpigmented melanoma, these lesions are very rare.

## Evaluation of Patients With Biopsy-Proved Melanoma

After melanoma is diagnosed by biopsy (Fig. 16-16), it is imperative to perform definitive surgery to ensure complete removal of the melanoma and adjacent tissue as soon as possible. Before surgery, the patient should be evaluated for evidence of regional lymph node metastasis. All patients with invasive melanoma have the potential for later recurrence or metastasis. These patients will therefore need follow-up examinations for life to check for evidence of local recurrence, new melanomas, or distant metastasis.

### Workup

Initial evaluation of all patients with invasive melanoma (Clark's Level 2 or greater [See Box 6-1]) should consist of a general skin examination, lymph node examination, and thorough history and physical examination. A chest x-ray and chemistry panel with LDH would be recommended for patients with melanoma greater than 0.76 mm in thickness because of the potential for metastasis. A surgical oncologist, medical oncologist, and/or a dermatologist should evaluate these patients.

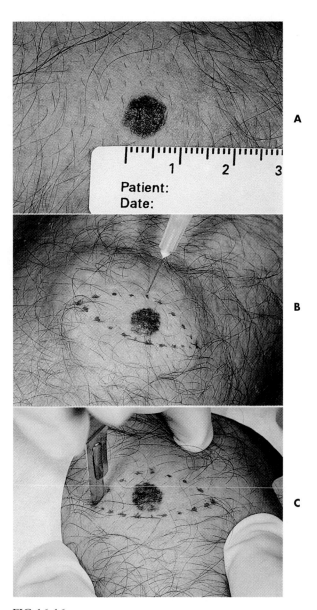

**FIG 16-16**

Excisional biopsy of suspected malignant melanoma. **A,** Pigmented lesion on the forearm of a 58-year-old man that satisfies all of the ABCDE criteria for the clinical diagnosis of malignant melanoma. **B,** An ellipse encompassing the entire lesion with small margins of normal skin is drawn with a surgical marking pen, and local anesthesia has been infiltrated beneath and around the lesion. **C,** The excision is begun with a No. 15 blade being held vertically. As it advances further, the scalpel will be brought closer to a 30-degree angle with the skin.

*Continued*

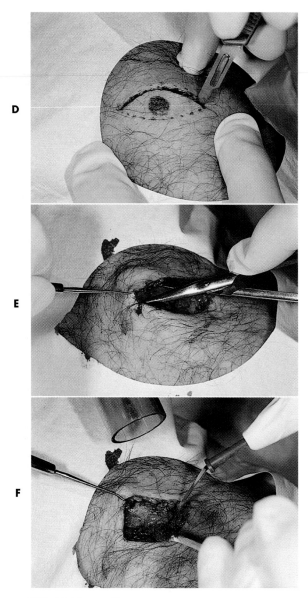

**FIG 16-16, cont'd**

Excisional biopsy of suspected malignant melanoma. **D,** The top half of the ellipse is cut, ending with the scalpel brought back to vertical. **E,** The wound is undermined with blunt scissors as wound edges are retracted with a skin hook. **F,** Small bleeding points are electrocoagulated with a Hyfrecator.

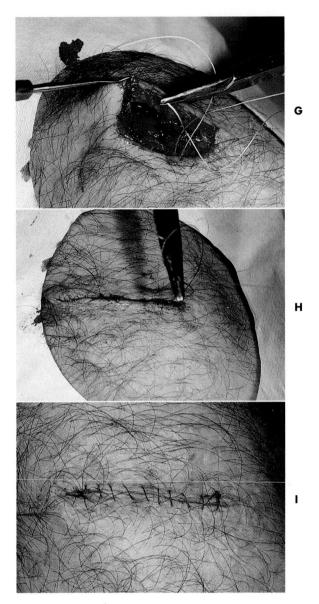

**FIG 16-16, cont'd**
Excisional biopsy of suspected malignant melanoma. **G,** A
subcutaneous 4-0 absorbable suture is placed. **H,** The
wound edges are approximated by pulling the subcutaneous
suture tight. This removes pressure on the cutaneous
sutures, leading to a more secure wound and a better cosmetic result. **I,** The cutaneous nylon sutures are placed, finishing the wound repair. The tissue specimen was sent for
histopathology. Diagnosis was malignant melanoma with a
depth of 0.4 mm.

## Treatment of Melanoma

Early surgical removal is the only definitive treatment of choice. It is curative if done before the melanoma has had time to metastasize.[11]

Melanomas can be divided into three prognostic categories: good, less favorable, and poor. The 1992 NIH Consensus Panel on Early Melanoma stated that melanomas can be treated with conservative surgical margins. The guidelines are 0.5-cm margins for melanoma in situ and 1-cm margins for malignant melanoma less than 1 mm in thickness. It is standard to use 2-cm margins for melanomas between 1 to 2 mm in thickness. For a lesion greater than 2 mm in depth, margins of at least 2 cm are called for (Table 16-1).

Melanomas falling into the less favorable and the poor prognostic categories require 2 cm or greater surgical margins, except in circumstances where margins this large would cause important functional impairment.[10] Certain patients in these categories may benefit from sentinel lymph node biopsy and/or lymph node dissection. In December 1995 adjuvant therapy with $\alpha$-interferon was approved for certain melanoma patients at high risk of recurrence.

**TABLE 16-1   Classification and Treatment of Melanoma**

| Melanoma | Depth | Clark | Breslow | Margin | Other therapy |
|---|---|---|---|---|---|
| **Good Prognosis** | | | | | |
| Melanoma in situ (lentigo maligna) | Confined to epidermis | I | | Small (usually ~5 mm) | None |
| Malignant melanoma without metastasis (thin) | Dermis | II | <1 mm | 1 cm | None |
| Intermediate | Dermis | III | 1-2 mm | 2 cm | None |
| **Less Favorable Prognosis** | | | | | |
| Intermediate | Deep dermis | IV | 2-4 mm | 2 cm or greater | Consider lymph node dissection, adjuvant chemotherapy or biologic therapy |
| **Poor Prognosis** | | | | | |
| Melanoma* | Deep subcutaneous fat | V | >4 mm | 2 cm or greater | Consider† |

*Clarks levels and Breslow levels do not always match up as shown in this table.*

*Melanoma any level with regional or distant metastasis, or deep melanoma without metastasis.

†Chemotherapy or biologic therapy, clinical trials including vaccines, and resection of isolated metastasis.

Treatment guidelines for patients in these categories is evolving, with new treatments offering promise for patients with advanced disease. All patients in these categories should be evaluated and managed by oncologic teams experienced with melanoma. Discussion of chemotherapy and other treatments for advanced melanoma and those lesions that have metastasized or have recurred despite previous treatment is beyond the scope of this book. However, excellent up-to-date, in-depth guidelines concerning treatment of advanced melanoma can be found on the website of the National Cancer Institute (http://www.nci.nih.gov).

## CONCLUSION

Early diagnosis of skin cancer can be lifesaving and can prevent local tissue destruction, which is particularly important on the face, where so many skin cancers arise. The incidence of skin cancer is high and is increasing. Familiarity with the essentials of skin cancer is helpful for all physicians responsible for patient care. The approach to the patient with potential skin cancer requires a knowledge of the clinical features, diagnosis, differential diagnosis, and treatment options for the most common skin cancers, including BCC, SCC, and melanoma.

It is important to understand the clinical features of common skin cancers to be able to perform the correct biopsy procedure. By doing a complete skin examination for all patients and performing a biopsy of suspicious lesions, physicians can improve the length and quality of life for all patients.

## REFERENCES

1. Miller DL, Weinstock MA: Nonmelanoma skin cancer in the United States: incidence, *J Am Acad Dermatol* 30(5):774-778, 1994.
2. Gumport SL et al: The diagnosis and management of common skin cancers, *Cancer* 31:79-90, 1981.
3. Salasche SJ, Amonette RA: Morpheaform basal cell epitheliomas, *J Dermatol Surg Oncol* 7: 387-394, 1981.
4. Lang PG: Variables to consider in the management of nonmelanoma skin cancer, *J Geriatr Dermatol* 4(7):231-237, 1996.
5. Parker SL et al: Cancer statistics, 1996, *CA Cancer J Clin* 46: 7-29, 1966.
6. Salopek TG et al: An estimate of the incidence of malignant melanoma in the United States: based on a survey of members of the American Academy of Dermatology, *Dermatol Surg* 21:301-305, 1995.
7. Parker SL et al: Cancer statistics, 1997, *CA Cancer J Clin* 47(1)5-27, 1997.
8. Balch CM, Houghton A, Peters L: Cutaneous melanoma. In DeVita VT, Heliman S, Rosenberg SA, editors: *Cancer: Principles and practice of oncology,* ed 3, Philadelphia, 1989, JB Lippincott.
9. Koh HK: Cutaneous melanoma, *New Engl J Med* 325(3):171-182, 1991.
10. Veronesi U et al: Thin stage I primary cutaneous malignant melanoma: comparison of excision with margins of 1 or 3 cm, *New Engl J Med* 318(18):1159-1162, 1988.
11. Johnson TM et al: Current therapy for cutaneous melanoma, *J Am Acad Dermatol* 32:689-707, 1995.
12. NIH Consensus Conference: Diagnosis and treatment of early melanoma, *JAMA* 268:1314-1319, 1992.

# CHAPTER 17

# When to Refer

*Richard P. Usatine    Ronald L. Moy*

This book is based on the premise that all physicians can learn to do simple skin surgery. With experience and training, most physicians (regardless of specialty) can learn to do more advanced skin procedures. In this chapter we will provide some guidelines to help assess when referral to a dermatologist or surgeon is necessary. There are five principal situations that should prompt a referral:

1. Aggressive skin cancer
2. A large lesion
3. A lesion located in a sensitive area (cosmetic or functional)
4. A lesion that is beyond the scope of one's skills
5. The patient has a higher chance than normal of having a complication or may require close monitoring during or after surgery

## AGGRESSIVE SKIN CANCER

We are defining aggressive skin cancer to include skin cancers with a predisposition to metastasis or local invasion. Melanoma is the skin cancer most likely to metastasize and can be fatal if it does. Squamous cell carcinoma (SCC) can metastasize and can also be locally invasive. Basal cell carcinomas (BCC) rarely metastasize but can recur or be locally invasive. Because of the lower malignant potential of a BCC, the diagnosis and primary treatment options will often be within the scope of this book. A recurrent BCC will usually warrant referral. Recurrence of a melanoma or SCC should always be referred to an appropriate specialist. In Fig. 17-1, *A*, a BCC on the patient's nose recurred after previous treatment. Fig. 17-1, *B* represents a pigmented, recurrent BCC on the back. These situations warrant referral for Mohs' micrographic surgery (Box 17-1). See Appendix D for further information on Mohs' surgery.

Although it is appropriate to do an elliptical excision or a punch biopsy to diagnose melanoma, often the definitive treatment will require a large excision. For melanoma between 1 to 2 mm in thickness, it is standard to excise the melanoma with 2-cm surgical margins. For a lesion greater than 2 mm in depth, margins of at least 2 cm are recommended. Usually, it is best to refer patients needing this procedure to a physician experienced in the treatment of melanoma. This might be a dermatologist, plastic surgeon, or general surgeon.

The deeper (>2 mm thick) and larger the melanoma, the more important this referral becomes. In Fig. 17-2, a large melanoma was diagnosed on the cheek of a woman (Clark's level IV). The deepest portion of the melanoma was 1.75 mm, and the lesion was excised with Mohs' surgery. In Fig. 17-3, a deep melanoma was diagnosed on the ear of a man (Clark's level IV). We recommend

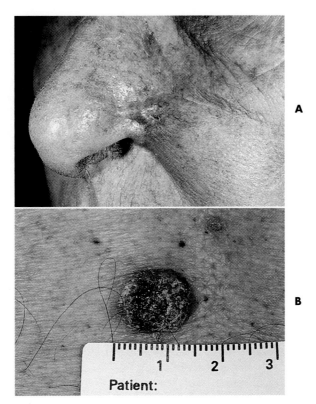

FIG 17-1
A, Recurrent BCC on a patient's nose. B, Recurrent BCC on the back (pigmented).

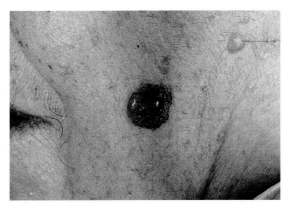

FIG 17-2
Melanoma on the face.

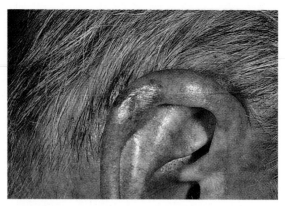

**FIG 17-3**
Melanoma on the ear (Clark's level IV).

---

**BOX 17-1    Indications for Referral for Mohs' Surgery**

Recurrent skin cancers
Primary lesions in locations with high lesion recurrence rates
   Posterior auricular area
   Nasolabial fold
   Temple
   Periauricular area
   Periocular area
   Scalp
   Nasal alae
   Center face
Anatomic areas where presentation of normal tissue is vital (for cosmetic
   and functional reasons)
   Nose
   Eyelids
   Lips
   Fingers
   Ears
   Penis
Sclerosing (morpheaform) BCC
Skin cancers known to be difficult to cure
   Melanoma, including lentigo maligna
   Poorly differentiated SCC
   Paget's disease of skin
   Verrucous carcinoma
   Microcystic adnexal carcinoma
   Dermatofibrosarcoma protuberans
   Sebaceous carcinoma
Malignant tumors with indistinct clinical margins
Large tumors greater than 2 cm
Skin cancers that have been present for many years

---

Modified from Moy RL, Zitelli JA: Mohs micrographic surgery for treatment of skin cancer in the
elderly, *Geriatric Med Today* 8(1), 1989.

referral for both of these patients. Even after the patient with the melanoma on the ear was treated by an experienced surgeon, the melanoma metastasized to the patient's brain.

The treatment of some melanomas will require lymph node dissection, a procedure that is far beyond the scope of this book.

SCCs or BCCs may warrant referral because of their size or location. In Fig. 17-4, the patient has a large BCC on the cheek. In addition, features that suggest an SCC or BCC is locally invasive or may have metastasized should prompt referral. For example, a physician should consider referring a patient with an SCC on the lips, temple, and ears because SCC has a 10% rate of metastasis from these locations. Also, SCC is more aggressive in the following circumstances:

- Size >2 cm
- SCC in a scar
- Patient is immunosuppressed
- Histology shows the lesion to be a poorly differentiated SCC or there is evidence of perineural invasion

In Chapters 11, 12, and 16 we covered various treatments for BCCs. Although cryotherapy and curettage and desiccation are convenient and easy methods to treat a BCC, recurrences can occur. The risk of recurrence is higher when a less skilled person performs the procedure. Sclerosing, morpheaform, or infiltrating BCC often recur. When a BCC recurs, consider referring your patient for Mohs' micrographic surgery or a large excision. If the BCC is in a cosmetically or functionally sensitive area, Mohs' surgery will provide the best result by maximizing the cure rate and tissue preservation. Some recurrent BCCs (e.g., on the back) may be treated with a wide and deep excision. Unless a physician is experienced in this type of surgery, a referral is prudent.

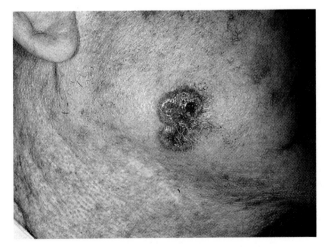

**FIG 17-4**
Large BCC over the mandible.

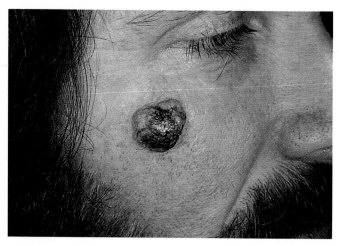

**FIG 17-5**
Large BCC on the cheek.

## LARGE LESION

Flaps and grafts are not within the scope of this book. Unless one has training in flaps and grafts, any lesion that would require a flap or graft will require referral. Such lesions are usually larger than 1.5 cm or are in areas where the skin is tight. Any surgical excision that will be difficult to close should prompt referral. For example, the large BCC on the cheek of the patient in Fig. 17-5 might warrant referral.

## LOCATION (COSMETIC)

The face is clearly the most cosmetically sensitive area. It is better to build up surgical experience working on areas such as the trunk and extremities. It is best to confine initial surgeries on the face to shave and punch biopsies. With experience, any physician may be able to handle elliptical excisions and cyst or lipoma excisions on the face.

In deciding whether to do surgery on a patient's face, consider the age, profession, and expectations of that person. An actor or model will likely have less tolerance for scarring on the face than a mineworker. A young person will probably live with the scar for more years and may have higher expectations for a cosmetic result than an older person. Because it is not good to generalize, it is always best to understand your patients' expectations by discussing these issues before undertaking the surgery.

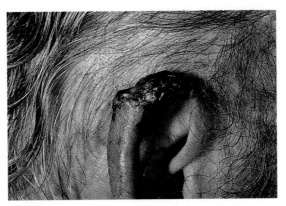

**FIG 17-6**
Large advanced BCC on the ear.

Finally, patients may ask to see a plastic surgeon or a dermatologist because they believe that only these specialists can produce a cosmetically acceptable outcome. A physician needs to weigh his or her experience and confidence with the patient's concerns and the external constraints of the prevailing health care system to make this decision. The patient's insurance status (capitated, HMO, fee-for-service indemnity plan, uninsured) will play a role in these decisions. In rural areas, limited access to specialists may also influence this decision.

One stated purpose of this book is to help all physicians maximize the cosmetic outcome of their biopsies and skin surgeries. It is not the specialty of the physician that determines the outcome of the procedure. We have shown a number of examples of skin surgery on the face because we believe that training and experience can lead to cosmetically excellent results in this area. There are limitations and risks to all surgical procedures, regardless of the training or specialty of the physician. Part of the process should always include obtaining informed consent so patients have a realistic understanding of the risks (including scarring) and benefits of the procedure. See Appendix A for an example of a consent form. Knowing a patient's previous history of keloid formation can help put risks and benefits into proper perspective for that individual.

In addition to the face, other cosmetically sensitive areas may include the hands, neck, genitalia, and a woman's breasts. Physicians should let preoperative discussions with patients guide them in determining the cosmetic significance of the area in question. In Fig. 17-6, the patient has a large BCC on the ear. Because there is a significant risk of deformity after removing this BCC, the procedure should be done by an experienced skin surgeon.

## LOCATION (FUNCTIONALLY SENSITIVE AREAS)

Functionally and cosmetically sensitive areas include the eyelids, alae of the nose, and corners of the mouth. Special expertise is needed to deal effectively with biopsies and excisions in these areas. Complications of inexperienced work in these areas include ectropion, entropion, and deformities of the nose and mouth. The BCC in Fig. 17-7 is on the lower eyelid, and the risk of treating this lesion is the development of entropion or ectropion. When the eyelid turns in or out, this can cause poor function, discomfort, and a poor cosmetic result.

In Fig. 17-8, the BCC is close to the nasal alae. Referral may avoid the production of a deformity of the nose.

Understanding the anatomic path of the temporal branch of the facial nerve is crucial to doing any deep surgical procedure in the temporal region (See Fig. 19-6, C). For this reason, it is prudent to refer a patient for excision of deep lesions in the temple area, such as epidermal cysts and lipomas. The complications of cutting this nerve are ptosis and inability to wrinkle the forehead. As described in Chapters 10 and 19 (See Fig. 19-7, B), care must be taken when performing procedures around the spinal accessory nerve (11th cranial nerve) where it runs superficially through the posterior triangle of neck. If this nerve it cut, the patient will lose major innervation to the trapezius muscle, resulting in impaired mobility of the scapula and shoulder.

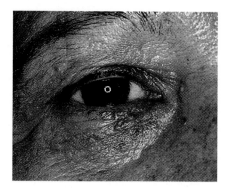

**FIG 17-7**
BCC on the lower eyelid.

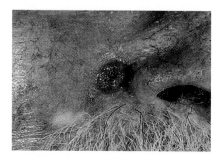

**FIG 17-8**
BCC on the nasal alae.

## DOUBTS ABOUT ONE'S OWN SKILLS

There is a first time for any procedure and it is healthy for a physician to have reservations before undertaking any new skin surgery. It is optimal to approach a new procedure with understanding and under adequate supervision. A number of the minor procedures described and illustrated in this book can be performed for the first time without supervision. By following our guidelines and using good judgment, a physician should be able to do high-quality skin surgeries. Whenever significant doubts arise about how to handle a specific skin surgery, do not hesitate to refer or get supervision. Skill also includes efficiency, and physicians must decide, after weighing their experience and confidence with the patient's concerns and the external constraints of the prevailing health care system, whether they should undertake any given procedure themselves or refer the patient to another physician.

Fig. 17-9 shows a keratoacanthoma on the back of the hand. Treatment options include a shave excision followed by curettage and desiccation or Mohs' surgery. For those who have never treated a keratoacanthoma, this is not the type to begin with because the vital structures of the hand are so close to the skin. This patient was referred for and underwent Mohs' surgery.

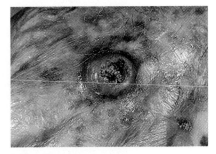

**FIG 17-9**
Keratoacanthoma on the back of the hand.

In Fig. 17-10, the condylomata on the penis have not responded to multiple applications of cryotherapy and various topical agents. This is a case of condylomata that are refractory to treatment, and large lesions that are located in a sensitive area. If the physician is not comfortable doing a shave excision in this area, it is appropriate to refer this patient for a shave biopsy to rule out Bowenoid papulosis. Bowenoid papulosis histologically resembles Bowen's disease (SCC in situ). However, evolution to invasive carcinoma is not observed.[1] This patient may need laser treatment or multiple large shave excisions. Conservative treatment with topical fluorouracil is an alternative treatment.[1]

Other examples of lesions that are difficult to excise even though they are benign include deep epidermal cysts and lipomas. A physician should not underestimate the difficulty of removing a simple epidermal cyst on certain portions of the body. These cysts are tricky to remove in many areas except for the scalp. On the scalp they tend to be easy to differentiate and separate from the surrounding tissue and are not deep in subcutaneous fat as they often are on the back and the neck. Lipomas on the forehead are particularly difficult because they can be deep and below the frontalis muscle in a subgaleal plane. Unless a physician is adept at dissecting lipomas from muscle and can do a good cosmetic closure on the forehead, a lipoma on the forehead is probably a good surgery for which to refer the patient.

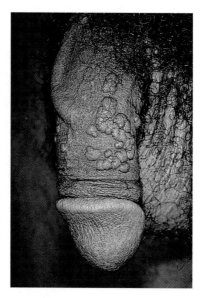

**FIG 17-10**
Severe case of condylomata acuminata on the penis that has not responded to cryotherapy and topical agents. Consider referral or perform shave biopsy to rule out Bowenoid papulosis.

## ECONOMIC AND LEGAL ISSUES

There are a number of economic disincentives for referring a patient to a specialist. With a fee-for-service patient, the physician will lose the compensation for the procedure. However, keep in mind that a cyst removed in 10 to 15 minutes can be cost effective, but the same procedure taking 60 to 90 minutes can be a money-loser in any setting. If the patient is enrolled in a capitated plan in which the primary care physician (or the group) will pay for the referral and procedure from the per-patient per-month revenue, the physician or group will directly spend money on such a referral. However, referrals may prevent costly complications. In many managed care settings, dermatology referrals will need to be approved by a utilization review committee. In this case, the final decision to approve a referral may be out of the primary care physician's hands. Regardless of the system, physicians should always remember the credo "do no harm" and should not do procedures for which they feel inadequately trained.

If a utilization review committee turns down a request for referral because the health plan does not cover a "cosmetic" procedure, a physician should not feel compelled to do a procedure that is too complicated. Legal consequences need to be weighed with financial concerns. Most of all, as physicians, we must make our patient's best interest our first priority.

## CONCLUSION

With the help of this book, all physicians should be able to extend their level of expertise in office skin surgery. The guidelines described in this chapter will help to assess the situations in which a patient should be referred to a physician with greater expertise. Discussing the procedure with the consultant or observing the actual procedure may allow a physician to further develop knowledge of and experience in skin surgery.

## REFERENCE

1. Habif T: *Clinical dermatology: a color guide to diagnosis and therapy,* ed 3, St. Louis, 1996, Mosby.

# CHAPTER 18

# Wound Care

*Daniel Mark Siegel    Ronald L. Moy    Richard P. Usatine**

There are different types of wound care procedures that are used, depending on the type and/or size of the wound. Sutured wounds are dealt with differently than wounds that are allowed to heal by secondary intention. Wound-care technique is a vital element in promoting new tissue growth. Similarly, the teaching of wound care to patients is an essential component of successful treatment.

Teaching wound care to the patient or a family member is best done after the surgical procedure is completed. The patient is usually worried before the procedure and will not be able to attend to information concerning postoperative care. Patients will appreciate receiving written postoperative instructions along with verbal explanations. Patients should be encouraged to look at the wound in the office so that they will not be frightened at home; a mirror can be used when the wound is on the face. If the patient feels faint at the sight of the affected area, it can be more safely managed in the office.

Quite often patients will not want to or cannot see the wound. In this case, wound care may be demonstrated to a family member or the person who is accompanying the patient. Patients are sometimes instructed to return for follow-up examinations so the physician will be able to assess the wound as well as the patient's ability to care for the wound. See Appendixes E and F for examples of wound-care instructions.

Techniques used for wound care promote wound healing and comfort by maintaining a moist environment, which usually yields better cosmetic results. A moist wound will generally not pull or feel tight and therefore will lead to more comfort for the patient during the healing process.

## WOUND-HEALING PHYSIOLOGY

### Re-epithelialization

It has been clearly demonstrated that the rate of re-epithelialization is directly related to moistness of the wound. Open, dry superficial wounds re-epithelialize significantly more slowly than occluded moist wounds.[1]

### Dermal Repair and Remodeling

Dermal healing is a slow process; animal studies suggest that 2 weeks postoperatively a sutured dermal scar possesses only 5% of the strength of normal skin. This emphasizes the importance of supporting these wounds by the use of buried sutures and adhesive wound-closure strips (especially at the time of suture removal).[1]

*We would like to acknowledge the assistance of Nitza Artman, RN, in writing this chapter.

## Bacterial Colonization and Wound Infection

It is impossible to completely sterilize human skin, and consequently all wounds rapidly become colonized by the local microbial flora. Clinical signs and symptoms of infection only occur when a critical number of pathogenic organisms accumulate within the wound and overwhelm local defenses. The presence of devitalized tissue and foreign material (such as sutures) may permit infection to develop with substantially fewer numbers of pathogens.[1]

# WOUND DRESSINGS

The selection and use of wound dressings can be highly personalized and modified by experience. Interestingly, not all physicians believe them to be necessary. Some studies suggest that in the short term the incidence of both infection and dehiscence of sutured wounds is no different between groups of dressed and undressed wounds.[2,3] For physicians who do prefer to use wound dressings, characteristics required for the ideal dressing are found in Box 18-1. Trade names of some commonly used dressings can be found in Box 18-2.

There are many types of wound dressings. Many of them have three layers: a contact layer, an absorbent layer, and an outer (secondary) layer.

## Contact Layer

The contact layer of a dressing is placed directly on the wound. It is usually selected for its nonadherent properties to limit the risk of sticking to the underlying wound. Plain gauze absorbs exudate but will readily stick to both open and sutured wounds. Specially designed nonadherent dressings may be applied either directly to the wound or after the application of an antibiotic ointment, which further minimizes the risks of adherence of the contact layer to the wound and

---

**BOX 18-1   Characteristics Required for the Ideal Dressing**

Handling of excess exudate
Removal of toxic substances
Maintenance of moist environment over wound
Barrier to microorganisms
Provides thermal insulation
Freedom from particulate contaminants
Removal without trauma to new tissue
Adheres well to a thin margin of surrounding skin
Does not adhere to the wound
Nontoxic and nonreactive
Conforms well to bodily contours and motion
Promotes patient comfort and is not bulky or conspicuous
Readily available and inexpensive
Long shelf life

Modified from Freitag DS: Surgical wound dressings. In Lask G, Moy R, editors: *Principles and techniques of cutaneous surgery*, New York, 1996, McGraw-Hill.

---

**BOX 18-2    Trade Names of Commonly Used Dressings**

**Transparent Films**
Tegaderm Transparent Dressing (3M)
Op-Site Wound Dressing (Smith &
    Nephew United)

**Gels and Hydrogels**
Vigilon (Bard Home Health)
IntraSite Gel Hydrogel (Smith &
    Nephew United)
2nd Skin Dressing (Spenco)

**Hydrocolloids**
Tegasorb Ulcer Dressing (3M)
Duoderm (Convatec)

**Calcium Alginates**
Kaltostat Wound Dressing (Calgon
    Vestal)
Sorbsan Absorbent Dressing (Dow B.
    Hickam, Inc.)
Algosteril (Johnson & Johnson)

---

Modified from Bernstein E et al: Wound healing. In Lask G, Moy R, editors: *Principles and techniques of cutaneous surgery,* New York, 1996, McGraw-Hill.

ultimately facilitates dressing removal. Plain gauze may be used if petrolatum or an antibiotic ointment is applied liberally to the wound to prevent sticking.

A variety of dressings are available for use as a nonadherent contact layer and include Vaseline impregnated gauze, Telfa, and a number of semipermeable dressings (e.g., Op-Site, Tegaderm, and Vigilon).

## Absorbent Layer

The absorbent layer of a dressing absorbs exudate and blood extruded from the wound and cushions the wound from outside trauma. Lying on top of the contact layer, it also presses this layer into contact with the wound or wound bed. The combination of both the contact and absorbent layers is referred to as the *primary dressing.* Many manufacturers have produced single dressings that combine both the contact and absorbent layer. For example, the widely used Telfa dressing consists of an absorbent layer of cellulose sandwiched between two layers of nonadherent polyester film.

## Outer (Secondary) Layer

The outer, or secondary, layer of dressing usually consists of gauze or cotton wadding. This layer is also referred to and acts as the *pressure dressing* and is secured in place with adhesive tape or bandage. Pressure dressings prevent hematomas by applying pressure to the subcutaneous dead space and immobilizing the underlying wound.

## Complete Dressing

The best example of a complete wound dressing involving all three layers is the ordinary household adhesive bandage (e.g., Band-Aid, Elastoplast, Telfa Ouchless Adhesive Pad) that combines contact, absorbent, and outer adhesive layers into a single sterile unit.

# TYPES OF SKIN WOUNDS

There are two common types of skin wounds that result from basic dermatologic surgery: a partial-thickness wound that heals by secondary intention and a full-thickness wound that is sutured.

## Secondary Intention Healing

Partial thickness wounds that heal by secondary intention are those wounds that result from shave biopsies and ablative procedures such as curettage and desiccation. The wound may be cleansed using a cotton-tipped swab dipped in hydrogen peroxide or tap water. The swab is gently rolled—not rubbed—over the wound to remove any loose debris and/or crusting. Recent laboratory studies have shown that hydrogen peroxide is toxic to epithelial cells, but ultimate clinical outcomes using the above technique are excellent.[4] Tap or distilled water may be substituted for the hydrogen peroxide.

### Topical antibiotics

After cleansing, the wound should be dressed with generous amounts of Bacitracin or Polysporin ointment. These ointments are over-the-counter products and are used to promote a moist environment for new tissue growth. If a patient has a known allergy to either of the antibiotic ointments, they are instructed to use plain petrolatum, such as Vaseline. In a recent study, Smack et al[5] showed that "white petrolatum is an effective, safe wound care ointment for patients after ambulatory surgery. In comparison with Bacitracin, white petrolatum possesses minimal potential for selection of resistant bacterial strains, no risk for induction of local and systemic allergic reactions, and an impressively lower cost. The incidence of infection and healing characteristics are not significantly affected by substituting white petrolatum for Bacitracin ointment."

When treating contaminated, dirty, or grossly infected wounds, data support the use of antibiotic-containing ointments in place of white petrolatum. However, the data to support for the use of antibiotic-containing ointments in the postprocedural care of clean wounds is lacking.[5] See Table 18-1 for information about the topical antibiotics most used for prophylaxis during wound healing.

**TABLE 18-1   Types of Antibacterial Ointments**

| Brand name | Active antimicrobial ingredients |
|---|---|
| Bacitracin | Bacitracin zinc |
| Polysporin | Bacitracin zinc, polymyxin B sulfate |
| Neosporin | Neomycin sulfate,* bacitracin zinc, polymyxin B sulfate |
| Gentamicin | Gentamicin sulfate |
| Ilotycin | Erythromycin |
| Aquaphor Faster Healing Ointment | Bacitracin zinc, polymyxin B sulfate |

From Freitag DS: Surgical wound dressings. In Lask G, Moy R, editors: *Principles and techniques of cutaneous surgery*, New York, 1996, McGraw-Hill.
*Avoid neomycin because it is a potent sensitizer.

### Dressings

If a wound is small, patients are encouraged to use adhesive bandages to cover the wound. When the wound is large, it may be covered with a nonstick dressing pad, such as Telfa, and secured with a hypoallergenic tape. This approach can be used for wounds of all depths in almost all locations.

Dressings should be changed once a day, preferably after a shower or bath. Patients can keep the dressing in place during bathing so that new tissue growth is not washed away with a forceful water stream. Alternatively, if the wound needs cleaning, the shower helps remove debris and exudate. For wounds in which the ointment will drain away because of gravity, the patient should be instructed to apply ointment more than once a day to ensure that the wound stays moist 24 hours per day. In this case, the patient is instructed to add ointment at some point during the day, but is also instructed that the wound is to be cleaned only once a day.

### Occlusive dressings

Deeper exudative or superficial slow-healing wounds such as leg ulcers can be treated with calcium alginate or hydrocolloid (Duoderm) dressings. The dressings are used in an occlusive fashion, minimizing the air penetration to the wound site.

Before applying an occlusive dressing, the wound is first cleansed with normal saline using a cotton-tipped swab. The dressing is then placed onto or into the wound. The calcium alginate dressing is either placed directly onto the wound bed or packed tightly into wounds that are deep. The wound can then be covered with a piece of Telfa. Then absorbent gauze is placed above the Telfa. The dressings are then cut down to the size of the wound. The area can be secured with a transparent dressing such as Tegaderm and covered with a nontransparent tape to camouflage the yellowish drainage that is produced by the dressing. It should be noted that although this drainage is foul-smelling, it is a normal result of using these dressings and is not a sign of infection.

The dressings are changed every 3 to 4 days, and patients are asked to return for follow-up examinations 3 to 4 days after they have changed the dressing so that their technique can be evaluated and a decision can be made as to whether the patient will continue using this type of dressing. An occlusive dressing is used for approximately 2 weeks.

The types of wounds effectively treated by occlusive dressings are determined by depth and anatomic location. The location is evaluated with respect to whether the dressings can be completely sealed without leakage and if they can stay in place for 3 to 4 days. When occlusive dressing is discontinued, the patient is instructed to use hydrogen peroxide or water to clean the wound and to apply Bacitracin ointment and a nonstick pad or Band-Aid as discussed above until complete healing has occurred.

## Sutured Wounds

One method of caring for sutured wounds is similar to that noted above for shave biopsies. A cotton-tipped swab is dipped in hydrogen peroxide and gently rolled—not rubbed—along the suture line to remove any loose debris and/or crusting. The wound is then dressed with ointment and covered with a nonstick dressing pad or Band-Aid.

Another dressing method involves using Steri-Strips and/or micropore tape over the incision site immediately after surgery. These are left in place until the sutures are removed. Semi-permeable tape strips (e.g., Steri-Strips) may be applied transversely across the wound, providing support and reducing tension across the suture line. Spaces left between the strips allow wound exudate and blood to escape and be absorbed by the overlying dressing. Tissue adhesives (e.g., tincture of benzoin, Mastisol) may be used to increase the adherence of tape strips to the skin. A nonadherent primary dressing may then be applied and taped in place, and a pressure dressing applied on top of that (Fig. 18-1). In most situations, pressure dressings consist of bulky gauze or cotton wadding secured in place by adhesive tape.

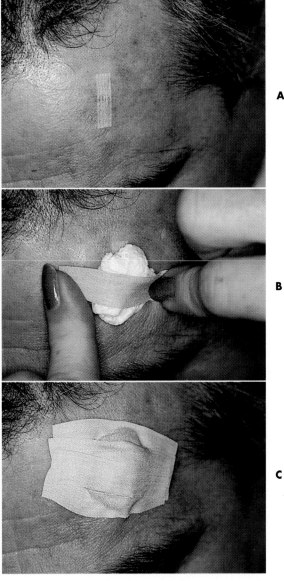

**FIG 18-1**
A, Steri-strip placed over incision closed with sutures.
B, Placing tape with pressure (micropore tape is generally preferred at this time). C, Final pressure dressing.

The use of pressure dressings to reduce the risk of hematoma formation is especially important after the excision of cysts or lipomas. Patients may be instructed to remove the bulky outer pressure dressing 24 to 36 hours after surgery, leaving the underlying primary dressing undisturbed. In view of the unique local vasculature, it is not advisable to apply pressure dressings to the digits.

After surgical procedures performed in the physician's office, the sutured wound should be cleaned with saline, hydrogen peroxide, or an antiseptic solution, with the specific exception of periorbital wounds. Small sutured wounds are easily dressed with the use of a sterile adhesive bandage (e.g., Band-Aid) with or without the use of topical antibiotic ointment.

### Hydrocolloid dressing

The dressings discussed above all require varying degrees of maintenance by the patients. One maintenance-free dressing for sutured wounds uses wound closure tape (Steri-Strips) or a hydrocolloid dressing (e.g., DuoDerm) cut to cover and extend beyond the suture line for 5 to 10 mm in all directions. This is then covered with Tegaderm, Op-Site, or a standard pressure dressing.[6] If the wound is deep and hematoma formation is a concern, a pressure dressing can be placed. This pressure dressing consists of generous amounts of absorbent gauze fluffs taped firmly over the Tegaderm to apply pressure. Instructions are given to the patient to remove the pressure dressing in 24 hours, leaving DuoDerm and Tegaderm dressing in place until a follow-up examination in 1 week, when the dressing is removed in the office by peeling it off parallel to the suture line. Absorbable sutures below the skin will be hydrolyzed and significantly weakened, whereas sutures above the surface will have melted into the Duoderm (Fig. 18-2). When the Duoderm is removed, the absorbable sutures come with it.[6]

Hydrocolloid dressing is unique in many ways. It is water resistant, maintenance free, and popular among patients because they do not have to do anything for its care. This type of dressing is ideal for wounds that are closed by 6-0 and 5-0 fast-absorbing plain or mild chromic gut suture on the surface. This dressing should not be used on contaminated wounds, such as dog bites. Also, if there is a higher risk of infection, such as in a diabetic patient, it is best to use a dressing that allows for daily observation.

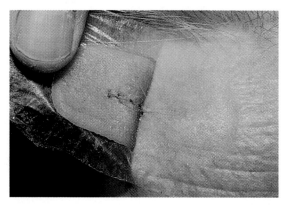

**FIG 18-2**
Removal of hydrocolloid/Op-Site dressing. Dressing is turned over showing the gut sutures incorporated into the hydrocolloid dressing.

## PATIENT INSTRUCTIONS FOR POSTOPERATIVE WOUND CARE

Overall, patients should be instructed to keep their wounds covered and moist to prevent the formation of any scabs and crusts. Specific advice on bathing and taking showers is necessary because this is a potential point of confusion for patients. It is generally acceptable for open, granulating wounds to become wet, and it seems reasonable to allow showers but to discourage prolonged immersion in water (baths and swimming). After a shower, patients may clean and redress their wounds. Many physicians advise patents with sutured wounds to keep their dressings dry until suture removal; however, there is evidence that undressed sutured wounds can be washed with soap and water twice a day, beginning the morning after surgery, without any increased risk of infection or wound dehiscence.[7]

At the time of suture removal, sutured wounds possess only a small fraction of the strength of normal skin, and the possibility of dehiscence, stretching, or splaying of the scar still exists. Therefore patients must be advised to limit physical activities that might place unnecessary stretching forces on the wound for a reasonable period after suture removal.

## DRESSING CHANGES

For uncomplicated sutured wounds, the primary dressing can remain in place until sutures are removed. The patient is told to remove the outer pressure bandage 24 to 48 hours postoperatively. The patient should be instructed not to allow the primary dressing to become wet, especially during the first 24 hours after surgery. Open wounds usually require dressing changes once or twice daily so the wound can be cleaned of exudate and debris and the moist environment that is conducive to rapid wound healing can be maintained.

If bandages become soaked with blood or exudate, the patient must be instructed to return promptly to the physician's office to have the dressing removed and the wound inspected for signs of active bleeding or hematoma formation before reapplication of a wound dressing.

Topical antiseptic solutions potentially interfere with wound healing; it has been reported that 1% povidone-iodine, 3% hydrogen peroxide, and 0.3% chlorhexidine solutions all produce toxic effects on fibroblasts and keratinocytes and may delay the formulation of granulation tissue.[8] Cleaning the wound with clean tap water or sterile saline may be most beneficial and avoid the tissue toxicity of antiseptic solutions.

## SPECIAL LOCATIONS

### The Digits

When applying dressings to a finger or toe, two main types may be used: a tubular dressing or a bandage applied obliquely and attached at the wrists. Excessive pressure should be avoided.

### Periorbital Wounds

Wounds that involve or approach the cutaneous-conjunctival junction should not be cleaned with either hydrogen peroxide or antiseptic solutions such as Hibiclens; these solutions are potentially oculotoxic. If the application of topical antibiotic ointment to the wound is likely to involve spread to the eye, it is preferable to select a preparation specifically formulated for ophthalmic use (e.g., Polysporin Ophthalmic Ointment).

## CONTACT DERMATITIS IN WOUND CARE

Eczematous eruptions have been associated with tissue adhesives, tapes, and antibiotic ointments. Erosions, bullae, and bruising may be associated with the use of adhesive tapes (particularly when used with tissue adhesives) and are most commonly seen on the facial skin of elderly patients and those patients on systemic steroid therapy. Avoiding the use of neomycin and using micropore tape can minimized the risk of contact dermatitis.

## CONCLUSION

There are many ways to dress a wound and obtain good wound healing. The physician can choose the wound dressing based on the characteristics of the surgery, the patient, and the availability of the needed resources. Using the principles discussed in this chapter will help produce optimal healing with a minimum of pain and scarring. For further information on potential complications of surgery and wound healing, see Chapter 19.

## REFERENCES

1. Telfer N, Moy R: Wound care after office procedures, *Dermatol Surg Oncol* 19:722-731, 1993.
2. Heifetz CJ, Richards FO, Lawrence MS: Wound healing without dressings: clinical study, *Arch Surg* 67661-669, 1953.
3. Palumbo LT, Monning PJ, Wilkinson DE: Healing of clean surgical wounds of thorax and abdomen with or without dressings, *JAMA* 160:553-555, 1956.
4. Niedner R, Schopf E: Inhibition of wound healing by antiseptics, *Br J Dermatol* 115:41-44, 1986.
5. Smack DP et al: Infection and allergy incidence in ambulatory surgery patients using white petrolatum vs bacitracin ointment: a randomized controlled trial, *JAMA* 276:972-977, 1996.
6. Siegel D et al: Surgical pearl: a novel cost-effective approach to wound closure and dressings, *J Am Acad Dermatol* 34(4):673-675, 1996.
7. Noe JM, Keller M: Can stitches get wet? *Plast Reconstr Surg* 81:82-84, 1988.
8. Lineaweaver W et al: Cellular and bacterial toxicities of topical antimicrobials, *Plast Reconstr Surg* 75:394-396, 1985.

# CHAPTER 19

# Complications and Their Prevention

*Ronald L. Moy    Richard P. Usatine*

It is important for every physician who performs skin surgery to be familiar with the gamut of complications that may occur because it is impossible to prevent every complication. It is important for the physician and the office staff to recognize potential complications. If postoperative patients have any complaint it is usually worthwhile for them to come into the office to be examined. Offering the patient the opportunity to be seen in the office that day is a good way of screening out the overly concerned patient from the patient who truly has a problem while also protecting yourself medicolegally. Another good tip for physicians is to make a postoperative call the evening after surgery to all patients who have undergone a significant procedure. The call between 6 PM and 9 PM usually eliminates the call between 9 PM and 6 AM! The incidence of severe complications can be decreased with surgical experience, good surgical techniques, and the recognition of problems before they become severe. Potential postoperative complications of skin surgery are listed in Box 19-1.

## SCARRING

Scarring is the most common complication resulting from skin surgery. Scarring can occur in any patient operated on by any physician. There are situations where scarring is predictable and cannot be prevented. The deltoid area, the chest, and the back are prone to scarring because of either the skin tension in these areas, the thicker skin in these areas, or some unknown factor. Surgery on sebaceous skin, such as the type that appears on the nose, often leads to obvious incisional scars. The most important point is to warn the patient that in these areas excisional surgery will often result in scarring no matter who does the surgery. Therefore on the back, chest, and deltoid areas, a shave technique should be used when it is an acceptable alternative because it can offer a better cosmetic result than an excision with stitches. If a patient is overly concerned about a scar or expresses the unrealistic desire to have absolutely no scar, it is better for them to find their way to a plastic surgeon's office before the procedure than after.

Excessive or increased skin tension leads to a widened scar. This is the reason that buried sutures that decrease tension can improve cosmetic results. The increased skin tension in younger patients probably contributes to the widened scars seen in young patients compared with the narrow, fine scars seen in older patients. In Fig. 19-1, a widened scar is seen on a young woman's back years after the wide excision of a melanoma.

Allowing sutures to remain in for too long can also increase scarring. Fig. 19-2 shows the scar that occurred when a patient did not keep his follow-up appointment and returned 2 weeks too late for suture removal.

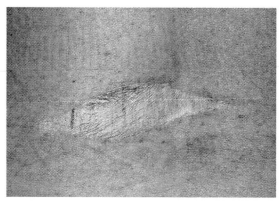

**FIG 19-1**
Widened scar on lower back years after wide excision of melanoma in a young woman.

---

**BOX 19-1   Possible Postoperative Complications of Skin Surgery**

**Within the First 2 Weeks**
Infection
Pain
Bleeding
Dehiscence
Hematoma
Bruising and swelling
Suture spitting

**Prolonged or Permanent**
Scarring
Hypertrophic scars
Keloid
Hyperpigmentation
Hypopigmentation
Nerve damage
Ectropion and entropion of eyelids
Notching and atrophy of tumors overlying cartilage
Tenting or notching of the vermilion border of the upper lip
Skin atrophy
Alopecia
Recurrence of the lesion

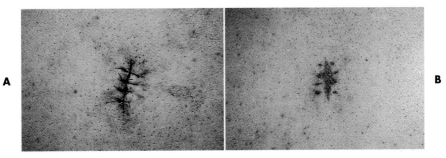

**FIG 19-2**
**A,** Primary closure of elliptical excision of an atypical nevus on the back. **B,** Scarring that resulted from patient returning for suture removal in 4 weeks rather than the recommended 10 to 14 days.

Complications such as infection, necrosis, or dehiscence can increase scarring. Excessive skin tension often leads to dehiscence and scarring. Infection or necrosis often leads to dehiscence. Infection may be prevented by using meticulous sterile surgical techniques. Dehiscence may be prevented by using good excision planning, undermining when necessary, and using deep absorbable sutures to decrease skin tension across a wound. Tying sutures too tightly can also cause scarring.

Depressed scars result when a deep shave biopsy is performed or when another complication leads to scarring within the dermal layer of the skin. These depressed scars need to be reexcised before a flat appearance can be obtained. Limiting the depth of a shave excision or curettage can prevent depressed scars.

The most important point when discussing potential scarring after surgery is to warn the patient about the risk of scarring or highly visible incision lines. The patient should understand that if scarring does occur, it can be treated with dermabrasion, intralesional cortisone, Cordran tape, laser resurfacing, or the yellow light laser used to treat persistent redness. It may be helpful to warn patients who want the optimal result that a dermabrasion approximately 8 weeks after the surgery will improve any incision line.

An informed consent of the potential complications should be discussed with and signed by the patient. The informed consent should at least discuss the possibility of scarring, bleeding, and infection. It may also include the possibility of nerve damage and tumor recurrence. No absolute guarantees of cosmetic results can be made. Specific possible complications related to the anatomic site should be discussed where appropriate. See the sample consent form in Appendix A.

## SCAR IMPROVEMENT WITH DERMABRASION

The optimal time to perform dermabrasion is approximately 8 to 12 weeks after the surgery. Dermabrasion performed in this early phase of wound healing has been shown to improve the cosmetic appearance of an incision scar more than if the dermabrasion is deferred until many months later. The reason may have to do with inducing collagen remodeling during the early phase of wound healing when new collagen is being formed.

The dermabrasion that we do is performed manually with the use of sterile, medium-grade, dry wall grid wrapped around the same syringe used for anesthetizing the area.[1] This medium-grade, dry wall grid can be found in most hardware stores in the sandpaper section. It can be cut into rectangles and sterilized in instrument bags.

Dermabrasion is performed after local anesthesia is achieved; it is carried down to the depth where bleeding starts. The objective is to smooth out the area but not to induce an indentation. Hemostasis is achieved with pressure alone for about 10 minutes or with a pressure bandage.

## WOUND DEHISCENCE

If a wound dehiscence (Fig. 19-3) occurs without evidence of infection (redness, warmth, pus), it might be advisable to resuture the wound with interrupted sutures and start the patient on antibiotics. The sutures may only have to be left in place for half the normal time because the fibroblasts have already initiated the wound site and the wound is partially healed. The cause of the dehiscence may need to be addressed if significant wound tension exists. A buried absorbable suture may decrease the wound tension.

If infection or a hematoma is the cause of dehiscence, the wound should be opened and irrigated, and the patient should be started on antibiotics. The wound should be cleansed daily and left to heal naturally. It will usually take at least 3 to 4 weeks before the wound healing is complete. The patient should be informed that a scar revision may be performed at a later time if desired.

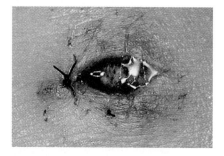

**FIG 19-3**
Dehiscence occurring at day 7 when the sutures where removed from an atypical nevus excised on the back. No buried sutures were used in this patient, and the nylon sutures should have been removed at day 10. Dehiscence occurred during suture removal. Wound-closure tape should be applied after suture removal.

# INFECTION

Infection (Fig. 19-4) is not very common with most skin surgery if good sterile technique and principles are applied. The infection rate for the type of skin surgery discussed in this book should be less than 1%. The head and neck area will have a lower infection rate because the blood supply is better than with the extremities. Surgery performed on the extremities may have a higher infection rate.

By the time that most patients are seen with an infection, the classic signs of redness, warmth, and pain are usually present. The patient may have a slight fever, and pus may be expressed from the wound. These symptoms usually become obvious around 5 to 7 days postoperatively or at the time of suture removal. Infections can manifest at postoperative day 2 to 4. If a patient has any complaints, it is best to examine the wound for evidence of infection. If the wound is tender and fluctuant, removal of one or more sutures to allow drainage will speed up resolution of the infection. If there is frank pus in the wound and it is not removed, antibiotics will be ineffective.

The use of prophylactic antibiotics is not usually recommended. Most studies have not proved the value of antibiotics in preventing infection. There are a number of situations where the use of antibiotics given just before or after a surgical procedure is performed may be advisable. Surgery performed on the extremities, the perineum or genitalia, the axilla, and the ear may benefit from the use of antibiotics because these anatomic areas may have a higher incidence of infection.[2] Examples of when a physician should consider providing prophylactic antibiotics to a patient are listed in Box 19-2.

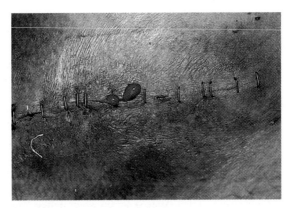

**FIG 19-4**
Wound infections usually manifest between 5 to 10 days after surgery. The usual clinical manifestations are redness, pain, warmth, swelling, and pus. This wound will need to be drained by removing enough staples (or sutures) to irrigate the wound. The wound should be cultured and the patient started on antibiotics.

---

**BOX 19-2   When to Consider Prophylactic Antibiotics**

**Location of surgery**
Extremities
Perineum or genitalia
Axilla
Ear

**Patient**
Immunosuppressed patient
Diabetic patient

**Timing/other**
Wound has been open more than 1 hour
Complete sterile technique was not optimal
Follow-up difficult

---

Cutaneous surgery on the ear can result in postoperative chondritis caused by trauma to the cartilage. The risk of chondritis may be decreased by having the patient take one to three aspirin (325 mg) per day with meals beginning 24 hours after surgery for 5 to 7 days.

Surgery in which the wound has been open more than 1 hour has a higher incidence of infection. Surgery on a patient in which an infection would be very dangerous, such as in an immunosuppressed patient, may require that the patient be given prophylactic antibiotics. The usual antibiotics given to patients include cephalexin 250 mg qid or 500 mg bid, dicloxacillin 250 mg qid, or erythromycin 250 mg qid in the penicillin-allergic patient. Newer cephalosporins and other drugs, such as ciprofloxacin, are not cost effective prophylactic agents and should be reserved for specific treatments where indicated. Prophylactic antibiotics do not need to cover methicillin-resistant *S. aureus* because it is very uncommon in the office surgery setting.

Suture reactions are frequently mistaken for infections and must be differentiated from them. These may arise in areas where buried sutures have been placed and can present as a small pustule or erosion in the suture line (Fig. 19-5). The patient can complain of a "pimple" on the suture line or a piece of suture extruding from the incision line. This can occur when a buried suture is placed too close to the skin surface. Purulent material from these sites is sterile.

Suture reactions can range from mild, with only a spicule of suture spitting, to more severe reactions in which the entire wound gets warm and boggy. These reactions are self limited and can be calmed with intralesional injections of triamcinolone 2.5 mg/ml and warm compresses. Removal of reacting and spitting sutures can speed up resolution. Antibiotics are frequently given with severe reactions to cover the chance that there is also an element of infection. Suture reactions rarely affect the ultimate cosmetic outcome.

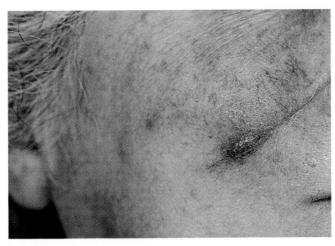

**FIG 19-5**
Suture abscess that can be drained with an 18-gauge needle or a No. 11 blade. Suture abscesses result from superficial placement of buried sutures.

# BLEEDING

Excessive bleeding during surgery often results from a patient who did not stop taking aspirin 2 weeks before surgery. This often results in the type of oozing that is hard to stop with electrocoagulation. Nonsteroidal antiinflammatory drugs can also cause excessive bleeding if they are not stopped 2 days before surgery.

Some patients will have a bleeding diathesis. It may not be necessary to order coagulation studies or platelet counts for the types of minor skin surgeries described in this book because the bleeding can be controlled with the hemostatic methods described in Chapter 4.

Patients who are on Coumadin do not bleed as much as those on aspirin. Most patients who are having limited skin excisions do not need their Coumadin stopped. If the planned surgery is "large" and the risk of bleeding is great, the Coumadin can be discontinued for 2 to 4 days before surgery and restarted about 2 days after surgery. The risk of bleeding can also be lessened by waiting 15 to 20 minutes before beginning the procedure after injecting an epinephrine-containing local anesthetic. This may make the procedure less bloody and decrease the chance of postoperative bleeding.

The risk of hematoma can be lessened with careful attention to hemostasis with conservative electrocoagulation. An appropriate pressure dressing can also prevent hematoma formation. Excessive electrocoagulation can damage tissue and impair wound healing. Although sutures that are placed tightly can cause suture marks, they can also stop bleeding. Tighter sutures might be used in a situation where the patient seems to be oozing or bleeding excessively. If the patient has a bleeding diathesis, undermining should be minimized to that which is absolutely necessary. This will also minimize potential dead space and the risk of hematoma.

Postoperative bleeding usually occurs within the first 24 hours after surgery. It will occur more in a patient who was taking aspirin but may also occur more often in a patient who has high blood pressure or who is physically active. Sometimes a bleeder can be missed during surgery. It was once argued that the use of epinephrine would mask the bleeding during surgery but then lead to postoperative bleeding. A recent study has shown that the use of epinephrine does not lead to postoperative bleeding or hematomas.

The usual scenario for post-operative bleeding is that the patient will call the physician and complain of blood soaking through the bandage. The physician must then determine whether this is the type of bleeding that will require electrocoagulation. The patient should be instructed to apply firm pressure for about 1 hour. This will usually stop the bleeding in a majority of situations. A good, firm pressure dressing will prevent many of these after-hour bleeding episodes. The pressure dressing should consist of gauze that is fluffed up and many layers of paper tape, resulting in very firm pressure being applied during the first 24 hours. Blood on the dressing is better than blood in the wound.

If the patient complains of increased pain and bulging around the surgical incision wound, the patient needs to be evaluated for a potential hematoma. If the hematoma is detected during the first 24 hours, the incision usually needs to be opened. All of the sutures should be removed, and the bleeding should be stopped with electrocoagulation. The wound can then be sutured again and the patient started on systemic antibiotics.

If the hematoma is detected after more than 24 hours postoperatively and there does not seem to be active bleeding or an expanding hematoma, the wound may not need to be opened. Instead, a syringe with an 18-gauge needle is used to extract the blood. A pressure dressing is applied, and the patient is started on antibiotics. The use of a needle to decrease the size of the hematoma may not work after 1 week, when the blood from the hematoma has organized and formed a clot. If the hematoma has clotted, this must resolve with time.

## NERVE DAMAGE

Numbness is a common complaint from patients after cutaneous surgery. It usually resolves in about 6 to 12 months after the nerves have regrown and arborized. The concern from cutaneous surgery is damaging a superficial motor nerve. The two nerves that can easily be damaged permanently are the temporal branch of the facial nerve and the spinal accessory nerve.

The temporal branch of the facial nerve can be damaged by any surgery of the temple area. The nerve lies very superficially within the fat layer. It can be impossible to see, and there is enough anatomic variation that it can be unpredictable in its location. The best way to locate the nerve is to draw an imaginary line from the tragus to the eyebrow and another imaginary line from the tragus to the upper forehead wrinkle area. The area between these two lines within the temple area is where the temporal branch of the facial nerve is most superficial. If this nerve is cut, the patient will not be able to wrinkle the forehead because the innervation to the frontalis muscle is lost. The patient will also likely have permanent drooping of the upper eyelid (Fig. 19-6), called *ptosis*. If any surgery is performed in this area, it is important that this risk is discussed with the patient. It is one reason that a superficial curettage and electrodesiccation may be a less risky procedure if it is appropriate on a superficial skin cancer. Mohs' micrographic surgery is also an appropriate technique in this area because the tissue is removed layer by layer.

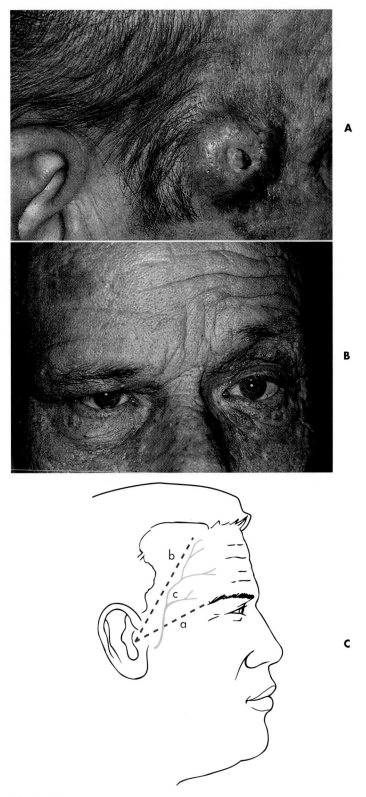

**FIG 19-6**
**A,** SCC on the temple area where the temporal branch of the facial nerve lies just under the dermis within the superficial fat. **B,** The temporal branch of the facial nerve was cut, resulting in the patient having a permanent ptosis. **C,** *a,* Line from tragus to eyebrow; *b,* line from tragus to upper forehead wrinkle area; *c,* temporal branch of facial nerve.

The spinal accessory nerve lies within the posterior triangle posterior to the sternocleidomastoid muscle (Fig. 19-7). The nerve can lie very superficially posterior to the sternocleidomastoid muscle at the level of the thyroid cartilage notch. If this nerve is cut, the patient will lose major innervation to the trapezius muscle, resulting in impaired mobility of the scapula and shoulder.

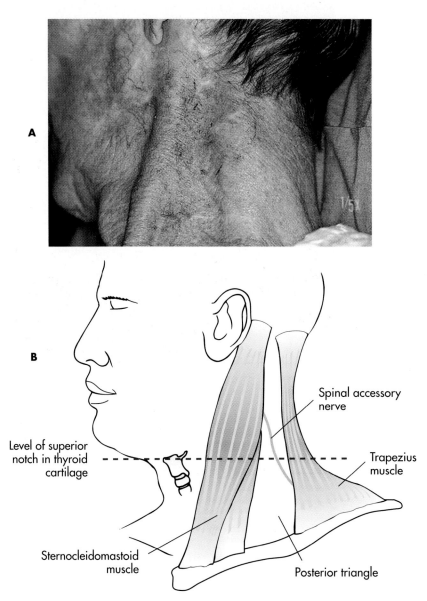

**FIG 19-7**
**A,** Recurrent sclerosing BCC in the region of the spinal accessory nerve. **B,** Using anatomic landmarks to identify the location of the nerve may prevent cutting the nerve during surgical removal of the BCC. The spinal accessory nerve lies within the posterior triangle at the level of the superior notch in the thyroid cartilage.

## SWELLING AND BRUISING

Patients should be warned that surgery performed around the nose or forehead can cause tremendous swelling and bruising around the eyes (Fig. 19-8). It is even possible that the eyes may swell shut. The use of ice may help prevent some of this edema if it is used during the first few hours after surgery. The lips can also stay swollen for many weeks or months after surgery.

## PAIN

Most patients do not complain of severe pain unless the wound is closed under tension. A majority of patients will require only acetaminophen after surgery. Acetaminophen with codeine can also be given to patients; however, the complications of nausea and constipation make this drug combination a second choice compared with acetaminophen alone. If a patient complains of increasing pain, a hematoma or infection should be considered in the differential diagnosis.

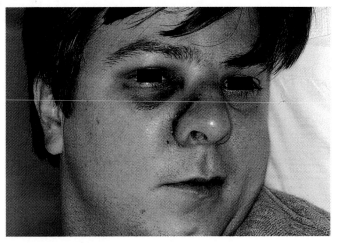

**FIG 19-8**
Bruising can occur after any surgery on the face, even in young individuals. Swelling of the eyes is common after excisions on the face.

# RECURRENCE OF THE LESION OR SKIN CANCER

There is almost nothing in the practice of medicine that is a 100% guarantee. Mohs' micrographic surgery for the removal of skin cancer has a cure rate of only 99% in primary skin cancers. Most other surgical techniques have cure rates of about 90%, depending on a number of factors. Lipomas, cysts, and nevi (especially if they are removed with a shave) can all recur. Although recurrent lesions may be considered a complication, it should be recognized by both the patient and physician that recurrences will occur in a small percentage of cases. When a recurrent lesion develops, the lesion will usually need to be excised again. In Fig. 19-9, a BCC recurred in the incision line after an elliptical excision.

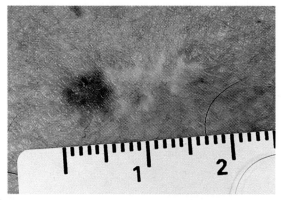

FIG 19-9
Recurrent BCC in the incision line after an elliptical excision.

## MAKING MISTAKES

As a physician, it feels awful to make a mistake that leads to harming a patient. It may also feel bad when a patient gets a less than optimal cosmetic result after a surgical procedure. We all took the oath "First, do no harm." In performing skin surgery it is inevitable that you will have wounds that dehisce, scars that are larger than expected, and infections and hematomas that will occur in surgical sites. These are known complications of skin surgery, and may not be caused by an error on your part. However, it is also possible for a scalpel to slip and cut a larger wound than intended. Postoperative infections and hematomas can occur even in the most carefully performed surgery. However, if a physician is in a rush and uses less careful sterile technique or pays less attention to possible bleeders, he or she may contribute to these complications. A physician may choose to take out sutures too soon and get dehiscence.

We have presented ways to minimize complications, but poor outcomes can and do happen to the patients of most practicing physicians. If the poor outcome is caused by the physician's mistake, he or she will face the ethical dilemma of whether to disclose the mistake to the patient. Although this discussion is beyond the scope of this book, Dr. Bernard Lo has a written an insightful and practical chapter on disclosing mistakes in his book entitled *Resolving Ethical Dilemmas: A Guide for Clinicians*.[3] In all cases, the goal will be to provide the patient with the best possible outcome.

## CONCLUSION

Careful planning and execution of surgery can prevent most complications. Early recognition of complications and rapid treatment can minimize the potential bad outcomes that can occur when complications are allowed to progress untreated.

## REFERENCES

1. Zisser M, Kaplan B, Moy RL: Surgical pearl: manual dermabrasion, *J Am Acad Dermatol* 33(1):105-106, 1995.
2. Haas AF, Grekin RC: Antibiotic prophylaxis in dermatologic surgery, *J Am Acad Dermatol* 32(2 Pt 1):155-176, 1995.
3. Lo B: Disclosing Mistakes. In *Resolving ethical dilemmas: a guide for clinicians*, Baltimore, 1995, Williams & Wilkins.

# Skin Surgery Consent Form

The surgical procedure or treatment to be performed is a:

- Skin biopsy_____
- Removal of lesion/tumor_____
- Other_____

I, _____ hereby consent to the surgical procedure or treatment that has been explained to me. I understand the following are possible risks involved:

- Pain
- Bleeding
- Infection
- Scar formation (which can sometimes look worse than the original lesion)
- Persistent redness
- Increase or decrease of my skin pigmentation
- Recurrence of the lesion
- Local nerve damage or numbness
- Severe allergic reaction to the local anesthesia, dressings, or medications

I understand there may be other methods to do this procedure, but agree to the procedure about to be done, understanding all risks. I have been given the opportunity to ask all my questions regarding the procedure and its risks. I agree that photographs may be taken. I understand that specimens may be sent for microscopic evaluation.

This is an elective procedure and is being done at my request. _____

Patient's initials

_____    _____
Patient's signature                 Guardian's signature, if applicable

Date_____    Witness_____

May be duplicated for use in clinical practice. From Usatine RP, Moy RL, Tobinick EL, Siegel DM: *Skin surgery: a practical guide*, St. Louis, 1998, Mosby.

# Outline of the Ellipse Procedure

1. Determine direction of ellipse.
2. Clean area with Hibiclens or Betadine on gauze. Wipe off skin twice.
3. Mark ellipse, 3:1 ratio.
4. Inject local anesthesia.
5. Cut with No. 15 blade.

    Keep blade at 90-degree angle to surface.

    Cut repeatedly until you feel the give that occurs when you cut through the dermis into the subcutaneous fat. Make sure that you have cut through the dermis around the full ellipse.
6. Lift up one corner of ellipse and cut off specimen flat in the fat layer.
7. Use sterile cotton-tipped swabs for hemostasis (better than gauze).

    Use electrocoagulation to produce a dry field. It is essential to stop all bleeding and have a dry field before suturing. This will prevent hematoma formation. Hematoma formation is a risk factor for infection and dehiscence.
8. Undermine if needed. Use cotton-tipped swabs and electrocautery for hemostasis if needed again.
9. Use skin hook to place buried vertical mattress suture (Vicryl or Dexon). An ellipse of 1 to 2 cm in length will need one to two of these absorbable sutures.

    Use a surgeon's knot (two throws) and pull tight with hands on suture, pulling perpendicular to suture direction (parallel to wound edges).

    This should close the deep space and approximate the wound edges.
10. Place simple interrupted sutures with nylon.
11. Clean blood off with hydrogen peroxide on cotton-tipped swabs.
12. Place micropore tape across the wound.
13. Apply pressure dressing.

May be duplicated for use in clinical practice. From Usatine RP, Moy RL, Tobinick EL, Siegel DM: *Skin surgery: a practical guide*, St. Louis, 1998, Mosby.

# Consent Form for Cryosurgery

The surgical procedure or treatment to be performed is called cryosurgery. I, _____ hereby consent to the surgical procedure or treatment that has been explained to me. I understand the following are possible risks involved:

- Pain
- Bleeding
- Infection
- Scar formation (which can sometimes look worse than the original lesion)
- Persistent redness
- Increase or decrease of my skin pigmentation
- Recurrence of the lesion
- Local nerve damage or numbness
- Fainting

I understand there may be other methods to do this procedure, but agree to the procedure about to be done, understanding all risks. I have been given the opportunity to ask all my questions regarding the procedure and its risks. I agree that photographs may be taken.

This is an elective procedure and is being done at my request._____

Patient's initials

_____  _____
Patient's signature         Guardian's signature, if applicable

Date_____   Witness_____

May be duplicated for use in clinical practice. From Usatine RP, Moy RL, Tobinick EL, Siegel DM: *Skin surgery: a practical guide,* St. Louis, 1998, Mosby.

# Description of Mohs' Micrographic Surgery

Mohs' surgery is a technique of microscopically controlled excision of cancer that produces the highest cure rates for skin cancer and maximal preservation of normal tissue by applying a precise mapping technique and obtaining frozen tissue sections for examination.[1] Mohs' surgery is performed under local anesthesia. The lesion is initially debulked. A thin layer of tissue around the margin of the wound is excised, creating a wafer-thin specimen. Landmarks (superficial incisional nicks made through the specimen and surrounding wound margin) on this thin specimen correspond to landmarks on the wound, so that exact orientation of the specimen can be maintained.

After the wafer is cut into pieces and its edges color-coded with dyes, a map is drawn so that the physician can mark areas of lesion seen when the sections are examined microscopically. The physician may then return to the patient and know the specific location of any remaining lesion.

To cut the sections for microscopic examination, the specimen is flattened, and frozen sections are performed on the undersurface of each section. The physician then reads each frozen-section specimen and marks any lesion that is found on the corresponding area of the map. Any remaining lesion that is present is removed by excising another thin layer of skin from the area of the wound that corresponds to the marked area on the map. During the processing and reading of the slides, the patient may wait in the waiting room. The processing is accomplished rapidly to prevent loss of anesthesia, thereby minimizing the discomfort of further anesthetic injections.

## ADVANTAGES OF MOHS' SURGERY

- Highest cure rate possible
- Conservation of normal tissue, allowing potentially better cosmetic results
- Use of local anesthesia
- Lower cost than in-patient surgery

For primary basal cell carcinomas (BCCs), the cure rate using Mohs' surgery is close to 99%, which is higher than any other treatment method available.[1,2] Cure rates for recurrent BCCs are greater than 96% with Mohs' surgery, compared with an approximate 50% cure rate when conventional surgical excision is used to guess the clinical margins of recurrent tumors.[2,3] The reason for these high cure rates is that Mohs' surgery allows for the complete examination of the surgical margins.

Mohs' surgery has the ability to conserve normal tissue. Conservation of a maximal amount of normal tissue allows for the best possible reconstructive repair procedure. Physicians that are well-trained in Mohs' surgery are adept at performing reconstructive surgery, including flaps, grafts, and primary closures. In addition, because only a minimal amount of normal tissue is sacrificed, some excisions result in only partial-thickness wounds, which allows for the best possible cosmetic result by the simple management of healing by granulation and epithelialization. Scar revision at a later date is still possible if the scar is unacceptable to the patient. Approximately 50% of surgical defects are managed by immediate postoperative reconstruction.

Mohs' micrographic surgery is more expensive than curettage and desiccation, cryosurgery, or simple excisional surgery. These other methods of lesion destruction are still cost effective in the treatment of primary lesions in areas where lesions have a tendency not to recur and where wide surgical margins would not compromise the cosmetic results.

## REFERENCES

1. Moy RL, Zitelli JA: Mohs' micrographic surgery for treatment of skin cancer in the elderly, *Geriatric Med Today* 8(1), 1989.
2. Mohs FE: *Chemosurgery: microscopically controlled surgery for skin cancer,* Springfield, Ill, 1978, Charles C. Thomas.
3. Menn H et al: The recurrent basal cell epithelioma: a study of 100 cases of recurrent retreated basal cell epitheliomas, *Arch Dermatol* 103:628, 1971.

# Home Wound Care Instructions for Naturally Healing Wounds After a Shave Excision, Cryotherapy, or Electrosurgery With No Sutures Used

## SUPPLIES NEEDED

- Hydrogen peroxide (alternatively, tap water can be used)
- Cotton-tipped swabs (applicators) or sterile gauze pads
- Polysporin, Bacitracin, or Vaseline ointment (not Neosporin)
- Band-Aids or generic equivalent or nonstick gauze pads (Telfa) and micropore paper tape

## INSTRUCTIONS

1. Remove the original dressing (bandages) after 24 hours.
2. Take a cotton-tipped swab and dip it into the hydrogen peroxide. Alternatively, you can use tap water with sterile gauze pads or cotton-tipped swabs.
3. Use the cotton-tipped swab or sterile gauze pad to gently clean the wound. Allow the peroxide to bubble and clean the wound until any loose material and crusts are removed. Dry with a cotton-tipped swab or sterile gauze pad. *Note: Never place a used swab back into the bottle of hydrogen peroxide.*
4. Apply antibiotic ointment such as Bacitracin or Polysporin to the wound (Vaseline is adequate if it is a clean wound). Do not use Neosporin.
5. Use a Band-Aid or cut a nonstick dressing to cover the wound. Change dressing once or twice a day. Although cleansing only need be done once or twice a day, additional Polysporin or Bacitracin may be added as needed to keep the wound moist and comfortable.
6. If drainage occurs, you may cut a gauze pad to the size of the wound and place it over the nonstick dressing. If drainage does not occur, a nonstick dressing is sufficient.
7. Use micropore paper tape to hold the dressing in place.
8. Tylenol (acetaminophen) can be taken for pain if needed. DO NOT start taking any medications with aspirin or aspirin products.

Repeat these instructions at least once a day until the wound has completely healed. *Note: It is an old wives' tale that a wound heals better when exposed to the air. The wound will actually heal faster and with a better cosmetic result if kept clean and covered with ointment and a fresh bandage.*

## Additional Information

1. You may shower daily before changing your dressing. Leave the dressing on during the shower to protect the wound from the forceful flow of water. Alternatively, if the wound needs cleaning, the shower is helpful to remove debris and exudate. Remove the dressing after the shower, dry gently, and then follow steps 2 through 7. We recommend not bathing (in a tub) until the wound is completely healed over to avoid infection.

2. During the healing process, you will notice a number of changes. During the first week or 10 days there will be little apparent progress. *All* wounds develop a small surrounding halo of redness that means healing is occurring. Extensive itching and severe redness usually indicate a reaction to the bandage tape or perhaps a sensitivity to the ointment used to dress the wound. You should call our office if this develops.

3. Swelling and/or discoloration around the surgical site is not uncommon, particularly if the surgery was on the face.

4. All wounds normally drain (the larger the wound, the more the drainage), which is why daily dressing changes are so important. This drainage becomes less apparent after the first week. After 1 to 2 weeks, the healing will become more rapid, and you will notice the wound beginning to shrink and new skin beginning to grow. A healed wound has a healthy, shiny look to the surface and is red to dark pink in color. Another way to know that your wound is healed is when the peroxide no longer bubbles when applied. Small wounds may heal in 2 to 3 weeks. Larger wounds may take 4 to 5 weeks total. After the wound is healed, you can stop daily dressing changes. The wound will remain quite red and will slowly fade over the next few weeks or months. Sometimes it can take 6 months to 1 year for the redness to fade completely.

5. You may experience a sensation of tightness as your wound heals. This is normal and will gradually subside. After the wound has healed, frequent, gentle massaging of the area will help to loosen the scar. Sometimes the surgery involves small nerves and it may take up to a year before feeling returns to normal. Only rarely will the area remain numb permanently.

6. Your healed wound may be sensitive to temperature changes (such as cold air). This sensitivity improves with time, but if you are experiencing a lot of discomfort, try to avoid temperature extremes.

7. You may experience itching after your wound appears to have healed. This is due to the healing that continues underneath the skin. Vaseline may help to relieve this itching.

May be duplicated for use in clinical practice. From Usatine RP, Moy RL, Tobinick EL, Siegel DM: *Skin surgery: a practical guide*, St. Louis, 1998, Mosby.

# Home Wound Care
# Instructions for Sutured Wounds

## GENERAL INSTRUCTIONS

1. After surgery, go home and take it easy (no exertion, lifting, bending, or straining).
2. Do not drink any alcoholic beverages or take any aspirin for 24 hours. If you require medication to control your pain, take only Tylenol or a similar aspirin-free pain reliever.
3. After 24 hours, remove the bulky top bandage. Leave the flat dressing on your skin until the sutures are removed.
4. If the flat dressing is soiled from drainage from the wound, you may cover it with another piece of paper tape. Do not remove the original piece of tape. If the dressing starts becoming loose, you will need to reinforce the tape.
5. Do not get the dressing wet for the first 24 hours. After the first 24 hours you may wash carefully around the dressing or allow clean shower water to run over the wound.
6. Do not do any heavy lifting or exercising until after the sutures are removed.

### Bleeding

Significant bleeding is rare. If it occurs, have someone apply firm pressure to the site. Direct pressure should be applied to the wound for 15 minutes, timed by looking at a clock. You are not to discontinue pressure to see if the bleeding has stopped until 15 minutes have elapsed. If the bleeding continues, remove the pad and press directly with a clean gauze pad over the bleeding site. If bleeding continues, call our office or go to your local emergency room.

### Infection

If you notice pus coming from the wound, this may be an infection. This is particularly worrisome if you develop a fever and the wound is red, swollen, and warm. If this occurs, call our office or go to your local emergency room.

## SPECIAL INSTRUCTIONS FOR SUTURED WOUNDS OF THE FACE

1. While sleeping, keep your head elevated for the first two nights.
2. Do not sleep on the same side of the body as the wound.
3. Do not bend over with your head lower than your heart level. Bend at the knees to stoop down. Be careful not to lift anything heavy or do anything that might cause strain on the sutures.
4. It is perfectly normal to have bruising or discoloration around the surgery site, especially if the wound is around the eye area. Do not be alarmed by this; it will eventually fade and return to normal color.

May be duplicated for use in clinical practice. From Usatine RP, Moy RL, Tobinick EL, Siegel DM: *Skin surgery: a practical guide*, St. Louis, 1998, Mosby.

# Index